SECOND EDITION

The Doctor *of* Nursing Practice

A Guidebook for Role Development and Professional Issues

Lisa Astalos Chism, DNP, GNP, BC, NCMP, FAANP
Nurse Practitioner
Alexander J. Walt Comprehensive Breast Center
High Risk Breast Clinic
Karmanos Cancer Institute
Detroit, Michigan

Certified Menopause Practitioner
North American Menopause Society

Adjunct Assistant Professor
Madonna University
Livonia, Michigan

JONES & BARTLETT
LEARNING

World Headquarters
Jones & Bartlett Learning
5 Wall Street
Burlington, MA 01803
978-443-5000
info@jblearning.com
www.jblearning.com

Jones & Bartlett Learning books and products are available through most bookstores and online booksellers. To contact Jones & Bartlett Learning directly, call 800-832-0034, fax 978-443-8000, or visit our website, www.jblearning.com.

Substantial discounts on bulk quantities of Jones & Bartlett Learning publications are available to corporations, professional associations, and other qualified organizations. For details and specific discount information, contact the special sales department at Jones & Bartlett Learning via the above contact information or send an email to specialsales@jblearning.com.

Production Credits

Publisher: Kevin Sullivan
Acquisitions Editor: Amanda Harvey
Editorial Assistant: Sara Bempkins
Production Manager: Carolyn F. Rogers
Marketing Manager: Elena McAnespie
V.P., Manufacturing and Inventory Control: Therese Connell
Composition: Arlene Apone
Cover Design: Kristin E. Parker
Cover Image: © Michal Duriník/ ShutterStock, Inc.
Printing and Binding: Malloy, Inc.
Cover Printing: Malloy, Inc.

Library of Congress Cataloging-in-Publication Data
Chism, Lisa Astalos.
  The doctor of nursing practice : a guidebook for role development and professional issues / Lisa Astalos Chism. — 2nd ed.
       p. ; cm.
  Includes bibliographical references and index.
  ISBN 978-1-4496-4560-1 (pbk.)
  I. Title.
  [DNLM: 1. Education, Nursing, Graduate—United States. 2. Advanced Practice Nursing—United States. 3. Professional Role—United States. WY 18.5]
  610.73071'1--dc23
                              2012001038

6048
Printed in the United States of America
16 15 14 13 12   10 9 8 7 6 5 4 3 2 1

Dedication

This book is dedicated to my father, Paul Astalos, and my mother, Judy Astalos. You were both my inspiration and my cheerleaders. Mom and Dad, you continue to guide me in spirit, and I know you are smiling down on us all.

This book is also dedicated to my husband, Bruce, and my daughter, Isabel. Your enduring love, support, and friendship mean more than you will ever know.

Contents

Foreword   xi
Preface   xv
Acknowledgments   xvii
Contributors   xix

■ **Part I: Role Transition**   1

1   **Overview of the Doctor of Nursing Practice Degree**   3
    Lisa Astalos Chism
    The Doctor of Nursing Practice Degree Defined   4
    The Research-Focused Doctorate and the Practice-Focused
        Doctorate Defined   4
    The Evolution of Doctoral Education in Nursing   5
    Why a Practice Doctorate in Nursing Now?   10
    What Is a DNP Degree Made Of? The Recipe for
        Curriculum Standards   13
    Role Transition Introduced   22
    Interview with a DNP Co-Founder: Then and Now   23
    Summary   30
    Reflection Questions   31
    References   31

2   **Leadership, Collaboration, and the DNP Graduate**   35
    Lisa Astalos Chism
    Curriculum Standards for Leadership and Collaboration   36
    What's a DNP-Prepared Leader Made Of? The Recipe
        for Success   37
    Collaboration: DNP Graduates Working with Others   43
    A Discussion About Change   46
    The Reluctant Leader: Unexpected Leadership   47
    Role Modeling: DNP Graduates Setting the Example   48
    Case Scenarios Related to the DNP Degree in Leadership
        and Collaboration   48
    Interview with a DNP Nurse Leader: Then and Now   51
    Summary   55
    Reflection Questions   56
    References   57

3 The DNP Graduate as Expert Clinician 59
Lisa Astalos Chism
Curriculum Standards Related to Clinical Practice 60
Advanced Nursing Practice and Advanced Practice Nursing:
    Let's Clear This Up 61
The APRN Consensus Model 63
Evidence-Based Practice 63
Information Technology 67
Interprofessional Collaboration in the Clinical Setting:
    More Than Just Getting Along 73
Mentoring: DNP Graduates Shaping the Future of
    Clinician Roles 78
Conclusion 81
Interviews with DNP Clinicians: Then and Now 82
A DNP Graduate's Personal Journey: Who, Me? 94
Why a DNP for Clinicians? 95
Summary 95
Reflection Questions 96
References 97

**4 The DNP: Expectations for Theory, Research,
and Scholarship** 101
Morris A. Magnan
The DNP and Theory 102
The DNP and Research 105
The DNP and Scholarship 108
Scholarship and Research Beyond Graduation 119
Building a Network for Research and Scholarship 123
Summary 125
Reflection Questions 125
References 126

5 DNP Involvement in Healthcare Policy and Advocacy 131
Marlene H. Mullin
Curriculum Standards 132
Historical Perspective 133
Tips for Becoming Informed and Involved 137
Interviews with Nurse Policy Makers and Advocates 145
Case Scenario: DNP Involvement in Healthcare Policy
    and Advocacy 151
Summary 153
Reflection Questions 154
Editor's Note 155
References 155

6   The DNP Graduate as Educator   157
Karen McBroom Butler
Curriculum Standards   158
The Nursing Faculty Shortage   159
DNP Graduates Can Fill the Nursing Faculty Gap   162
Promotion and Tenure   166
Conclusion   169
Case Scenarios: The DNP Graduate as Nurse Educator   169
Summary   174
Reflection Questions   175
Author's Note   176
References   176

7   The DNP Graduate as Ethical Consultant   179
Lisa Astalos Chism
First a Story . . .   180
Back to the Basics   181
Bioethics: Expanding the Basics   185
Nursing Ethics   187
Ethical Leadership Tools for the Ethical Leader   192
Telehealth Ethics: Ethical Concerns in the 21st Century   195
Ethical Decision-Making Model   198
Putting It All Together: Ethical Scenarios with Discussion   199
Interviews with Nurse Ethicists: Wisdom from the Field   204
Summary   209
Reflection Questions   211
References   212

■ Part II: Professional Issues Related to the
Doctor of Nursing Practice Degree   215

8   So You Want to Go Back to School? Exploring How to
Make the Big Decision   217
Elizabeth Johnston Taylor
To Be a DNP or Not to Be: Relevant Facts   218
Decision-Making Research   219
Practical Tools for Decision Making   220
Spiritual Approaches to Decision Making   224
Living with the Decision   229
Conclusion   230
Summary   230
Reflection Questions   231
References   232

9 **The Dr. Nurse: Overcoming Title Issues** 233
Lisa Astalos Chism
History of *Docere*: The First Teachers 234
Parity Among Healthcare Professionals: One of the DNP
Drivers Revisited 234
Review of "The Pearson Report" Regarding Title Protection 236
The Debate 237
Case Scenario: A Dr. Nurse's Story 243
Interview with a "Doctor Nurse" Champion: Then and Now 245
Interview with a "Doctor Nurse" Advocate and DNP Program
Director: Then and Now 251
Tips for Using the Title "Doctor" 257
Summary 259
Reflection Questions 260
References 260

10 **Why Didn't You Just Become a Doctor? Educating
Others About the DNP Degree** · 263
Lisa Astalos Chism
Definitions Revisited: Know Who You Are 264
Current DNP Trends: A DNP, LLC/DNPPD Outcome Study 266
Go Forth and Teach 270
Speaking Publicly About the DNP Degree 276
Interview with a Co-Founder of DNP, LLC: Then and Now 279
Summary 286
Reflection Questions 286
References 287

11 **Shaping Your Brand: Marketing Yourself as a
DNP Graduate** 289
Lisa Astalos Chism
Marketing vs. Branding 289
DNP Graduates as "Marketpreneurs" 291
Mission Statement 291
Vision Statement 291
Marketing Strategies 292
Unique Strategies for DNP Graduates 294
Interview with Dr. Margaret Fitzgerald, Owner, Fitzgerald
Health Associates 300
Summary 302
Reflection Questions 304
References 304
Appendix 11-A: Sample Marketing Pamphlet Describing the
DNP-Prepared Nurse Practitioner 305

12 **Where Do We Go From Here? The Future of the**
DNP Degree 309
Lisa Astalos Chism
Nursing's Debate Regarding the DNP Degree 310
The Future of the DNP Degree 314
A Word About Nurse Residencies 316
An Update from the AACN 316
The DNP Degree and Societal Needs 317
Interview with an Innovative DNP Program Director:
    Then and Now 318
Summary 324
Reflection Questions 326
References 326

Appendix A: The Certification Question: Where Are We? 329
Karen McBroom Butler
Introduction 329
ANCC DNP Survey Results 330
American Board of Comprehensive Care 331
Conclusion 331
References 332

Appendix B: Relevant Doctor of Nursing Practice Websites 333

Index 335

Foreword

They say that time changes things. But you
actually have to change them yourselves.
—*Andy Warhol*

For over a decade warnings and calls have been made by such notable authorities as the American Hospital Association (2002), Institute of Medicine (IOM, 2001; Kohn, Corrigan, & Donaldson, 2000), and Joint Commission (2002) to improve the way care is delivered in this country, focus on quality improvement and patient safety, improve access to high-quality care, and address healthcare inequities. In 2003, the IOM reported that health professions education was in need of an overhaul and identified five areas of competence in which *all* health professionals should be prepared: patient-centered care, interdisciplinary team care, evidence-based practice, quality improvement, and informatics (Greiner & Knebel, 2003). In 2002, in response to these calls, the American Association of Colleges of Nursing (AACN) initiated a dialogue among nursing leaders, stakeholder organizations, and other health professional representatives focused on what nursing education should and could do and what nurses needed to know to address immediate and future healthcare needs. Two of the most critical responses that grew out of this dialogue were the approval by the AACN Board of Directors to develop and pilot a new nursing role, the first in over 35 years, titled the Clinical Nurse Leader (CNL). The CNL is a master's-prepared nurse with preparation focused on quality improvement, evidence-based practice, interprofessional communication, and care coordination. The second major outcome of the dialogue was the approval in 2004 of the *Position Statement on the Practice Doctorate in Nursing* (AACN, 2004) by the AACN membership, which established the doctorate of nursing practice (DNP) as the highest level of preparation for clinical nursing practice and set in motion the transition of all advanced nursing practice from the master's degree to the doctoral level. In a separate motion and to galvanize the profession into action, the year 2015 was set as the targeted date for this transition to occur.

More recently, the Institute of Medicine report, *The Future of Nursing: Leading Change, Advancing Health*, has brought to the forefront the role nursing should play in addressing this country's healthcare needs, particularly quality of care and improved patient outcomes. The report's four key messages include the following: nurses should practice to the full extent of their education and training; nurses should achieve higher levels of education and training through an improved education system that promotes seamless academic profession; nurses should be full partners, with physicians and other health professionals, in redesigning health care in the United States; and effective workforce planning and policy making require better data collection and an improved information infrastructure (IOM, 2010, p. 4). To achieve these outcomes the report recommends the need to double the number of doctorally prepared nurses, including both practice- and research-focused doctorates, by 2020.

These reports and efforts to reform healthcare delivery over the past decade provide a strong impetus for the development and expansion of the DNP. The growth in the number and size of programs from 2 programs with 70 enrollees in 2002 to 153 programs with 7,034 enrollees in 2010 reflects the demand from both employers and nurses (AACN, 2011); and this exponential growth is expected to continue. Graduates of DNP programs are being sought for their leadership and for the new knowledge and skill mix they bring to the practice environment.

This timely book, now in its second edition, provides a contemporary and practical perspective on the transition of advanced nursing education and practice to the DNP degree. Questions about the degree, the need for the transition, and future directions frequently heard from prospective students, new graduates, faculty, employers, and other healthcare professionals are addressed in a straightforward and easy to understand manner. The chapters in this book address a wide array of topics, including the DNP curriculum; the DNP graduate as clinician, scholar, policy advocate, and educator; and professional issues. Written and edited by individuals who have lived the experiences, the book provides a guide to the what, why, who, and how for the Doctor of Nursing Practice. Each chapter ends with a summary of issues and reflection questions, which will be particularly helpful to students and faculty. Case scenarios provide real-life experiences of students, graduates, and faculty that demonstrate what others may be experiencing as well. Another particularly innovative aspect of the book is the inclusion of interviews with nurse leaders and early advocates of the DNP movement. For this second edition, the interviews have been updated to provide insight into changes that have occurred in opinions and DNP-related experiences over the past 3 years.

The DNP degree provides the credential, but the knowledge and skills that graduates bring to the table and practice arena will be the real reason that nursing will have a significant impact on the future of health care.

Joan M. Stanley, PhD, RN, CRNP, FAAN, FAANP
Senior Director of Education Policy
American Association of Colleges of Nursing

REFERENCES

American Association of Colleges of Nursing. (2004). *Position statement on the practice doctorate in nursing.* Retrieved from http://www.aacn.nche.edu/dnp/position-statement

American Association of Colleges of Nursing. (2011). *Institutional data system.* Washington, DC: Author.

American Hospital Association Commission on Hospitals and Health Systems. (2002). *In our hands: How hospital leaders can build a thriving workforce.* Chicago: American Hospital Association.

Greiner, A. C., & Knebel, E. (Eds.). (2003). *Health professions education: A bridge to quality.* Washington, DC: National Academies Press.

Institute of Medicine. (2001). *Crossing the quality chasm: A new health system for the 21st century.* Washington, DC: National Academies Press.

Institute of Medicine. (2010). *The future of nursing: Leading change, advancing health.* Washington, DC: National Academies Press.

Joint Commission. (2002). *Health care at the crossroads: Strategies for addressing the evolving nursing crisis.* Chicago, IL: Author.

Kohn, L. T., Corrigan, J. M., & Donaldson, M. S. (Eds). (1999). *To err is human: Building a safer health system.* Committee on Quality of Health Care in America, Institute of Medicine. Washington, DC: National Academies Press.

Preface

I had recently graduated from a Doctor of Nursing Practice program in 2007 when I woke up in the middle of the night and thought, now what? I had just spent the last 3 years researching, finding, applying, and finally completing a DNP program. I realized at 2:00 a.m. that day, 2 months after graduation, that I wasn't sure how to integrate my new degree into my professional life. I felt that if I wasn't sure how to transition into my new role/roles, then my colleagues probably had the same concerns, questions, and issues.

Since that time, I have received wonderful feedback from colleagues and nursing faculty that this was indeed true. The previous edition of this book has served as a resource for everyone from prospective and current students to those who have completed their DNP degree. I am very pleased this book has been helpful for so many. Writing and editing the second edition was just as rewarding as the first edition. From my first query letter to the development of the second edition, this book has been a wonderful adventure.

The American Association of Colleges of Nursing (AACN) continues to recommend that by 2015, the terminal degree in nursing practice will transition from the traditional master's degrees in nursing to the Doctor of Nursing Practice degree (AACN, 2004). With the growth of this innovative degree comes the challenge for students and graduates to be able to synthesize the new knowledge and skills they garner in a DNP program and transition into DNP-prepared nurses. What does this mean? That is the question I have attempted to continue to answer in the second edition of this book. I also strived to share valuable insights pertinent to DNP students, graduates, nurses, and other healthcare professionals who are impacted by the development of this degree.

This book is organized into two parts. Part I reviews the DNP degree as well as the various roles DNP graduates may assume and integrate. DNP graduates may find themselves developing roles in leadership, clinical practice, research, health policy and advocacy, education, and ethics. No doubt many nurses who return to school for a DNP degree already possess expertise in these roles. Therefore, the challenge lies in the integration of new knowledge and skills obtained through a DNP program with the intent to improve healthcare delivery in the 21st century.

Part II describes the unique issues DNP graduates may find themselves facing, such as deciding whether or not to return to graduate school for a DNP degree , the use of the title "doctor," educating others about the degree, marketing oneself as a DNP graduate, and finally, the future of the DNP degree. Case scenarios are used throughout the book to illustrate further the unique situations that DNP graduates may encounter. The interviews have been updated and are included to bring life to the book and describe the wonderful contributions made by many DNP graduates as well as the anecdotal accounts of those who helped bring the DNP degree into fruition.

Healthcare delivery and nursing education are evolving, and nursing has responded with the development of the DNP degree. We are practice professionals, and we now have a practice doctorate that is reflective of our heritage. The knowledge and expertise garnered through a DNP program have equipped DNP graduates with the skills and perspective necessary to continue to provide high-quality health care and proactively advocate for patients and the nursing profession. DNP graduates will further contribute to health care and nursing in the 21st century through leadership, use of evidence-based practice, expertise in information technologies, involvement in health policy, and the mentoring and education of future generations of nurses and healthcare professionals. Whether you are deciding if this degree is right for you, assimilating into your new role as a Doctor of Nursing Practice, or simply seeking information about this innovative degree, it is my hope that this book will prove to be a valuable resource.

REFERENCE

American Association of Colleges of Nursing (AACN). (2004). *AACN position statement on the practice doctorate in nursing.* Retrieved from http://www.aacn.nche.edu/dnp/position-statement

Acknowledgments

I wish to first acknowledge God. I am sure that without Your guidance and inspiration, I would not have succeeded in this endeavor. Although I thought this project was bigger than me, You proved to me again that once You planted the seed, You would be with me through it all.

I wish to acknowledge Dr. Elizabeth Johnston Taylor for her immediate encouragement. Dr. Taylor helped me write my first query letter and edited my proposal for the first edition. Her faith and encouragement instilled in me the confidence to push forward with my ideas. She has been a mentor and a friend, and I am thankful for her unending guidance and encouragement. It was so appropriate that Dr. Taylor, a spiritual care expert, wrote a chapter about weighing the decision to go back to school. Her perception regarding decision making is uncanny. She expertly integrated her expertise in spiritual care, which only added to a wonderful, insightful chapter.

I wish to also acknowledge my first mentor, Dr. Morris Magnan. Prior to returning to graduate school for my DNP degree, I am quite sure I had never had a mentor. I initially met Dr. Magnan during my interview for the DNP program. Needless to say, my initial intimidation has grown to true admiration. He is a nursing scholar who impresses me with his level of clinical expertise and overall commitment to the profession of nursing. Through his mentorship, I have developed a much broader understanding of nursing as a discipline, science, and profession. Dr. Magnan has not only inspired me to grow as a nurse, but he has also taught me what a true mentor is and should be. I am so thankful to call him a mentor and a friend. It was an honor to have Dr. Magnan write the chapter regarding DNP graduates' expectations for theory, research, and scholarship. He clearly understands the benefit of DNP/PhD partnerships and has supported the need for a practice doctorate in nursing.

I would also like to acknowledge Dr. Karen McBroom Butler. Dr. Butler was an original reviewer of the proposal for this book and not only offered wonderful feedback but also graciously volunteered to assist me with this project. It was an honor that she accepted the task to write the DNP as educator chapter. She is a perfect example of the impact DNP graduates are making in the role of educator. She beautifully articulated the issues and transitions necessary to move nursing education into the 21st century. Her insights into the role of university faculty member through the eyes of a DNP graduate are invaluable. I am so thankful for her contributions both to the book and to nursing education.

I would also like to acknowledge my good friend and colleague, Dr. Marlene Mullin. Dr. Mullin is a champion for the nursing profession. Her commitment to issues such as the homeless crisis and the number of uninsured individuals in this country has motivated her to get involved on a grassroots level by volunteering at a homeless shelter and become politically involved. Her dedication to health care and nursing inspires me. I am honored and thankful that she contributed to this project by writing the health policy and advocacy chapter. Dr. Mullin wonderfully describes the rich history of nursing's involvement in policy and political issues. Dr. Mullin exemplifies the importance of addressing healthcare policy issues and continues to be a strong advocate for nursing and for her patients.

I also wish to acknowledge my wonderful friends and colleagues at Karmanos Cancer Institute, especially Ms. Christine Rymal MSN, APRN, BC, CLT, and Ms. Cathy Nichols MS, APRN, BC, DNP student. You are both incredible examples of exemplary advanced practice nurses. Your friendship and support are invaluable to me.

I also want to acknowledge by beautiful "sisters," Ms. Jill Frieders, BSN, RN, and Ms. Tonya Schmitt, MS, APRN, BC. You inspired me to make sure this book was a practical, useful resource for nurses in every area of practice. I am so thankful for your wisdom, expertise, humor, and, most of all, your friendship.

Thank you to a future nurse, Ms. Suzanne Molter. I appreciate you giving your point of view from a future nurse perspective. I truly appreciate your commitment to pursue your dream to become a nurse.

I also thank Ms. Andrea Rogers, MILS, reference librarian at Beaumont Hospitals. I would not have been able to revise this book without your expert literature searches and research.

I would also like to thank the editorial and production staff at Jones & Bartlett Learning for their support, expertise, and encouragement, especially Ms. Amanda Harvey, Ms. Sara Bempkins, Ms. Carolyn Rogers, and Mr. Kevin Sullivan. Thank you especially to Kevin for your immediate interest and continued support for this project.

Most important, I would like to acknowledge my family. Thank you to my beautiful daughter, Isabel, who is the greatest joy of my life. Your wisdom and humor are beyond your 11 years. Thank you, Izzy, for your patience and for cheering me on. I am so proud to be your mom. Finally, I would like to thank my husband, Bruce, for being my best friend, my cheerleader, and my champion. I am thankful for your support and guidance and for keeping me on track. Thank you for teaching me to be true to myself and for believing in me.

In closing, I would like to acknowledge all the readers of the previous and current editions of the book. This book is for you. My hope is that the practical, real-life tips, case scenarios, interviews, and information provided in this book will inspire you and guide you on your path.

Contributors

Karen McBroom Butler, DNP, RN
Assistant Professor and Course Coordinator
Faculty Associate, Tobacco Research Policy Program
University of Kentucky School of Nursing
Lexington, Kentucky

Morris A. Magnan, PhD, MSN, RN
St. Joseph Mercy Hospital
Pontiac, Michigan

Marlene H. Mullin, DNP, APRN, BC
Nurse Practitioner
Adjunct Faculty
Wayne State University School of Nursing
Detroit, Michigan

Elizabeth Johnston Taylor, PhD, RN
Associate Professor
Loma Linda University School of Nursing
Loma Linda, California
Research Director
Mary Potter Hospice
Wellington, Aotearoa, New Zealand

PART I

Role Transition

The evolution of a Doctor of Nursing Practice (DNP) degree continues to be a fascinating journey for the profession of nursing.
As DNP graduates begin their own journeys, many challenges
and issues related to role transition are likely to be presented.
While reading the chapters in Part I, it is indeed apparent that
today's DNP graduate will engage in a variety of roles that will
include leadership, evaluation and translation of research, practice, education, health policy, and ethics. Often, these roles will
be integrated and adapted to meet the current needs of healthcare delivery.

As a practice-focused profession, nursing is responding to
the healthcare needs of individuals, communities, and systems
by developing a practice-focused doctorate. Most assuredly, as
the demands of a complex healthcare environment continue to
evolve, nursing will continue to evolve as well. The Doctor of
Nursing Practice degree truly exemplifies this evolution and nursing's commitment to the future of health care. The following
chapters specifically discuss the various roles DNP graduates may
fulfill to meet the current and future needs of a complex healthcare environment.

CHAPTER 1

Overview of the Doctor of Nursing Practice Degree

■ LISA ASTALOS CHISM ■

> "You cannot hope to build a better world without improving the individual. To that end each of us must work for his own improvement, and at the same time share a general responsibility for all humanity, our particular duty being to aid those to whom we think we can be most useful."
>
> —*Marie Curie (1867–1934)*

What exactly is a Doctor of Nursing Practice (DNP) degree? As enrollment to this innovative practice doctorate program increases, this question is frequently posed by nurses, patients, and other healthcare professionals both in and out of the healthcare setting. Providing an explanation to this question requires not only defining the DNP degree but also reflecting on the rich history of doctoral education in nursing. Doctoral education in nursing is connected to our past and influences the directions we may take in the future (Carpenter & Hudacek, 1996). The development of the DNP degree is a tribute to where nursing has been and where we hope to be in the future of doctoral education in nursing.

Understanding what a DNP degree is requires developing an awareness of the rationale for a practice doctorate. This rationale illustrates the motivation behind the evolution of doctoral education in nursing and provides further explanation of this contemporary degree. The need for parity across the healthcare team, the Institute of Medicine's call for safer healthcare practices, and the need for increased preparation of advanced practice registered nurses to meet the changing demands of health care are all contributing antecedents of the development of the practice doctorate in nursing (American Association of Colleges of Nursing [AACN], 2006a; AACN, 2006b; Apold, 2008; Dracup, Cronenwett, Meleis, & Benner, 2005; Roberts & Glod, 2005). Becoming familiar with the motivating factors behind the DNP degree will add to the understanding of the development of this innovative degree.

This chapter provides a definition of the DNP degree as well as a discussion of the evolution of doctoral education in nursing. The rationale for a practice doctorate is also described. The recipe for the DNP degree, which includes the *Essentials of Doctoral Education for Advanced Nursing Practice* degree outlined by the American Association of Colleges of Nursing (AACN, 2006b) and the *Practice Doctorate Nurse Practitioner Entry-Level Competencies* outlined by the National Organization of Nurse Practitioner Faculties (NONPF, 2006), is provided in this chapter as well. The pathway to the DNP degree is also discussed. Providing a discussion regarding these topics will equip one with the information necessary to become familiar with this innovative degree.

■ The Doctor of Nursing Practice Degree Defined

The DNP degree has been adopted as the terminal practice degree in nursing (AACN, 2004; AACN, 2006b). The AACN (2004) position statement specifically defines the DNP degree as a "practice focused" doctorate degree with nursing practice defined as:

> any form of nursing intervention that influences health care outcomes for individuals or populations, including the direct care of individual patients, management of care for individuals and populations, administration of nursing and health care organizations, and the development and implementation of health policy. (p. 3)

Preparation at the practice doctorate level is considered to be the highest level of preparation for nursing practice, hence, the terminal degree for nursing practice (AACN, 2004).

The DNP degree curriculum is focused on, although not limited to, evidence-based practice, scholarship to advance the profession, organizational and systems leadership, information technology, healthcare policy and advocacy, interprofessional collaboration across disciplines of health care, and advanced nursing practice (AACN, 2006b). It is projected that by 2015, the DNP degree will be the terminal preparation for advanced practice nursing, and current master's degree options for advanced nursing practice will be replaced by the DNP degree (AACN, 2006a). A newly developed master's degree, the Clinical Nurse Leader (CNL) degree, will be offered for those who wish to provide healthcare services at the point of care to individuals and cohorts of clients within a healthcare unit or setting (AACN, 2007). This degree prepares the graduate as "a leader in the health care delivery system, not just in the acute care setting but in all settings in which health care is delivered" (AACN, 2007, p. 10). Details regarding the content of the DNP degree curriculum are provided later in this chapter.

■ The Research-Focused Doctorate and the Practice-Focused Doctorate Defined

The question, What is a Doctor of Nursing Practice degree? is often followed by the question, What is the difference between a Doctor of Philosophy (PhD) and a DNP degree? Nurses now have a choice between a practice-focused or research-focused doctorate as a terminal degree. Although the academic or research degree, once the only terminal preparation in nursing, has traditionally been the Doctor of Philosophy (PhD), the American Association of Colleges of Nursing has included the Doctor of Nursing Science (DNS, DNSc, DSN) as a research-focused degree as well (AACN, 2004). Further, the AACN Task Force on the Practice Doctorate in nursing has recommended that the practice doctorate be the DNP degree, which will replace the traditional Nursing Doctorate (ND) degree (AACN, 2006a). Currently, nursing doctorate programs are taking the necessary steps to adjust their programs to fit the curriculum criteria of DNP degree programs.

The practice- and research-focused doctorates in nursing share a common goal regarding a "scholarly approach to the discipline and a commitment to the advancement of the profession" (AACN, 2006b, p. 3). The differences in these programs include differences in preparation and expertise. The practice doctorate curriculum places more emphasis on practice and less on theory and research methodology (AACN, 2006b; AACN, 2004). The final scholarly project differs as well in that a dissertation required of a PhD degree should document development of new knowledge, and a final scholarly project required of a DNP degree should be grounded in clinical practice and demonstrate ways in which research has an impact on practice.

The focus of the DNP degree is expertise in clinical practice. Additional foci include the *Essentials of Doctoral Education for Advanced Nursing Practice* as outlined by the AACN (2006b), which includes leadership, health policy and advocacy, and information technology. The focus of a research degree is the generation of new knowledge for the discipline and expertise as a principal investigator. However, although the research degree prepares the expert researcher, it should be noted that frequently DNP research projects will also contribute to the discipline by generating new knowledge related to clinical practice as well as demonstrate the use of evidence-based practice.

Please refer to **Table 1-1** for AACN's comparison of DNP and PhD/DNS/DNSc programs.

■ The Evolution of Doctoral Education in Nursing

To appreciate the development of doctoral education in nursing, one must understand where nursing has been with regard to education at the doctoral level. Indeed, nursing has been unique in the approach to doctoral preparation since nurses began to earn doctoral degrees. Even today nurses are prepared at the doctoral level through varying degrees, which include Doctor of Education (EdD), Doctor of Philosophy (PhD), Doctor of Nursing Science (DNS), and more recently, the Doctor of Nursing Practice degree. Prior to the development of the DNP degree, the Nursing Doctorate was also offered as a choice for nursing doctoral education.

Examining the chronological development of doctoral education in nursing is somewhat complicated due to the fact that early doctorates were offered outside of nursing. These included the EdD degree and the PhD degree in basic science fields,

Table 1-1 **AACN Contrast Grid of the Key Differences Between DNP and PhD/DNS/DNSc Programs**

	DNP	*PhD/DNS/DNSc*
Program of study	*Objectives:* ■ Prepare nurse specialists at the highest level of advanced practice *Competencies:* ■ Based on *Essentials of Doctoral Education for Advanced Nursing Practice* (AACN, 2006b)	*Objectives:* ■ Prepare nurse researchers *Content:* ■ Based on *Indicators of Quality in Research-Focused Doctoral Programs in Nursing* (AACN, 2001)
Students	■ Commitment to a practice career ■ Oriented toward improving outcomes of care	■ Commitment to a research career ■ Oriented toward developing new knowledge
Program faculty	■ Practice doctorate and/or experience in area in which teaching ■ Leadership experience in area of specialty practice ■ High level of expertise in specialty practice congruent with focus of academic program	■ Research doctorate in nursing or related field ■ Leadership experience in area of sustained research funding ■ High level of expertise in research congruent with focus of academic program
Resources	■ Mentors and/or precepts in leadership positions across a variety of practice settings ■ Access to diverse practice settings with appropriate resources for areas of practice ■ Access to financial aid ■ Access to information and patient-care technology resources congruent with areas of study	■ Mentors/preceptor in research settings ■ Access to research settings with appropriate resources ■ Access to dissertation support dollars ■ Access to information and research technology resources congruent with program of research
Program assessment and evaluation	*Program outcome:* ■ Healthcare improvements and contributions via practice, policy change, and practice scholarship ■ Oversight by the institution's authorized bodies (i.e., graduate school) and regional accreditors ■ Receives accreditation by specialized nursing accreditor ■ Graduates are eligible for national certification exam	*Program outcome:* ■ Contributes to healthcare improvements via the development of new knowledge and other scholarly projects that provide the foundation for the advancement of nursing science ■ Oversight by the institution's authorized bodies (i.e., graduate school) and regional accreditor

Source: Reprinted with permission from *AACN DNP Roadmap Task Force Report*, October 20, 2006.

such as anatomy and physiology (Carpenter & Hudacek, 1996; Marriner-Tomey, 1990). The first nursing-related doctoral program was originated in 1924 at Teachers College, Columbia University and was an EdD designed to prepare nurses to teach at the college level (Carpenter & Hudacek, 1996). Teachers College was unique in that its program was the first to combine both the "nursing and education needs of leaders in the profession" (Carpenter & Hudacek, 1996, p. 5). Doctor of Education (EdD) degrees continued well into the 1960s to be the mainstay of doctoral education for nursing (Marriner-Tomey, 1990).

The first PhD in nursing was offered in 1934 at New York University. Unfortunately, the next PhD in nursing was not offered until the 1950s at the University of Pittsburgh and focused on maternal and child nursing. Incidentally, this degree was the first to recognize the importance of clinical research for the development of the discipline of nursing (Carpenter & Hudacek, 1996). The PhD degrees earned elsewhere continued to be in nursing-related fields, such as psychology, sociology, and anthropology. This trend continued until actual nursing PhD degrees became more popular in the 1970s (Grace, 1978).

Grace (1978) summarized the progression of nursing education over time. During the time between 1924 and 1959, doctoral education in nursing focused on preparing nurses for "functional specialty" (p. 22). In other words, nurses were prepared to fulfill functional roles as teachers and administrators to lead the field of nursing toward advancement as a profession. The problem noted with these programs is that they lacked the substantive content necessary to develop nursing as a discipline, as well as a profession. The next shift in doctoral education attempted to fulfill this need and took place between 1960 and 1969. Within this time period, popularity increased for doctoral programs that were nursing related. This included doctorates (PhDs) that were related to disciplines such as sociology, psychology, and anthropology. Grace (1978) noted that the development of these types of programs provided the basic science and research input necessary for the development of future nursing doctorate programs. Murphy (1981) concurred that this stage in the development of doctoral education in nursing led to pertinent questions for the discipline of nursing, such as: "(1) What is the essential nature of professional nursing? (2) What is the substantive knowledge base of professional nursing? (3) What kind of research is important for nursing as a knowledge discipline? As a field of practice? (4) How can the scientific base of nursing knowledge be identified and expanded?" (p. 646).

In response to these questions, nursing doctoral education again progressed in the 1970s to include doctorate degrees that are actually in nursing (Grace, 1978). This stage also supported the growth of nursing's substantive structure, hence, the growth of the discipline of nursing.

Now, this is where nursing's history of doctoral education becomes more complex. In 1960, the Doctor of Nursing Science (DNS) degree originated at Boston University and "focused on the development of nursing theory for a practice discipline" (Marriner-Tomey, 1990, p. 135), hence, the development of the first practice doctorate. The notion of a practice-focused doctorate in nursing is not new. Even as early as the 1970s, it was proposed that the research doctorate (PhD) should focus on preparing nurses to contribute to nursing science, and the practice (or professional) doctorate (DNS) should focus on expertise in clinical practice (Cleland, 1976). Newman (1975) also suggested a practice doctorate as the preparation of "professional practitioners" (p. 705) for entry into practice. Grace (1978) noted that it was not sufficient to have a core of nursing researchers building the knowledge base (discipline) without also giving attention to the clinical field. It was also suggested by Grace (1978) that nurses prepared through a practice doctorate be titled "social engineers" (p. 26). This seems appropriate given what expert clinicians in nursing are called upon to do.

Although the DNS degree was initially proposed as a practice or professional doctorate, over time the curriculum requirements have become very similar to those for a PhD degree (AACN, 2006a; Apold, 2008; Marriner-Tomey, 1990). Research requirements for this degree have eventually become indistinguishable from that of a PhD in nursing. Because of this, it is not surprising that the American Association of Colleges of Nursing has characterized all DNS degrees as research degrees (AACN, 2004).

With the DNS and PhD degrees so similar in content and focus, the challenge to develop a true practice doctorate remained. An attempt toward this was made in 1979 when the Nursing Doctorate (ND) originated at Case Western Reserve University, followed by the University of Colorado, Rush University, and South Carolina University. The first ND program was developed by Rozella M. Schlotfeldt, PhD, RN. The Nursing Doctorate was different in that the research component was not the general focus of the degree. This degree was designed to be a "pre-service nursing education which would orient nursing's approach to preparing professionals toward competent, independent, accountable nursing practice" (Carpenter & Hudacek, 1996, p. 42). This general theme for a practice doctorate remains consistent even today. Unfortunately, this program did not share the same popularity of DNS or PhD degrees in nursing, and it was less common to find a clinician with this preparation. Further, the curricula in these programs were varied and lacked a uniform approach toward a practice doctorate (Marion, et al., 2003).

In 2002, the AACN board of directors formed a task force to examine the current progress of practice doctorates in nursing. Their objective also included comparing proposed curriculum models and discussing recommendations for the future of a practice doctorate (AACN, 2004). To accomplish their mission, the AACN task force (2004) took part in the following activities:

- Reviewed the literature regarding practice doctorates in nursing and other disciplines.
- Established a collaborative relationship with the National Organization of Nurse Practitioner Faculties (NONPF).
- Interviewed key informants (deans, program directors, graduates, and current students) at the eight current or planned practice-focused doctoral programs in the United States.

- Held open discussions regarding issues surrounding practice-focused doctoral education at AACN's Doctoral Education Conference (January 2003 and February 2004).
- Participated in an open discussion with NONPF along with representatives from key nursing organizations and schools of nursing that were offering or planning a practice doctorate.
- Invited an External Reaction Panel, which involved participation from 10 individuals from various disciplines outside of nursing. This panel responded to the draft of the *AACN Position Statement on the Practice Doctorate in Nursing*.

In 2004, the AACN published a *Position Statement on the Practice Doctorate in Nursing* and recommended that the Doctor of Nursing Practice degree would become the terminal degree for nursing practice by 2015. According to NONPF, the purpose of the Doctor of Nursing Practice degree is to prepare nurses to meet the changing demands of health care today by becoming proficient at the following (Marion, et al., 2003):

- Evaluating evidence-based practices for care.
- Delivering care.
- Developing healthcare policy.
- Leading and managing clinical care and health systems.
- Developing interdisciplinary standards.
- Solving healthcare dilemmas.
- Reducing disparities in health care.

Not only is the development of the DNP degree a culmination of today's emerging healthcare demands, this degree also provides a choice for nurses who wish to focus their doctoral education on nursing practice.

Since its inception, the growth of this degree has been astonishing. The University of Kentucky's College of Nursing was the pioneer for this innovative degree and admitted the first DNP class in 2001. In spring of 2005, eight DNP programs were offered, with over 60 in development. By summer of 2005, 80 DNP programs were being considered. In the fall of 2005, 20 programs offered DNP degrees, and 140 programs were in development. Currently, approximately 130 DNP degree programs exist, and 100 are being considered (AACN, 2011a).

It should also be mentioned that in 1999, Columbia University's School of Nursing was formulating plans for a Doctor of Nursing Practice degree (DrNP) that would build on a model of "full-scope, cross-site primary care that Columbia had developed and evaluated over the past ten years" (Goldenberg, 2004, p. 25). This degree was spearheaded by Mary O. Mudinger, DrPH, RN, dean of Columbia University's School of Nursing. The curriculum of a DrNP program is clinically focused with advanced preparation designed to teach "cross-site, full-scope care with content in advanced differential diagnosis skills, advanced pathophysiology and microbiology, selected issues of compliance, management of health care delivery and reimbursement, advanced emergency triage and management, and professional role collaboration and referrals" (Goldenberg, 2004, p. 25). This expanded clinical component is what seems to differentiate a DrNP degree from a DNP degree. The first DrNP class graduated from Columbia University in 2003.

Since the development of the DrNP degree, the Commission on Collegiate Nursing Education (CCNE), the autonomous accrediting body of the American Association of Colleges of Nursing, has decided that only practice nursing doctorate degrees with the Doctor of Nursing Practice title will be eligible for CCNE accreditation (AACN, 2005). This decision was reached unanimously by the CCNE Board of Directors on September 29, 2005 in an effort to develop a process for accrediting only clinically focused nursing doctorates (AACN, 2005). The CCNE's decision is consistent with accrediting organizations for other health professions and helps to ensure consistency with degree titling and criteria. Specific criteria for the DNP degree, including the AACN's *Essentials of Doctoral Education for Advanced Nursing Practice* (2006b) and the *Practice Doctorate Nurse Practitioner Entry-Level Competencies* (NONPF, 2006), are discussed later in this chapter.

■ Why a Practice Doctorate in Nursing Now?

It has already been mentioned that the notion of a practice doctorate is not new, so why the development of the DNP degree now? It has been noted that the development of the DNP is "more than a mere interruption but rather a response to the need within the healthcare system for expert clinical teachers and clinicians" (Marion, O'Sullivan, Crabtree, Price, & Fontana, 2005, para. 1). The needs of health care are also not new, yet the growth of this program has been escalating. The question is therefore posed, What are the drivers of this DNP degree, and why such urgency?

The Institute of Medicine's Report and Nursing's Response

In 2000, the Institute of Medicine (IOM) published a report titled *To Err Is Human*. This report summarized information regarding errors made in health care and offered recommendations to improve the overall quality of care. It was found that "preventable adverse events are a leading cause of death in the United States" (Kohn, Corrigan, & Donaldson, 2000, p. 26). Out of over 33.6 million admissions to U.S. hospitals in 1997, 44,000 to 98,000 people died as a result of medical-related errors (American Hospital Association, 1999). It was estimated that deaths in hospitals by preventable adverse events exceed the amount attributable to the eighth leading cause of death in America (Centers for Disease Control and Prevention, 1999b). These numbers also exceed the number of deaths attributable to motor vehicle accidents (43,458), breast cancer (42,297), or AIDS (16,516) (Centers for Disease Control and Prevention, 1999a). The total cost of health care is greatly affected by these errors as well, with estimated total national costs (lost income, lost household production, disability, healthcare costs) reported as being between $29 billion and $36 billion for adverse events and between $17 billion and $29 billion for preventable adverse events (Thomas, et al., 1999).

As a follow-up to the *To Err Is Human* report, in 2001 the IOM published *Crossing the Quality Chasm: A New Health System for the 21st Century*. In an effort to improve health care in the 21st century, the IOM proposed six specific aims for improvement. According to the IOM (2001), these six aims deem that health care should be:

1. Safe in avoiding injuries to patients from the care they receive.
2. Effective in providing services based on scientific knowledge to those who could benefit but refraining from providing services to those who may not benefit.
3. Patient centered in that provided care is respectful and responsive to individual patient preferences, needs, and values. Also, all patient values should guide all clinical decisions.
4. Timely in that wait time and sometimes harmful delays are reduced for those who give and receive care.
5. Efficient in that waste is avoided, particularly waste of equipment, supplies, ideas, and energy.
6. Equitable in that high-quality care is provided to all regardless of personal characteristics, such as gender, ethnicity, geographic location, and socioeconomic status.

The IOM (2001) emphasized that to achieve these aims, additional skills may be required of the healthcare team. This includes all individuals who care for patients. The new skills needed to improve health care and reduce errors are, ironically, many skills that nurses have long been known to exemplify. Some examples of these skills include using electronic communications, synthesizing evidence-based practice information, communicating with patients in an open manner to enable their decision making, understanding the course of illness that specifically relates to the patient's experience outside of the hospital, working collaboratively in teams, and understanding the link between health care and healthy populations (IOM, 2001). Developing expertise in these areas required curriculum changes in healthcare education as well as addressing how healthcare education is approached, organized, and funded (IOM, 2001).

In 2003, the Health Professions Education Committee responded to the IOM's *Crossing the Quality Chasm* report by publishing *Health Professions Education: A Bridge to Quality* (Greiner & Knebel, 2003). The committee recommended that "all health professionals should be educated to deliver patient-centered care as members of an interdisciplinary team, emphasizing evidence-based practice, quality improvement approaches, and informatics" (Greiner & Knebel, 2003, p. 45). To meet this goal, the committee proposed a set of competencies to be met by all healthcare clinicians, regardless of disciplines. These competencies include the following: provide patient-centered care, function in interdisciplinary teams, employ evidence-based practice, integrate quality improvement standards, and utilize various information systems (Greiner & Knebel, 2003).

As part of the continued effort to advance the education of healthcare professionals, the Robert Wood Johnson Foundation (RWJF) and the IOM specifically addressed advancing nursing education. In 2008, the RWJF and the IOM "launched a two-year initiative to respond to the need to access and transform the nursing profession" (IOM, 2010a, p. 1). The IOM appointed the Committee on the RWJF Initiative on the Future of Nursing. This committee published a report titled *The Future of Nursing: Focus on Education.*

Within this report, the IOM (2010a) concluded that the "the ways in which nurses were educated during the 20th century are no longer adequate for dealing with the realities of healthcare in the 21st century" (p. 2). The IOM reiterated the need for the aforementioned competencies such as leadership, health policy, system improvement, research and evidence-based practice, and teamwork and collaboration. In response to the increasing demands of a complex healthcare environment, the IOM recommended higher levels of education for nurses as well as new ways to educate nurses to better meet the needs of this population.

The IOM (2010a) included recommendations within this report that specifically address the number of nurses with doctorate degrees. It was noted that, although 13% of nurses hold a graduate degree, less than 1% hold doctoral degrees (IOM, 2010a). The IOM (2010a) concluded that "nurses with doctorates are needed to teach future generations of nurses and to conduct research that becomes the basis for improvements in nursing science and practice" (p. 4). Therefore, Recommendation 5 states that "schools of nursing, with support from private and public funders, academic administrators and university trustees, and accreditation bodies, should double the number of nurses with a doctorate by 2020 to add to the cadre of nurse faculty and researchers, with attention to increasing diversity" (IOM, 2010b, p. 4).

The development of the DNP degree is one of the answers to the call proposed by both the IOM's Health Professions Education Committee and the IOM's and the RWJF's Initiative on the Future of Nursing Committee to redefine how healthcare professionals are educated. Nursing has always had a vested interest in improving quality of care and patient outcomes. Since Nightingale, "nursing education has been directed toward the individualized, personalized care of the patient, not the disease" (Newman, 1975, p. 704). To further illustrate nursing's commitment to improve quality of care and patient outcomes, the competencies described by the Health Professions Education Committee are reflected in the AACN's *Essentials of Doctoral Education for Advanced Nursing Practice* and the NONPF's *Practice Doctorate Nurse Practitioner Entry-Level Competencies.* Preparing nurses at the practice doctorate level who are experts at using information technology, synthesizing and integrating evidence-based practices, and collaborating across healthcare disciplines will further enable nursing to meet the challenges of health care in the 21st century.

Additional Drivers for a Practice Doctorate in Nursing

In 2005, the National Academy of Sciences also recommended that nursing develop a nonresearch doctorate in a report entitled *Advancing the Nation's Health Needs: NIH*

Research Training Programs (National Academy of Sciences, 2005). The rationale for this initiative included increasing the numbers of expert practitioners who can also fulfill clinical nursing faculty needs (AACN, 2011b). The report specifically states that "the need for doctorally prepared practitioners and clinical faculty would be met if nursing could develop a new non-research clinical doctorate, similar to the MD and PharmD in Medicine and Pharmacy, respectively" (National Academy of Sciences, 2005, p. 74). The initiatives of the National Academy of Sciences regarding doctoral education in nursing are reflected in the American Association of Colleges of Nursing's development of the DNP degree.

Additional rationale for a practice doctorate is reflected in nursing's educational history when the practice doctorate was first proposed. Newman (1975) noted that "nursing lacked the recognition for what it has to offer and authority for putting that knowledge into practice" (p. 704). Starck, Duffy, and Vogler (1993) stated that "for nursing to be accountable to the social mandate, the numbers as well as the type of doctorally prepared nurses need attention" (p. 214). The NONPF Practice Doctorate Task Force summarized the most frequently cited additional drivers for a practice doctorate in nursing (Marion, et al., 2005):

- Parity with other professionals who are prepared with a practice doctorate. Disciplines such as audiology, dentistry, medicine, pharmacy, psychology, and physical therapy require a practice doctorate for entry into practice.
- A need for longer programs that both reflect the credit hours invested in master's degrees as well as accommodate additional information needed to prepare nurses for the demands of health care. Most master's degrees require a similar number of credit hours for completion to the number required for that of practice doctoral degrees.
- Fulfill the current needs for nursing faculty shortages. The development of a practice doctorate will help meet the needs for clinical teaching in schools of nursing.
- The increasing complexity of healthcare systems requires additional information to be included in current graduate nursing programs. Rather than further burden the amount of information needed to prepare nurses at the graduate level for a master's degree, a practice doctorate allows for additional information to be provided as well as afford a practice doctorate to prepare nurses for the changing demands of society and health care.

▪ What Is a DNP Degree Made Of? The Recipe for Curriculum Standards

The standards of a DNP program have been formulated through a collaborative effort among various consensus-based standards. These standards reflect collaborative efforts among the AACN as the *Essentials of Doctoral Education for Advanced Nursing Practice*, NONPF as the *Practice Doctorate Nurse Practitioner Entry-Level Competencies*, and most recently, the National Association of Clinical Nurse Specialists (NACNS) as *Core*

Practice Doctorate Clinical Nurse Specialist (CNS) Competencies. These organizations' strategies for setting the standards of a practice doctorate in nursing demonstrate interrelated criteria that are congruent with all rationales for a practice doctorate in nursing. It should be noted, however, that while maintaining these consensus-based standards, there may be some variability in content within DNP curricula.

The AACN Essentials of Doctoral Education for Advanced Nursing Practice

In 2006, the AACN published the *Essentials of Doctoral Education for Advanced Nursing Practice.* These Essentials are the "foundational outcome competencies deemed essential for all graduates of a DNP program regardless of specialty or functional focus" (AACN, 2006b, p. 8). Nursing faculties have the freedom to creatively design course work to meet these Essentials, which are summarized as follows:

Essential I: Scientific Underpinnings for Practice

This Essential describes the scientific foundations of nursing practice, which are based on the natural and social sciences. These sciences may include human biology, physiology, and psychology. In addition, nursing science has provided nursing with a body of knowledge to contribute to the discipline of nursing. This body of knowledge or discipline is focused on the following (adapted from AACN, 2006b; Donaldson & Crowley, 1978; Fawcett, 2005; Gortner, 1980):

■ The principles and laws that govern the life process, well-being, and optimal functioning of human beings, sick or well

■ The patterning of human behavior in interaction with the environment in normal life events and critical life situations

■ The processes by which positive changes in health status are affected

■ The wholeness of health of human beings, recognizing that they are in continuous interaction with their environments

Nursing science has expanded the discipline of nursing and includes the development of middle-range nursing theories and concepts to guide practice. Understanding the practice of nursing includes developing an understanding of scientific underpinnings for practice (the science and discipline of nursing). Specifically, the DNP degree prepares the graduate to:

■ Integrate nursing science with knowledge from the organizational, biophysical, psychological, and analytical sciences as well as ethics as the basis for the highest level of nursing practice.

■ Develop and evaluate new practice approaches based on nursing theories and theories from other disciplines.

■ Utilize science-based concepts and theories to determine the significance and nature of health and healthcare delivery phenomena, describe strategies used to enhance healthcare delivery, and evaluate outcomes

(Adapted from AACN, 2006b)

Essential II: Organizational and Systems Leadership for Quality Improvement and Systems Thinking

Preparation in organizational and systems leadership at every level is imperative for DNP graduates to have an impact on and improve healthcare delivery and patient care outcomes. DNP graduates are distinguished by their ability to focus on new healthcare delivery methods that are based on nursing science. Preparation in this area will provide DNP graduates with expertise in "assessing organizations, identifying systems' issues, and facilitating organization-wide changes in practice delivery" (AACN, 2006b, p. 10). Specifically, the DNP graduate will be prepared to:

- Utilize scientific findings in nursing and other disciplines to develop and evaluate care delivery approaches that meet the current and future needs of patient populations.
- Guarantee accountability for the safety and quality of care for the patients they care for.
- Manage ethical dilemmas within patient care, healthcare organizations, and research, including developing and evaluating appropriate strategies.

(Adapted from AACN, 2006b)

Essential III: Clinical Scholarship and Analytical Methods for Evidence-Based Practice

DNP graduates are unique in that their contributions to nursing science involve the "translation of research into practice and the dissemination and integration of new knowledge" (AACN, 2006b, p. 11). Further, DNP graduates are in a distinctive position to merge nursing science, practice, human needs, and human caring. Specifically, the DNP graduate is expected to be an expert in the evaluation, integration, translation, and application of evidence-based practices. Additionally, DNP graduates are actively involved in nursing practice, which allows for practical, applicable research questions to arise from the practice environment. Working collaboratively with experts in research investigation, DNP graduates can also assist in the generation of new knowledge and affect evidence-based practice from the practice arena. To achieve these goals, the DNP program prepares the graduate to:

- Analytically and critically evaluate existing literature and other evidence to determine the best evidence for practice.
- Evaluate practice outcomes within populations in various arenas, such as healthcare organizations, communities, or practice settings.
- Design and evaluate methodologies that improve quality in an effort to promote "safe, effective, efficient, equitable, and patient-centered care" (AACN, 2006b, p. 12).
- Develop practice guidelines that are based on relevant, best-practice findings.
- Utilize informatics and research methodology to collect and analyze data, design databases, interpret findings to design evidence-based interventions,

evaluate outcomes, and identify gaps within evidence-based practice, which will improve the practice environment.

■ Work collaboratively with research specialists and act as a "practice consultant" (AACN, 2006b, p. 12).

(Adapted from AACN, 2006b)

Essential IV: Information Systems/Technology and Patient Care Technology for the Improvement and Transformation of Health Care

DNP graduates are cutting edge in their ability to use information technology to improve patient care and outcomes. Knowledge regarding the designing and implementing of information systems to evaluate programs and outcomes of care is essential for preparation as a DNP graduate. Expertise is garnered in information technology, such as web-based communications, telemedicine, online documentation, and other unique healthcare delivery methods. DNP graduates must also develop expertise in utilizing information technologies to support practice leadership and clinical decision making. Specific to information systems, DNP graduates are prepared to:

■ Evaluate and monitor outcomes of care and quality of care improvement by designing, selecting, using, and evaluating programs related to information technologies.

■ Become proficient at the skills necessary to evaluate data extraction from practice information systems and databases.

■ Attend to ethical and legal issues related to information technologies within the healthcare setting by providing leadership to evaluate and resolve these issues.

■ Communicate and evaluate the accuracy, timeliness, and appropriateness of healthcare consumer information.

(Adapted from AACN, 2006b)

Essential V: Healthcare Policy for Advocacy in Health Care

Becoming involved in healthcare policy/advocacy has the potential to affect the delivery of health care across all settings. Thus, knowledge and skills related to healthcare policy are central to nursing practice and therefore essential to the DNP graduate. Further, "health policy influences multiple care delivery issues, including health disparities, cultural sensitivity, ethics, the internalization of health care concerns, access to care, quality of care, health care financing, and issues of equity and social justice in the delivery of health care" (AACN, 2006b, p. 13). DNP graduates are uniquely positioned to be powerful advocates for healthcare policy through their practice experiences. These practice experiences provide rich influences for the development of policy. Nursing's interest in social justice and equality requires that DNP graduates become involved in and develop expertise in healthcare policy and advocacy.

Additionally, DNP graduates need to be prepared in leadership roles with regard to public policy. As leaders in the practice setting, DNP graduates frequently assimilate research, practice, and policy. Therefore, DNP preparation should include experience in recognizing the factors that influence the development of policy across various settings. The DNP graduate is prepared to:

- Decisively analyze health policies and proposals from the points of view of consumers, nurses, and other healthcare professionals.
- Provide leadership in the development and implementation of healthcare policy at the institutional, local, state, federal, and international levels.
- Actively participate on committees, boards, or task forces at the institutional, local, state, federal, and international levels.
- Participate in the education of other healthcare professionals, patients, or other stakeholders regarding healthcare policy issues.
- Act as an advocate for the nursing profession through activities related to healthcare policy.
- Influence healthcare financing, regulation, and delivery through the development of leadership in healthcare policy.
- Act as an advocate for ethical, equitable, and social justice policies across all healthcare settings.

(Adapted from AACN, 2006b)

Essential VI: Interprofessional Collaboration for Improving Patient and Population Health Outcomes

This Essential specifically relates to the IOM's mandate to provide safe, timely, equitable, effective, efficient, and patient-centered care. In a multitiered, complex healthcare environment, collaboration among all healthcare disciplines must exist to achieve the IOM's and nursing's goals. Nurses are experts at functioning as collaborators among multiple disciplines. Therefore, as nursing practice experts, DNP graduates must be prepared to facilitate collaboration and team building. This may include both participating in the work of the team and assuming leadership roles when necessary.

With regard to interprofessional collaboration, the DNP graduate must be prepared to:

- Participate in effective communication and collaboration throughout the development of "practice models, peer review, practice guidelines, health policy, standards of care, and/or other scholarly products" (AACN, 2006b, p. 15).
- Analyze complex practice or organizational issues through leadership of interprofessional teams.
- Act as a consultant to interprofessional teams to implement change in healthcare delivery systems.

(Adapted from AACN, 2006b)

Essential VII: Clinical Prevention and Population Health for Improving the Nation's Health

Clinical prevention is defined as health promotion and risk reduction/illness prevention for individuals and families, and population health is defined as including all community, environmental, cultural, and socioeconomic aspects of health (Allan, et al., 2004; AACN, 2006b). Nursing has foundations in health promotion and risk reduction and is therefore positioned to have an impact on the health status of people in multiple settings. The further preparation included in the DNP curriculum will prepare graduates to "analyze epidemiological, biostatistical, occupational, and environmental data in the development, implementation, and evaluation of clinical prevention and population health" (AACN, 2006b, p. 15). In other words, DNP graduates are in an ideal position to participate in health promotion and risk reduction activities from a nursing perspective with additional preparation in evaluating and interpreting data pertinent to improving the health status of individuals.

(Adapted from AACN, 2006b)

Essential VIII: Advanced Nursing Practice

Because one cannot become proficient in all areas of specialization, DNP degree programs "provide preparation within distinct specialties that require expertise, advanced knowledge, and mastery in one area of nursing practice" (AACN, 2006b, p. 16). This specialization is defined by a specialty practice area within the domain of nursing as well as a requisite of the DNP degree. Although the DNP graduate may function in a variety of roles, role preparation within the practice specialty, including legal and regulatory issues, is part of every DNP curriculum. With regard to advanced nursing practice, the DNP graduate is prepared to:

- Comprehensively assess health and illness parameters while incorporating diverse and culturally sensitive approaches.
- Implement and evaluate therapeutic interventions based on nursing and other sciences.
- Participate in therapeutic relationships with patients and other healthcare professionals to ensure optimal patient care and improve patient outcomes.
- Utilize advanced clinical decision-making skills and critical thinking, as well as deliver and evaluate evidence-based care to improve patient outcomes.
- Serve as a mentor to others in the nursing profession in an effort to maintain excellence in nursing practice.
- Participate in the education of patients, especially those in complex health situations.

(Adapted from AACN, 2006b)

A Note About Specialty-Focused Competencies According to the AACN

The purpose of specialty preparation within the DNP curricula is to prepare graduates to fulfill specific roles within health care. Specialty preparation, along with the DNP Essentials I–VIII, prepares DNP graduates for roles in two different domains. The first domain includes roles that involve specialization as advanced practice registered nurses who care for individuals (including, but not limited to: clinical nurse specialist, nurse practitioner, nurse anesthetist, nurse–midwife). The second domain includes roles that involve specialization in advanced practice at an organizational or systems level. Because of this variability, specialization content within DNP programs differs (AACN, 2006b).

The NONPF Practice Doctorate Nurse Practitioner Entry-Level Competencies

NONPF has developed specific *Practice Doctorate Nurse Practitioner Entry-Level Competencies* for nurse practitioner/DNP graduates. These Competencies differ somewhat from the AACN's Essentials in that they are particular to nurse practitioner roles. However, these Competencies are also reflective of the AACN's Essentials. These Competencies are as follows:

I.   Competency Area: Independent Practice
   - Practices independently by assessing, diagnosing, treating, and managing undifferentiated patients.
   - Assumes full accountability for actions as a licensed practitioner.

II. Competency Area: Scientific Foundation
   - Critically analyzes data for practice by integrating knowledge from arts and sciences within the context of nursing's philosophical framework and scientific foundation.
   - Translates research and data to anticipate, predict, and explain variations in practice.

III. Competency Area: Leadership
   - Assumes increasingly complex leadership roles.
   - Provides leadership to foster intercollaboration.
   - Demonstrates a leadership style that uses critical and reflective thinking.

IV. Competency Area: Quality
   - Uses best available evidence to enhance quality in clinical practice.
   - Evaluates how organizational, structural, financial, marketing, and policy decisions affect cost, quality, and accessibility of health care.
   - Demonstrates skills in peer review that promote a culture of excellence.

V.   Competency Area: Practice Inquiry
   - Applies clinical investigative skills for evaluation of health outcomes at the patient, family, population, clinical unit, systems, and/or community levels.

- Provides leadership in the translation of new knowledge into practice.
- Disseminates evidence from inquiry to diverse audiences using multiple methods.

VI. Competency Area: Technology and Information Literacy
- Demonstrates information literacy in complex decision making.
- Translates technical and scientific health information appropriate for user need.

VII. Competency Area: Policy
- Analyzes ethical, legal, and social factors in policy development.
- Influences health policy.
- Evaluates the impact of globalization on healthcare policy.

VIII. Competency Area: Health Delivery System
- Applies knowledge of organizational behavior and systems.
- Demonstrates skills in negotiating, consensus building, and partnering.
- Manages risks to individuals, families, populations, and healthcare systems.
- Facilitates development of culturally relevant healthcare systems.

IX. Competency Area: Ethics
- Applies ethically sound solutions to complex issues.[1]

Core Practice Doctorate Clinical Nurse Specialist (CNS) Competencies

In 2006, the National Association of Clinical Nurse Specialists (NACNS) consulted with various nursing organizations and nursing accrediting entities regarding the implications of the DNP degree for CNS practice and education (NACNS, 2009). A formal task force, including representatives from NACNS and 19 other nursing organizations, was charged with developing competencies for the CNS at the doctoral level (NACNS, 2009). Because traditional CNS education has included a master's degree, the *Core Practice Doctorate Clinical Nurse Specialist Competencies* should be used with the National CNS Competency Task Force Organizing Framework and Core Competencies (2008) and the AACN *Essentials of Doctoral Education for Advanced Nursing Practice* (2006) to inform educational programs and employer expectations" (NACNS, 2009, p. 10). The NACNS core competencies can be accessed at http://www.nacns.org/docs/CorePracticeDoctorate.pdf.

The foci of the *Core Practice Doctorate Clinical Nurse Specialist Competencies* are congruent with the AACN's *Essentials of Doctoral Education for Advanced Nursing Practice* and the NONPF's *Practice Doctorate Nurse Practitioner Entry-Level Competencies*. (See **Figure 1-1**.) Specifically, graduates of CNS-focused DNP programs should be prepared beyond traditional CNS competencies to "strengthen the already significant contribution that CNSs make in ensuring quality patient outcomes through

---

[1]Competencies provided courtesy of the National Organization of Nurse Practitioner Faculties (NONPF). Available at www.nonpf.org.

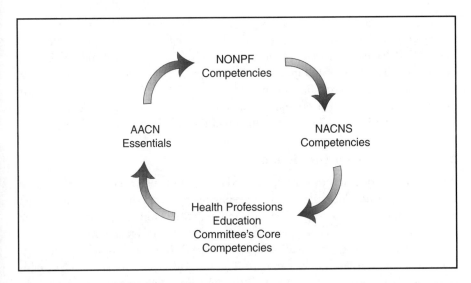

■ **Figure 1-1** Relationship among the DNP Essentials, the NONPF Competencies, the NACNS Competencies, and the Core Competencies Needed for Healthcare Professionals per the Committee on Health Professions Education.

establishing a practice foundation based on advanced scientific, theoretical, ethical, and economic principles" (NACNS, 2009, p. 11). These competencies ensure that doctoral-prepared CNS graduates are prepared to:

- Generate and disseminate new knowledge
- Evaluate and translate evidence into practice
- Employ a broad range of theories from nursing and related disciplines
- Design and evaluate innovative strategies to improve quality of care and safety in all settings
- Improve systems of care
- Provide leadership that promotes interprofessional collaboration
- Influence and shape health policy

(Adapted from NACNS, 2009)

The Path to the DNP Degree: Follow the Academic Road

The path to the DNP degree is currently in transition. It should be mentioned that while the transition toward DNP preparation as entry into advanced nursing practice is taking place, current DNP programs are being offered as a post-master's degree. Many prospective students will have already fulfilled several of the criteria listed in the *Essentials of Doctoral Education for Advanced Nursing Practice* as well as the

Practice Doctorate Nurse Practitioner Entry-Level Competencies in their master's degree curricula. Further, as mentioned earlier, the specialization content included in the DNP degree curriculum is currently being fulfilled within the master's degree curriculum. Therefore, each individual's path to the DNP degree may be unique. Prospective students' program content may be individualized to include the learning experiences necessary to incorporate the described requirements for the DNP degree. Please refer to **Figure 1-2** for an illustration of the pathways to the DNP degree.

■ Role Transition Introduced

As explained earlier in the chapter, the DNP is currently not a specialization degree but rather a practice doctorate for advanced nursing practice. This degree builds upon advanced nursing practice specialization and provides additional preparation in the formulation, interpretation, and utilization of evidence-based practices, health policy, information technology, and leadership. Although DNP graduates may function as evaluators and translators of research, health policy advocates, nursing leaders, educators or clinicians, it is entirely likely that these roles will be integrated as well. One DNP graduate may participate in research in addition to practicing as a nurse anesthetist. Another DNP graduate may be a nurse executive in addition to developing health policy. Nursing has always been a profession that involves juggling multiple roles (Dudley-Brown, 2006; Jennings & Rogers, 1988; Sperhac & Strodtbeck, 1997).

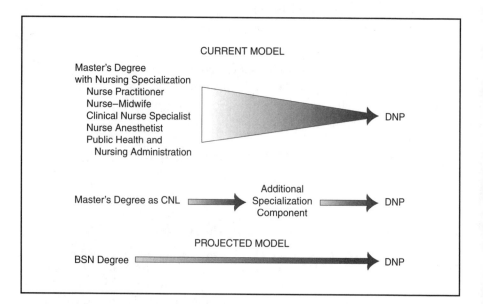

■ **Figure 1-2** Pathways to the DNP Degree.

Within these multiple roles, the fundamental goal of the DNP graduate remains the development of expertise in the delivery of high-quality, patient-centered care, which utilizes the necessary avenues to provide that care.

Interview with a DNP Co-Founder: Then and Now

Carolyn A. Williams, PhD, RN, FAAN, is Professor and Dean Emeritus of the University of Kentucky. She was president of the American Association of Colleges of Nursing from 2000 to 2002 and Scholar-in-Residence at the Institute of Medicine from 2007 to 2008.

Then . . . 2008

Dr. Williams, could you please describe your background and current position?

I began my nursing career as a public health nurse at a public health department in a rural area and practiced for 2 years before returning to graduate school. I then received my master's degree in public health nursing. This was a joint master's degree from both the School of Nursing and the School of Public Health from the University of North Carolina at Chapel Hill (UNC, CH). I then went on to earn a PhD in epidemiology from the School of Public Health at UNC, CH. This was met with some controversy in that I did not have a large amount of nursing experience before returning to graduate school. Interestingly, the School of Public Health was supportive of my doctoral studies whereas the School of Nursing seemed to think I needed more nursing experience. This is what I call a "pernicious pattern" in nursing education. I actually had to talk faculty (in nursing) into supporting me to earn a doctorate. However, faculty from other disciplines, e.g., medicine, psychology, and sociology in the School of Public Health, were very supportive. This is where nursing differs from medicine: We don't build in the experience into our educational programs.

Upon finishing my PhD in epidemiology, I took a faculty position at Emory University's School of Nursing. From there, I was asked to return to Chapel Hill to participate in the development and evaluation of a family nurse practitioner program in the School of Nursing and to teach epidemiology in the School of Public Health. The program in the School of Nursing was one of the first six federally funded family nurse practitioner programs in the country. I remained at Chapel Hill for 13 years before accepting an appointment as dean of the College of Nursing at the University of Kentucky. Last year I retired as dean after 22 years in that position and remained as a faculty member.

This year (2007 to 2008) I am a Scholar-in-Residence at the Institute of Medicine in Washington, DC. My role here includes development of a project, which happens to be interprofessional collaboration. This stems from the view that improvement in quality care depends on people working together in interprofessional teams. Interprofessional collaboration is happening around the margins of education for health care instead of in the mainstream, particularly core clinical components of undergraduate and graduate education for health care. It may be picked up in passing, but frequently it is not a formal part of the curriculum. Part of my project involves identifying the policy changes [that] are needed at the university level to integrate interprofessional collaboration as part [of] an integral component of education in the health professions. Interprofessional collaboration is a necessary part of practice and therefore needs to be integrated into the preparation of healthcare professionals. This leads me to an issue I have always struggled with: Too few clinical faculty in nursing actually practice. This is a problem due to the fact that a practice culture is not as visible as I believe it needs to be in most schools of nursing. Some progress in having nursing faculty engaged in practice was achieved with the nurse practitioner movement that started in the 1970s, but it is still a struggle for nursing faculty to engage in practice as part of their faculty role in a manner similar to what happens in medical education. Some faculty attempt to practice on their own, not as a part of their faculty role, and usually faculty practice is not viewed as a priority in schools of nursing. I feel if we want nursing faculty to provide leadership in practice and develop leaders for practice, each school of nursing needs to have a core group of faculty who actually engage in practice as part of their faculty role.

Dr. Williams, could you please describe how your vision for a Doctor of Nursing Practice became a reality?

While on the faculty at the University of North Carolina at Chapel Hill and consulting with a number of individuals in practice settings, I developed some ideas of what nursing education to prepare nurse leaders needs to be. Initially, I viewed the degree as what public health nurses could earn to prepare them to face the challenges of public health nursing. I didn't feel that the master's degrees in nursing offered at that time (1970s through early 1980s) were sufficient for the kind of leadership roles nurses were moving into. I felt a true practice degree at the doctoral level was needed.

When I went to the University of Kentucky as the dean of nursing, I was charged with developing a PhD in nursing program. While at Chapel Hill I had been very involved in research activity, doctoral education in epidemiology, and was active nationally in research development and advocacy in nursing as chair of the American Nurses Association's Commission on Nursing Research and as the president of the American Academy of Nursing. I proceeded to work with the faculty at the University of Kentucky, and we developed the PhD program in nursing. However, I was still interested in the concept of a practice doctorate and promoting stronger partnerships between nursing practice and nursing education.

As time went on it became clearer and clearer to me that to prepare nurses for leadership in practice, something more in tune with preparing nurses to utilize knowledge, not necessarily generate new knowledge, which was expected in PhD programs, was needed. Thus, I began to talk with and work with my faculty colleagues on the concept of a new practice degree for nurses to prepare for leadership in practice, not in education or research.

I saw practice as the focus with this degree, not research. Working with my University of Kentucky faculty colleagues, particularly Dr. Marcia K. Stanhope and Dr. Julie G. Sebastian, we developed the initial conceptualization of the degree. These foci included four themes that I feel should be central to a practice doctorate in nursing:

- Leadership in practice, which included leadership at the point of care. This also includes leadership at the policy level to impact care.
- A population approach and perspective. This involves a broader view of health care, which recognizes the importance of populations when planning and evaluating care processes.
- Integration of evidence-based practice to make informed decisions regarding care.
- The ability to understand change processes and institute positive changes in health care.

These four themes guided the development of the curriculum of the first DNP program at the University of Kentucky, which when we instituted it was the first in the United States. These themes also influenced and are incorporated in what became the AACN's *Essentials of Doctoral Education in Advanced Nursing Practice*.

To expand on the development of the DNP program at University of Kentucky, the following is the timeline:

1994–1998	Informal conversations among faculty, people in practice, and others regarding a practice doctorate in nursing.
1998	Professional Doctorate Task Force Committee formed.
May 1999	Approval of DNP program by total college faculty.
July 1999	Medical Center Academic Council approval.
January 2000	University of Kentucky Board of Trustees approved the program.
May 2000	Approval by the Kentucky Council of Postsecondary Education.
January 2001	The first national paper on the DNP degree at the AACN's National Doctoral Education Conference (Williams, Stanhope, & Sebastian, 2001).
Fall 2001	Students admitted to the first DNP program in the country.

In 1998, when the University of Kentucky's DNP task force was created, we decided we didn't want this degree to look like anything else currently in nursing education. We also decided on the name of this degree in this committee. We wanted the degree and the name to focus on nursing practice, and we did not want the degree to be limited to preparing for only one particular type of nursing practice. We decided on the Doctor of Nursing Practice because that describes what the degree is: a practice degree in nursing.

One of the most important things that happened during my presidency of the American Association of Colleges of Nursing was the appointment [of] a task force to look at the issue of a practice doctorate. The task force committee was carefully planned. I wanted to have a positive group of people as well as major stakeholders represented. These stakeholders were credible individuals who had an interest in the development of a practice doctorate. Members of the committee included representatives from Columbia University, the University of Kentucky, a representative from an ND program, as well as a representative from schools that did not have nursing doctoral programs. This committee was chaired by Dr. Elizabeth Lentz, who has written extensively on doctoral education in nursing. As this task force began sorting out the issues, it became the goal that by 2015, the DNP would become the terminal degree for specialization in nursing.

From this point, a group to develop both the essentials of doctoral education in nursing and a roadmap task force were formed. These committees worked together, and we presented together nationally in a series of regional forums. We invited others to engage in discourse regarding the essentials as well as ask questions about the DNP degree. As our presentations across the country came to a conclusion, we noticed an obvious transformation. The DNP degree was beginning to gain more acceptance. By the time we were done, the argument of whether to adopt a practice doctorate in nursing had given rise to how to put this degree in place.

Dr. Williams, are you surprised by the acceptance of the degree and speed with which programs are being developed?

Yes, I am surprised. I thought the DNP degree would be an important development for the field of nursing, and I thought some would adopt a practice doctorate. I certainly did not think things would move so fast. The idea of a DNP really struck a chord with many people.

Dr. Williams, do you think the history of doctoral education in nursing has influenced the development of a practice doctorate in nursing?

Well, we need to have scientists in our field. However, we also need to come to grips with the fact that we are a practice discipline. Over the years, since the late 1970s, many of the leading academic settings in nursing have become increasingly research intensive and [have] not spent as much effort on developing a complementary practice focus. I feel the development of a practice doctorate has more to do with our development as a discipline than the history of doctoral nursing education. Attraction and credibility from the university setting stem from involvement in research. Therefore, it becomes a struggle when handling this practice piece. If nursing wants acceptance as a discipline, we must have research. But we are a practice discipline, and all practice disciplines struggle to some extent in research-intensive university environments.

Dr. Williams, do you agree that nursing should have both a research- and a practice-focused doctorate?

Of course. The ratio between research-focused and practice-focused doctorates may be tipped toward the practice focused due to the practice focus of our discipline.

Dr. Williams, could you describe what you feel is the future of doctoral education in nursing?

Down the pike, some people may move into DNP programs and then discover they want to be researchers and end up also getting a PhD. This would be very healthy for our profession. Essentially, we have lost talented folks due to offering only a research-focused terminal degree. The DNP allows us to accommodate those folks who don't want a research-focused degree.

I also feel we need a more intensive clinical component integrated into the degree. This may be in the form of residency programs integrated within nursing degrees or as a postdoctorate option.

Dr. Williams, could you expand on the grandfathering of advanced practice registered nurses (APRN) who don't wish to pursue a DNP degree?

The DNP degree will not be required to practice anytime soon. It took a while to require a master's degree to practice as an APRN. There will be a similar transition regarding the DNP degree. If someone is certified and successful as an APRN without a DNP, they should continue to be successful.

Dr. Williams, do you believe the DNP will continue to flourish as a degree option for nursing? If so, what would your advice be regarding nurses earning a DNP degree?

Yes, I do. My advice regarding nurses earning a DNP degree is that it depends on their career choice. Some have been looking for this option for a long time. This may be the right degree for some no matter where they are in practice.

Now . . . 2011

Dr. Williams, we discussed your nursing background and education last time we spoke. Could you please describe your current position and what types of projects you are currently involved in?

After leaving the deanship at the University of Kentucky I continued my role as a professor on the faculty. Throughout my time as dean of the college I always had a teaching assignment, although limited but usually one course a year. I now have a full-time teaching commitment and teach several courses in the DNP Program including one course that both DNP and PhD students take. In addition, I am working on a project to try to enhance the role of nursing faculty in clinical practice and decision-making roles in academic health science centers. This is the environment where many of our graduate students in nursing in North America are prepared, as well as a large proportion of our undergraduates. Yet, the way nursing education has been involved in clinical matters is very different from the role medicine plays. There are many reasons for this. I am evaluating this in an effort to understand and identify options for change.

Last time we talked, you were working at the Institute of Medicine on a special project regarding interprofessional collaboration. Did this project include any implications for DNP graduates?

While I was at the IOM I spent some time looking at interprofessional collaboration and how to enhance it. There is much written about preparing health professionals to value interprofessional collaboration and engage with other health professionals as they care for patients. However, innovative learning opportunities to expose students to interprofessional experiences represent a major challenge for educators in all of the health professions. Creating such experiences are particularly important for those preparing DNP students because of the role DNP graduates will play in working with and coordinating with other health professionals. But the educational model many DNP programs have developed involving distant learning strategies means that DNP faculty members have to be both highly committed to the importance of such learning experiences and extremely creative as they design them.

What is your impression of the progress of the DNP degree? How does the current progress of the DNP degree compare to your original vision of the DNP degree?

Our original vision at the University of Kentucky was that the DNP would be a doctoral degree for leadership in practice. The first program was set up as a post-master's offering. When AACN's Doctoral Task Force, that I appointed while I was AACN's President, proposed that preparation for specialization in nursing should be at the DNP level, I supported the proposal and worked to implement it as chair of the Roadmap Task Force and in other ways. I am still supportive of the concept.

I am surprised about how many programs have developed in a relatively short time. And, I admit to being somewhat concerned about what seems to be an effort in some programs to make the program as short as possible. Of course, we do not want to have unnecessarily long programs, but the DNP is a doctoral degree and there needs to be time for in-depth doctoral-level work. The challenge the discipline faces is to make sure that all DNP programs are high-quality doctoral programs. As more schools develop BSN to DNP programs, this challenge will be felt to a greater extent. Faculty will be challenged to prepare, in a very limited time frame, beginning specialists in an area of practice who also possess the broader analytical skills necessary for leadership.

I am aware that there are those in nursing who argue we should retreat back to the master's in order to respond to human resources concerns. I do not agree. I believe the history of nursing is replete with examples of compromising the education of nurses to deal with human resources issues. I think the momentum of the DNP, a concept that has "clicked" with so many young nurses, is strong enough to overcoming the backtracking of some.

Why do you think the DNP degree continues to gain acceptance and momentum?

In my view the reason is that the DNP was conceived to prepare nurses to move with and lead the kind of system changes necessary in health care. The first DNP program at Kentucky had four key concepts which formed the foundation for the program: a population-system perspective, evidence-based decision making, leadership, and facilitating change. These concepts remain as important components of the DNP essentials and as curricular components in DNP programs. I believe that young nurses who want to make a difference in their career in nursing realize that they will need additional knowledge, skills, and approaches to be successful in the complex arena of health care and they see that the DNP program can help provide what is needed.

When we last spoke in 2008, you agreed that nursing needed both a research- and practice-focused doctorate. Do you still agree that a research- and practice-focused doctorate are beneficial to the profession?

Absolutely YES!!!! We are a practice discipline and we need some of those in practice to be prepared with a focus on practice at the doctoral level. Had we had a practice-focused second professional degree earlier in our history I believe our discipline would be in a very different place today. We have a lot of ground to make up when we consider that as a health professional group, professional nurses are the least educated of the health professionals and each year the majority of those who sit for the licensure examination are not prepared at the baccalaureate level. Yes, we desperately need as many nurses with a practice doctorate that we can produce in order to change the world of nursing practice.

Do you believe that a partnership is currently forming between PhD and DNP graduates?

I believe this is coming. I think it will be most evident in schools that offer both programs. I think it will become clear to thoughtful faculty in such schools that there are some commonalities to both programs and we will see some creative curricular plans that allow students in both programs to work together at various points in their programs of study. The faculty at the University of Iowa has developed an innovative curricular model that brings together both student groups for selected experiences and has excellent potential for facilitating collaboration. A key factor at Iowa is that the faculty who teach in both programs are modeling what collaboration looks like for the students of both programs. This is very innovative and very inspiring.

How would you recommend we continue to move forward with the AACN's recommended target date of the DNP for entry into practice by 2015?

My answer is very simple, KEEP PRESSING FORWARD, DON'T MISS A BEAT!

SUMMARY

- The DNP degree is defined as a practice-focused doctorate degree that prepares graduates as experts in nursing practice.
- Nursing practice is defined by the AACN as "any form of nursing intervention that influences health care outcomes for individuals or populations, including direct care of individual patients, administration of nursing and health care organizations, and the implementation of health policy" (AACN, 2004, p. 3).
- According to the AACN's (2004) position statement, the DNP degree is proposed to be the terminal degree for nursing practice by 2015.
- A nursing PhD degree is a research-focused degree, and the DNP degree is a practice-focused degree.
- The evolution of doctoral education in nursing illustrates where we have been in doctoral education and the direction nursing is taking in the development of doctoral education.
- The concept of a practice doctorate is not new. The idea began in the 1970s with the development of the DNS degree.
- The AACN now designates the DNS and PhD degrees as research-focused degrees, with the DNP/DrNP being the designated practice-focused degrees.
- In 2002, the AACN board of directors formed a task force to examine the current progress of proposed doctorates in nursing.
- In 2000, the Institute of Medicine published a report titled *To Err Is Human*, which summarized errors made in the healthcare system and proposed recommendations to improve the overall quality of care.
- In 2003, the Health Professions Education Committee published *Health Professions Education: A Bridge to Quality*, which outlined a specific set of competencies that should be met by all clinicians.
- In 2008, the IOM appointed the Committee on the RWJF Initiative on the Future of Nursing. This committee published a report in 2010 titled *The Future of Nursing: Focus on Education*, which concluded that the "the ways in which nurses were educated during the 20th century are no longer adequate for dealing with the realities of healthcare in the 21st century" (IOM, 2010, p. 2). This committee also recommended doubling the number of nurses with doctorates by the year 2020.
- In 2004, the AACN published a position statement regarding a practice doctorate in nursing and recommended that by 2015 all nurses pursuing advanced practice degrees will be prepared as DNP graduates.
- In 2005, the National Academy of Sciences also recommended that a nonresearch nursing doctorate be developed to meet nursing faculty needs.
- In 2006, the AACN described the *Essentials of Doctoral Education for Advanced Nursing Practice*, which represents the standards for DNP curricula.
- NONPF outlined the *Practice Doctorate Nurse Practitioner Entry-Level Competencies* as standards for DNP curricula.

■ In 2009, the NACNS developed *Core Practice Doctorate Clinical Nurse Specialist Competencies.*

■ The DNP degree is currently a post-master's degree program while the transition to the doctoral preparation for advanced nursing practice is taking place.

■ Graduate students may follow an individualized path to the DNP degree depending on their current master's degree preparation.

■ DNP graduates may be involved in many different roles that may include, but are not limited to, evaluation and translation of research, leader, health policy advocate, educator, and clinician.

REFLECTION QUESTIONS

1. How do you think nursing's history has contributed to the development of the DNP degree?
2. How do you think the IOM report *To Err Is Human*, along with the follow-up report *Crossing the Quality Chasm*, contributed to the development of the DNP degree?
3. Explain why you think the IOM and the RWJF concluded in their report *The Future of Nursing: Focus on Education* that nurses need improvement in their educational preparation.
4. Do you think a struggle still exists within nursing today regarding whether doctoral education should be research or practice focused?
5. Do you think nursing doctoral education should be research focused, practice focused, or both?
6. Do you think a DNP degree is the right degree for you?

REFERENCES

Allan, J., Barwick, T., Cashman, S., Cawley, J. F., Day, C., Douglass, C. W., et al. (2004). Clinical prevention and population health: Curriculum framework for health professions. *American Journal of Preventive Medicine, 27*(5), 471–476.

American Association of Colleges of Nursing (AACN). (2001). *Indicators of quality in research-focused doctoral programs in nursing.* Washington, DC: Author.

American Association of Colleges of Nursing (AACN). (2004). *AACN position statement on the practice doctorate in nursing.* Retrieved from http://www.aacn.nche.edu/DNP/pdf/DNP.pdf

American Association of Colleges of Nursing (AACN). (2005). *Commission on Collegiate Nursing Education moves to consider for accreditation only practice doctorates with the DNP degree title.* Retrieved from http://www.aacn.nche.edu/Media/NewsReleases/Archives/2005/CCNEDNP.htm

American Association of Colleges of Nursing (AACN). (2006a). *Doctor of nursing practice roadmap task force report.* Retrieved from http://www.aacn.nche.edu/dnp/roadmapreport.pdf.

American Association of Colleges of Nursing (AACN). (2006b). *Essentials of doctoral education for advanced nursing practice.* Retrieved from http://www.aacn.nche.edu/publications/position /DNPEssentials.pdf

American Association of Colleges of Nursing (AACN). (2007). *AACN white paper on the education and role of the clinical nurse leader.* Retrieved from http://www.aacn.nche.edu/publications/white-papers/cnl

American Association of Colleges of Nursing. (2011a). *DNP program schools.* Retrieved from http://www .aacn.nche.edu/dnp/program-schools

American Association of Colleges of Nursing (AACN). (2011b). *Fact sheet: The doctor of nursing practice.* Retrieved from http://www.aacn.nche.edu/media-relations/fact-sheets/dnp

American Hospital Association. (1999). *Hospital statistics.* Chicago: Author.

Apold, S. (2008). The doctor of nursing practice: Looking back, moving forward. *Journal for Nurse Practitioners, 4*(2), 101–107.

Carpenter, R., & Hudacek, S. (1996). *On doctoral education in nursing: The voice of the student.* New York: National League for Nursing Press.

Centers for Disease Control and Prevention, National Center for Health Statistics. (1999a). Births and deaths: Preliminary data for 1998. *National Vital Statistics Reports, 47*(25), 1–45.

Centers for Disease Control and Prevention, National Center for Health Statistics. (1999b). Deaths: Final data for 1997. *National Vital Statistics Reports, 47*(19), 1–104.

Cleland, V. (1976). Developing a doctoral program. *Nursing Outlook, 24*(10), 631–635.

Donaldson, S., & Crowley, D. (1978). The discipline of nursing. *Nursing Outlook, 26*(2), 113–120.

Dracup, K., Cronenwett, L., Meleis, A., & Benner, P. (2005). Reflections on the doctorate of nursing practice. *Nursing Outlook, 53*(4), 177–182.

Dudley-Brown, S. (2006). Revisiting the blended role of the advanced practice nurse. *Gastroenterology Nursing, 29*(3), 249–250.

Fawcett, J. (2005). *Contemporary nursing knowledge: Analysis and evaluation of nursing models and theories* (2nd ed.). Philadelphia: F. A. Davis.

Goldenberg, G. (2004). The DrNP degree. *The Academic Nurse: The Journal of the Columbia University School of Nursing, 21*(1), 22–26.

Gortner, S. (1980). Nursing science in transition. *Nursing Research, 29*(3), 180–183.

Grace, H. (1978). The development of doctoral education in nursing: In historical perspective. *Journal of Nursing Education, 17*(4), 17–27.

Greiner, A. C., & Knebel, E. (Eds.). (2003). *Health professions education: A bridge to quality.* Washington, DC: National Academies Press.

Institute of Medicine (IOM). (2001). *Crossing the quality chasm: A new health system for the 21st century.* Washington, DC: National Academies Press.

Institute of Medicine. (2010a). *The future of nursing: Focus on education.* Retrieved from http://www .iom.edu/~/media/Files/Report%20Files/2010/The-Future-of-Nursing/Nursing%20Education %202010%20Brief.pdf

Institute of Medicine. (2010b). *The future of nursing: Leading change, advancing health.* Report recommendations. Retrieved from http://www.iom.edu/Reports/2010/The-Future-of-Nursing-Leading-Change-Advancing-Health.aspx

Jennings, B., & Rogers, S. (1988). Merging nursing research and practice: A case of multiple identities. *Journal of Advanced Nursing Research, 13*(6), 752–758.

Kohn, L. T., Corrigan, J. M., & Donaldson, M. S. (Eds.). (2000). *To err is human: Building a safer health system.* Committee on Quality of Health Care in America, Institute of Medicine. Washington, DC: National Academies Press.

Marion, L., O'Sullivan, A., Crabtree, M. K., Price, M., & Fontana, S. (2005). Curriculum models for the practice doctorate in nursing. *Topics in Advanced Practice Nursing eJournal, 5*(1). Retrieved from http://www.medscape.com/viewarticle/500742_print

Marion, L., Viens, D., O'Sullivan, A., Crabtree, M. K., Fontana, S., & Price, M. (2003). The practice doctorate in nursing: Future or fringe. *Topics in Advanced Practice Nursing eJournal, 3*(2). Retrieved from http://www.medscape.com/viewarticle/453247_print

Marriner-Tomey, A. (1990). Historical development of doctoral programs from the middle ages to nursing education today. *Nursing and Health Care, 11*(3), 132–137.

Murphy, J. (1981). Doctoral education in, of, and for nursing: An historical analysis. *Nursing Outlook, 29*(11), 645–649.

National Academy of Sciences. (2005). *Advancing the nation's health needs: NIH Research Training Programs*. Washington, DC: National Academies Press. Retrieved from http://www.nap.edu/openbook .php?isbn=0309094275

National Association of Clinical Nurse Specialists (NACNS). (2009). *Core practice doctorate clinical nurse specialist competencies*. Retrieved from http://www.nacns.org/docs/CorePracticeDoctorate.pdf

National Organization of Nurse Practitioner Faculties (NONPF). (2006). *Practice doctorate nurse practitioner entry-level competencies*. Retrieved from http://www.nonpf.com/associations/10789/files /DNP%20NP%20competenciesApril2006.pdf

Newman, M. (1975). The professional doctorate in nursing: A position paper. *Nursing Outlook, 23*(11), 704–706.

Roberts, S., & Glod, C. (2005). The practice doctorate in nursing: Is it the answer? *The American Journal for Nurse Practitioners, 9*(11/12), 55–65.

Sperhac, A., & Strodtbeck, F. (1997). Advanced practice nursing: New opportunities for blended roles. *The American Journal of Maternal Child Nursing, 22*(6), 287–293.

Starck, P., Duffy, M., & Vogler, R. (1993). Developing a nursing doctorate for the 21st century. *Journal of Professional Nursing, 9*(4), 212–219.

Thomas, E., Studdert, D., Newhouse, J., Zbar, B., Howard, K., Williams, E., et al. (1999). Costs of medical injuries in Utah and Colorado. *Inquiry, 36*(3), 255–264.

Williams, C. A., Stanhope, M. K., & Sebastian, J. G. (2001). Clinical nursing leadership: One model of professional doctoral education in nursing. In *Envisioning Doctoral Education for the Future. Proceedings of the American Association of Colleges of Nursing's 2001 Doctoral Education Conference* (pp. 85–91). Washington, DC: AACN.

CHAPTER 2

Leadership, Collaboration, and the DNP Graduate

■ LISA ASTALOS CHISM ■

"You can't give people pride, but you can provide the kind of understanding that makes people look to their inner strengths and find their own sense of pride."
—*Charleszetta Waddles (1912–)*

Leadership and collaboration are integral aspects of every potential role a Doctor of Nursing Practice (DNP) graduate may assume. It is well documented in the literature that nurses in all advanced nursing practice roles exhibit leadership and collaboration, whether they are in nurse executive positions, education, or clinical practice (Buonocore, 2004; Carroll, 2005; Joyce, 2001; Mastal, Joshi, & Schulke, 2007). Moreover, leadership is noted to be embedded within less obvious leadership roles, such as advocate, problem solver, idealist, and role model (Garrison & McBryde-Foster, 2004). The changing demands of a complex healthcare environment, the Institute of Medicine's (IOM) call for improved healthcare standards (IOM, 2001; Kohn, Corrigan, & Donaldson, 2000), and the Health Professions Education Committee's recommendations (Greiner & Knebel, 2003) collectively support the notion that nurses in all advanced nursing practice roles exemplify leadership across various healthcare settings (American Association of Colleges of Nursing [AACN], 2006; Greiner & Knebel, 2003).

The Health Professions Education Committee has suggested the need for healthcare professionals to exhibit increased collaboration across healthcare disciplines by leading and functioning in interdisciplinary teams (IOM, 2003). Moreover, a systematic review conducted by Wong and Cummings (2007) found that positive leadership behaviors, styles, and practices were significantly associated with increased patient satisfaction as well as a reduction of adverse events. Therefore, role development as a leader is essential for the DNP graduate. To better prepare nurses as leaders, current DNP curricula include additional preparation in leadership and collaboration. This is evidenced by the standards outlined in the AACN Essentials and the NONPF Competencies.

This chapter provides a review of the AACN's and the National Organization of Nurse Practitioner Faculties' (NONPF's) curriculum standards for preparation in leadership and collaboration. Leadership attributes and styles relevant to the DNP leadership role are also discussed. Collaboration and team styles also have relevance for successful leadership and are reviewed as well. Change as it relates to the DNP graduate is briefly discussed. The reluctant DNP leader—leadership even when one doesn't expect or want it—will also be reviewed. Finally, the responsibility of role modeling and portraying leadership and collaboration is addressed. Specific case scenarios related to the DNP graduate are included to illustrate how leadership and collaboration may be used to further enhance healthcare delivery at the patient and systems/organizational level.

■ Curriculum Standards for Leadership and Collaboration

The AACN has outlined curriculum standards through the *Essentials of Doctoral Education for Advanced Nursing Practice* (2006). Essential II: Organizational and Systems Leadership for Quality Improvement and Systems Thinking and Essential VI: Interprofessional Collaboration for Improving Patient and Population Health Outcomes describe specific curriculum requirements that intend to enhance DNP graduates' leadership and collaboration skills. In summary, the purpose of Essential II is to promote leadership skills to effectively manage patient safety issues, eliminate health disparities, and promote excellence in practice by evaluating evidence-based best practices for healthcare delivery. Further, DNP graduates must become proficient at quality improvement strategies that improve patient outcomes at every level in healthcare delivery (AACN, 2006). Course work that addresses these objectives will enable DNP graduates to gain a broader understanding of leadership attributes and styles. The purpose of Essential VI involves developing expertise in collaborating across the healthcare team to create effective solutions and overcome impediments to healthcare delivery (AACN, 2006). The DNP graduate's proficiency in leadership is also necessary to effectively lead interprofessional teams and promote collaboration within the healthcare team. Therefore, the course work that attends to collaboration will enhance the skills necessary to communicate between various professionals in multiple disciplines. Because leadership depends on effective collaboration, the skills that improve leadership and collaboration are often interrelated.

NONPF has developed specific *Practice Doctorate Nurse Practitioner Entry-Level Competencies* for nurse practitioner/DNP graduates to help guide curriculum standards as well. The Competency area "Leadership" specifically addresses the need for proficiency in leadership skills for DNP graduates. This Competency addresses the DNP graduate garnering increased proficiency in assuming additional leadership, fostering interprofessional collaboration, and demonstrating a reflective, appropriate leadership style (NONPF, 2006).

■ What's a DNP-Prepared Leader Made Of? The Recipe for Success

Successful leadership encompasses certain individual attributes and qualities, and Doctor of Nursing Practice graduates are encouraged to develop their own unique blends of leadership style. The following section reviews successful leadership qualities that may enable DNP graduates to thrive in leadership roles.

Leadership Attributes

Although it has been agreed upon that a single definition of leadership may not be sufficient, leadership has been described as "the art and science of influencing a group toward achievement of a goal" (McArthur, 2006, p. 8). It has also been found that a single set of attributes cannot be defined as the exclusive characteristics of an effective leader (Feltner, Mitchell, Norris, & Wolfle, 2008). Although DNP graduates are challenged to lead in a healthcare environment that is rapidly changing due to increased technology, population growth, disparity issues, ethical concerns, and political and economical changes, certain attributes may enhance the DNP graduate's leadership role (Jooste, 2004). Interestingly, research has shown that nurses themselves consider certain attributes to be valuable for effective leadership (Feltner, et al., 2008; Joyce, 2001; O'Connor, 2008). It is therefore safe to assume that DNP graduates will have insight regarding the various attributes that are valuable in a leadership role.

Feltner, Mitchell, Norris, and Wolfle (2008) conducted a descriptive study to evaluate what attributes nurses felt were important for effective leadership. Overall, nurses considered communication skills to be the most important attribute of an effective leader. It was found that if communication was effective, the perception of leadership was effective. Additionally, communication should be honest, approachable, open, trustworthy, and reciprocal. Additional attributes noted to be important for leadership were (in rank order): fairness, job knowledge, role model, dependable, participative partnership, confidence, positive attitude, motivating, delegation, flexibility, compassionate, employee loyal, and sets objectives (Feltner, et al., 2008). Nurses also mentioned that a leader should be "visionary and give staff members common, challenging, and achievable goals" (Feltner, et al., 2008, p. 368). It is interesting that the nurses in this study were able to easily articulate what attributes were valuable in an effective leader. This reinforces the notion that DNP graduates will have insight regarding what attributes are important for leadership.

In a related study, Joyce (2001) evaluated perceptions of leadership among nurse practitioners and described the attributes that were considered to be relevant for leadership. Joyce (2001, p. 24) stated that the "leadership experiences of nurse practitioners provide a better understanding of the attributes seen as most important for patient care, interacting with colleagues, and influencing health care delivery systems." The four themes that emerged from this study were facilitator, professional, role model, and visionist (Joyce, 2001).

"Facilitator" was further defined as "the ability to enable individuals or groups to move through tasks" (Joyce, 2001, p. 28). Additional attributes associated with "facilitator" were effective listener, communicator, collaborator, and decision maker. These attributes were demonstrated by the nurse practitioner to achieve mutual goals with clients in the practice setting, in the community, and in the organization (Joyce, 2001).

The attribute "professional" was also found to describe an effective leader. "Professional" was defined as the ability to inspire and enable others to achieve high standards (Joyce, 2001). Additional attributes associated with "professional" were integrity, accountability, competency, capable of managing time, confidence in judgment, ability to set standards, and resourcefulness (Joyce, 2001).

"Role model" was described as the "ability to demonstrate their profession to others" (Joyce, 2001, p. 28). Interestingly, role model was also noted as a leadership attribute by Feltner, Mitchell, Norris, and Wolfle (2008). Associated attributes were described as abilities to mentor, motivate, and teach. Role modeling is also discussed later in the chapter.

Finally, "visionist" was defined as the "ability to be future oriented" (Joyce, 2001, p. 28). The attributes associated with "visionist" included one who is able to "see the whole picture, take risks, and seek challenges" (Joyce, 2001, p. 28). Visionists also attract others toward their vision and work with others to achieve goals.

Interestingly, the leadership perceptions noted by nurse practitioners to be relevant for leadership also described how the nurse practitioners defined themselves as leaders. This provides support for the notion that DNP graduates in clinician roles will engage in leadership, sometimes without realizing it. Moreover, Joyce's research demonstrated that nurses have insight regarding the leadership attributes necessary for the delivery of health care.

O'Connor (2008) described a set of attributes developed by the Center for Nursing Leadership and further identified these attributes as "the caring competencies" (p. 21). These attributes are as follows: holding the truth, intellectual and emotional self, discovery and potential, quest for the adventure toward knowing, diversity as a vehicle to wholeness, appreciation of ambiguity, knowing something in life, holding multiple perspectives without judgment, and keeping commitments to oneself (O'Connor, 2008). O'Connor further expanded on these attributes and identified them as the "caring competencies" by identifying specific caring attributes associated with these competencies. For example, the competency "holding the truth" is further described by O'Connor as honest, trustworthy, reliable, and credible. O'Connor also stated that this attribute spoke to the "leader's internal truth" and described the "integrity and authenticity with which he or she does the job" (p. 22). The attribute "intellectual and emotional self" is described by O'Connor as the balance between intellect and emotional intelligence. Emotional intelligence is considered to be more important than intellect and a learned behavior that can be developed and practiced (Goleman, 1995). Emotional intelligence is discussed further in this chapter.

"Discovery of potential" is described as mentoring by O'Connor. Mentoring encourages others to discover their own path and share their own talents at work. "Quest for adventure toward knowing" is described by O'Connor as passion, curiosity, and enthusiasm. "Diversity as a vehicle to wholeness" requires the nurse leader to be open minded and committed to improving diversity within an organization (O'Connor, 2008). "Appreciation of ambiguity" is described as sharing in the decision making with others. This requires the nurse leader to exhibit empowerment, faith, trust, and importantly, caring (O'Connor, 2008). "Knowing something in life" relates to a nurse leader having had many experiences that may be shared with others to encourage and offer support (O'Connor, 2008). "Holding multiple perspectives without judgment" speaks to respecting the differences in people with regard to culture, values, beliefs, and ways of life (O'Connor, 2008). Further, Joyce related that the nurse leader must see the differences in people as strengths that can make groups stronger and more diverse. "Keeping commitments to oneself" requires the nurse leader to care for the self. Caring for one's self allows one to be ready and able to care for others.

The "caring competencies" described by O'Connor (2008) are practical and pertinent to nursing leadership. Further, they speak to the nature of nursing, which is to care (Shelly & Miller, 2006). As nurses, DNP graduates may already possess many of these valuable attributes or competencies, which can further foster their development as nurse leaders.

A discussion regarding leadership attributes for DNP graduates would not be complete without discussing emotional intelligence. Interestingly, emotional intelligence principles were included in this author's leadership and collaboration DNP course work. Further, it has been noted that nurses are perceived as having high levels of emotional intelligence (Grossman & Valiga, 2005). Emotional intelligence has been suggested to be more important in promoting excellence in leadership than intellect and expertise (Goleman, 1995). Emotional intelligence is defined as "an awareness of and ability to manage emotions and create motivation" (Emotional intelligence, n.d.). Although the definition of emotional intelligence is constantly changing, the basic premise has remained the same. Goleman, Boyatzis, and McKee (2002) expanded on emotional intelligence and described five specific attributes of an emotionally intelligent leader. These attributes are described within four leadership competencies that include self-awareness, self-management, social awareness, and relationship management (Goleman, Boyatzis, & McKee, 2002). Please refer to **Table 2-1.**

Table 2-1 Emotional Intelligence Leadership Competencies

- Self-awareness
- Self-management
- Social awareness
- Relationship management

Source: Used with permission from *Primal Leadership: Realizing the Power of Emotional Intelligence*, by Daniel Goleman, Richard Boyatzis, & Annie McKee, Harvard Business Review Press, 2002.

The attribute "self-awareness" describes leaders who have emotional self-awareness and possess the ability to speak openly about emotions regarding their vision. Leaders who possess self-awareness are able to accurately self-assess areas in need of improvement and pursue self-improvement with grace. The self-aware leader is also self-confident and able to stand out in the group (Goleman, Boyatzis, & McKee, 2002).

"Self-management" describes leaders who exhibit emotional self-control by maintaining a calm demeanor even in crisis situations. Self-managed leaders also exhibit transparency, which allows them to openly admit faults or mistakes as well as remain open to others' feelings and beliefs (Goleman, Boyatzis, & McKee, 2002). These leaders are also able to juggle multiple demands without losing focus or energy. Finally, these leaders are optimistic and see the glass as half full, not half empty (Goleman, Boyatzis, & McKee, 2002).

The emotional intelligence competency "social awareness" describes leaders who express empathy toward others. These leaders are able to "feel the room" and tune into what others are thinking or feeling, which allows them to appreciate others' perspectives. Additionally, socially aware leaders have organizational awareness and are able to understand unspoken values of others in the organization. This competency also describes leaders who believe in service-oriented behaviors (Goleman, Boyatzis, & McKee, 2002).

Finally, the competency "relationship management" describes leaders who inspire others to be involved in a shared mission. These leaders use influence to engage a group and create enthusiasm. Relationship management includes the ability to promote and facilitate change, especially in an environment with barriers to change. These leaders also are skilled at conflict management. Although conflict management may be uncomfortable, these leaders handle it by viewing all sides of an issue then redirecting the energy toward a solution. Finally, these leaders encourage close relationships within the group, which fosters collaboration and the development of strategies and solutions (Goleman, Boyatzis, & McKee, 2002).

Following a discussion of the pertinent leadership attributes, it becomes clear what leadership attributes DNP graduates should foster (please refer to **Table 2-2**). Most, if not all, of these attributes are known by nurses to be valuable attributes for leadership. Further, DNP graduates can develop these leadership attributes by drawing on their previous experiences in leadership and healthcare delivery. This is further elaborated on in the case scenarios provided at the end of the chapter.

Although it is important to discuss what leadership attributes are germane and perhaps even instinctive to DNP graduates, it is also necessary to explore the leadership styles that may be employed by DNP graduates. Styles of leadership may vary depending on the venue in which they are applied. DNP graduates may also find that their leadership styles fluctuate as they become more experienced leaders. It has been suggested that emotional intelligence is essential for effective leadership; therefore, the leadership styles congruent with emotionally intelligent leadership are reviewed next.

Table 2-2 Leadership Attributes Relevant for DNP Graduates

Leadership Attributes	Examples
Ability to communicate effectively	Communicate effectively across multiple disciplines or teams, such as evaluation of evidence-based practice patterns for development of practice protocols.
Fearlessness	Step into leadership roles when needed, such as instituting and leading a journal club in a practice setting. Also advocate for patients or team members when necessary.
Motivating	Inspire teams/colleagues, such as motivating the team/colleagues to participate in patient satisfaction surveys.
Visionary toward the future	Project where the goals of a healthcare setting are headed, such as initiating a practice group to include a dietician for onsite consultations for patients.
Role model	Set an example for others, such as mentoring other nurses in the practice setting and encouraging further education.
Knowledge and clinical competence	Maintain and expand current clinical knowledge, such as attending conferences or review journals.
Compassion	Exhibit compassion toward patients and others even when caring for a difficult patient.
Trustworthy	Maintain confidences in a practice setting, such as not sharing information about other team members when issues arise.
Participate in partnerships	Participate in partnerships with patients and others by negotiating with patients when developing a plan of care. Also, partner with other team members to share in the responsibility of problem solving when a difficult patient or team member situation arises.
Honesty about self and others	Openly admit weaknesses and mistakes to others on the team or practice setting, such as admitting to avoiding conflict with others. Also, openly admit areas that need improvement, such as difficulty initiating insulin therapy for patients.
Empathy	Express empathy to patients and team members and share all perspectives. Sense when empathy or understanding is needed in particular situations among team members.

Leadership Styles

Goleman, Boyatzis, and McKee (2002) described several styles of leadership and categorized them as resonant or dissonant styles. Goleman describes resonant styles as styles that encourage the group members to feel connected to each other and reflect the leader's enthusiasm. These types of leadership styles come naturally to emotionally intelligent leaders; hence, these styles may be easy for nurses to adopt. The resonant styles are as follows: visionary, coaching, affiliative, and democratic.

When engaged, the visionary style motivates the group to a shared dream while allowing others to be free to "innovate, experiment, and take calculated risks" (Goleman, Boyatzis, & McKee, 2002, p. 57). This type of style encourages people to stay with the group and the group's mission. The emotional intelligence competency empathy is most important to a visionary leader. Empathy allows a leader to sense how others feel and understand their perspectives. Interestingly, empathy has long been considered essential to a therapeutic nurse–patient relationship (Bennet, 1995; Kalish, 1973; LaMonica & Karshmer, 1978). One may assume that the visionary style is practiced regularly by nurses. DNP graduates may therefore draw from previous experiences and engage this style of leadership.

The coaching style is another style of leadership that may come naturally to nurses. The coaching style involves connecting others to the shared goals of the organization or group. The coaching leader helps others identify what their strengths and weaknesses are and apply them to their own aspirations (Goleman, Boyatzis, & McKee, 2002). Coaches also delegate tasks to others that will allow them to be innovative and expand on their potential. This in turn builds confidence in others and helps foster professional development (Goleman, Boyatzis, & McKee, 2002). Nurses regularly engage patients in coaching when providing counseling about health maintenance and prevention (Cook, Ingersoll, & Spitzer, 1999; Lambing, Adams, Fox, & Divine, 2004). Therefore, coaching is another leadership style that may be employed easily by the DNP graduate.

The affiliative style is considered to be the relationship-builder style. This style emphasizes connections between people to bring focus toward a shared goal (Goleman, Boyatzis, & McKee, 2002). Nurses are experts at this leadership style. This style is employed whenever nurses share personal stories with each other, as well as when they listen to their patients' and families' concerns. The affiliative leadership style can easily be utilized by DNP graduates when interacting with members of a group or organization.

Occasionally, it may not be enough to share with others to create harmony when trying to lead. The democratic leader is one who considers all views when there is conflict or a disagreement about what direction to take next (Goleman, Boyatzis, & McKee, 2002). This style of leadership is fostered through good communication, which stems from the ability to collaborate, resolve conflict, and influence others (Goleman, Boyatzis, & McKee, 2002). Each time a nurse listens to a patient's concerns and considers his or her viewpoint, a democratic style is employed. DNP graduates can draw on their past experiences with this style and employ a democratic style of leadership.

At times, leadership may be more challenging for the DNP graduate. This is when the more difficult styles or the dissonant styles may need to be employed. Dissonant styles may make a group feel "off-key" and produce a "lack of harmony" in a group (Goleman, Boyatzis, & McKee, 2002, p. 21). These styles include pacesetting and commanding. Further, Goleman, Boyatzis, and McKee (2002) relate that these styles should be "applied with caution" (p. 53). Although these styles may be less familiar and comfortable for nurses, the DNP graduate may need to employ them when necessary.

Pacesetting refers to a style that exhibits extremely high expectations when getting a task accomplished is the essential goal. This style can be useful in early phases of organizing a group toward shared goals. However, if employed too rigidly and too frequently, this style can backfire and create feelings of mistrust in a group (Goleman, Boyatzis, & McKee, 2002). When a plan of care is initially developed for a patient, goals are mutually set for the patient. However, if the patient's healthcare needs change, the plan of care will have to be adjusted in an effort to provide safe, effective care. Similarly, this leadership style may be used by DNP graduates, especially in early planning phases of goal setting or when goals need to be reassessed.

The final leadership style, the commanding style, is also a dissonant style. The commanding style must also be used with caution but may be necessary for specific goals of the group (Goleman, Boyatzis, & McKee, 2002). The commanding style involves the leader taking control of a situation and using a "do it because I said so" motto (Goleman, Boyatzis, & McKee, 2002, p. 76). This style must be used sparingly or goals will not be met. Nurses who have participated in code blue or other emergency situations, whether in or out of the healthcare setting, have experienced or even employed this type of leadership style. In crisis situations, nurses often take charge. DNP graduates will know how to employ this style, but experience will allow them to know when to employ it.

Please refer to **Table 2-3** for a summary of leadership styles.

■ Collaboration: DNP Graduates Working with Others

Ken Blanchard related a quotation in his book, *The Heart of a Leader* (1999), that "No one of us is as smart as all of us" (quotation originally from Blanchard, Carew, & Parisi-Carew, 1990). This quotation describes the true purpose of collaboration. The ability to collaborate, defined as working together, especially in a joint intellectual effort (Merriam-Webster, 1983), has been identified by the AACN, NONPF, and the Health Professions Education Committee as an essential skill of DNP graduates. Collaboration has been more specifically defined in relation to nursing and health care as "a dynamic, interpersonal process in which two or more individuals make a commitment to each other to interact authentically and constructively to solve problems and to learn from each other to accomplish identifiable goals, purposes, or outcomes" (Hamric, Spross, & Hanson, 2005, p. 344). Given this definition, DNP graduates may build alliances across teams and disciplines in an effort to solve problems, accomplish

Table 2-3 Leadership Styles

Resonant Styles	Dissonant Styles
Visionary	Pacesetting
Coaching	Commanding
Affiliative	
Democratic	

Source: Used with permission from *Primal Leadership: Realizing the Power of Emotional Intelligence*, by Daniel Goleman, Richard Boyatzis, & Annie McKee, Harvard Business Review Press, 2002.

goals, and improve outcomes. Certain characteristics that promote collaboration will be discussed further.

Qualities for Successful Collaboration

Hamric, Spross, and Hanson (2005) described common purpose as a characteristic that may promote collaboration. Common purpose is similar to the visionary leadership style (Goleman, Boyatzis, & McKee, 2002). If the group is striving toward a similar purpose or vision, they will likely be motivated to work together more effectively. Nurses and physicians often work together toward the common purpose of improved patient care. If the DNP graduate can establish a common purpose or vision for the group, the interactions will be more successful and the goals will likely be achieved.

Clinical competence was also identified by Hamric, Spross, and Hanson (2005) as the "most important characteristic underlying a successful collaborative experience among clinicians" (p. 360). These authors related that without this characteristic, trust among collaborative team members is difficult to establish. This can be seen in collaborative relationships between advanced practice registered nurses and collaborating physicians. A trust in each other's knowledge and abilities must be present for the collaborative relationship to be successful. Therefore, DNP graduates must establish reciprocal trust regarding the clinical competence between team members to ensure effective collaboration.

Interpersonal competence and communication skills were also noted by Hamric, Spross, and Hanson (2005) to be necessary characteristics for effective collaboration. These characteristics are similar to Goleman, Boyatzis, and McKee's (2002) leadership competencies social awareness and relationship management. As mentioned earlier in the chapter, social awareness includes the ability to exhibit empathy toward others. Relationship management describes leaders who are good at teamwork and collaboration. Therefore, collaboration should include communication between group members that is open, empathic, and cohesive. Nurses are often very effective communicators and exhibit this type of communication. DNP graduates can draw on these communication skills to promote effective collaboration among team members as well as across disciplines.

Hamric, Spross, and Hanson (2005) also found trust to be an essential characteristic of effective collaboration. This is evidenced by the collegial relationships across disciplines in the hospital setting. Pharmacy departments trust that nurses are properly dispensing the medications that they deliver to the unit. Surgeons trust that nurses are properly assessing patients after a procedure. Nurses trust that physical therapists provide appropriate therapy to a patient after hip replacement surgery. Without trust in each other's knowledge, collaboration and patient care would be compromised. DNP graduates are in a unique position to promote trust within a group. Because nurses are often experts at interacting across disciplines to ensure high-quality care, DNP graduates can lead by example in establishing trust among team members, especially when multiple disciplines are represented.

Valuing and respecting of diverse, complimentary knowledge is related to trust in that although team members must trust each other's knowledge, this knowledge should also be mutually respected. Hamric, Spross, and Hanson (2005) related that each discipline complements the other through mutual respect. DNP graduates can promote this characteristic by demonstrating that patient care is centered on the collaborative efforts of multiple disciplines. While working together across disciplines, the common goal of optimal healthcare delivery can be achieved.

Finally, Hamric, Spross, and Hanson (2005) identified humor as a necessary characteristic for effective collaboration. Interestingly, Goleman, Boyatzis, and McKee (2002) also found that humor was an important attribute of an emotionally intelligent leader and key for effective leadership. Hamric, Spross, and Hanson (2005) stated "when used with collaboration, humor serves to decrease defensiveness, invite openness, relieve tension, and deflect anger" (p. 362). Further, conflict can be defused and communication enhanced when humor is used effectively. DNP graduates are encouraged to recall their own experiences and employ humor to reduce tensions or resolve conflict.

Team Styles

Although the preceding characteristics can enhance collaboration, it is also promoted by team interdependence, which is mutually satisfying, positive, and oriented toward problem solving (Smith & Vezina, 2004). Therefore, it is prudent for the DNP graduate to have awareness about the styles of teams that will promote collaboration and effective results. These types of teams are fostered by leaders who employ the leadership competencies outlined by Goleman, Boyatzis, and McKee previously in this chapter. The team styles that enable a team to build and maintain effective relationships with each other and the rest of the organization are identified by Goleman, Boyatzis, and McKee (2002) as the self-aware team, the self-managed team, and the empathic team (see **Table 2-4**).

The self-aware team members share an awareness of the underlying emotions in the group as a whole. The leader of this group could be a role model for the group by employing empathy toward the emotions of the group, which builds trust and a sense of belonging. This type of scenario sends the message "we are all in this together" (Goleman, Boyatzis, & McKee, 2002, p. 178). This type of team also prioritizes listening to everyone's perspective before decisions are made and stepping in when other members are having difficulty with a task (Goleman, Boyatzis, & McKee, 2002). The

Table 2-4 Team Styles

- Self-aware team
- Self-managed team
- Empathic team

Source: Used with permission from *Primal Leadership: Realizing the Power of Emotional Intelligence*, by Daniel Goleman, Richard Boyatzis, & Annie McKee, Harvard Business Review Press, 2002.

DNP graduate may foster this type of team by employing the emotional intelligence competencies previously described.

The self-managed team manages itself when led by an emotionally intelligent leader. Further, this type of team will hold each member accountable to the positive norms already set in place (Goleman, Boyatzis, & McKee, 2002). The DNP graduate can promote this type of team style by clarifying the team's mission and practicing the team's norms.

The empathic team style is more than just members being nice to each other. The empathic team "figures out what the whole system really needs and goes after it in a way that makes all those involved more successful and satisfied with the outcomes" (Goleman, Boyatzis, & McKee, 2002, p. 182). For the DNP graduate, employing empathy across the boundaries between teams, groups, organizations, or disciplines can promote this type of team.

■ A Discussion About Change

A discussion about DNP graduates and leadership would not be inclusive without a discussion about change. Every DNP graduate, whether he or she is a nurse leader, clinician, researcher, health policy advocate, or educator, will deal with change at some point in his or her career. Obtaining a DNP degree alone presents change for the graduate and his or her colleagues due to the newness of the DNP degree. This author dealt with change simply by being a new DNP graduate in a clinic where she started as a master's degree-prepared nurse practitioner. Her colleagues viewed her a certain way prior to graduating with a DNP degree. Transitioning her colleagues to adjust to the differences, which included adjusting to the title "Dr.," in addition to educating others about her preparation, was a transition that could have gone poorly if dealt with the wrong way. This situation is perhaps a common one given the number of master's degree-prepared nurses who are returning to school for a DNP degree. Therefore, tips for smooth transitions as well as promoting change are discussed next.

Effective change has been discussed widely in the literature. One of the most mentioned change theories is Lewin's (1951) process of change, which involves three steps: unfreezing, which occurs as people prepare for change; moving, which occurs when people start to accept and move toward the change; and refreezing, which occurs when people accept the new change and integrate it as the norm. This can best describe the way in which change eventually becomes what is accepted rather than what is rejected.

How do DNP graduates get to the refreezing phase when instituting change? Porter-O'Grady (1998) described certain steps for leaders to apply to the change process that are reflective of the emotional intelligence competencies reviewed previously in the chapter. These steps include the following: (1) be aware of the signs and trends in and out of the organization; (2) construct a vision that will motivate others to become involved in the change process and promote unity; (3) empower others in the group/organization by encouraging all to become involved in the process; (4) provide the support others will need to institute the change and integrate the change as the norm; (5) have a plan of action that will ensure collaboration within and among groups/teams/organizations; and (6) evaluate the change and be able to adjust the process as necessary (Porter-O'Grady, 1998). These steps are employed every day by nurse leaders, possibly without them realizing it. This author employed these steps in this way: (1) knew the trends in doctoral education in nursing; (2) shared the benefits of having a DNP-prepared nurse practitioner working in the clinic; (3) educated staff members about the DNP degree; (4) provided education materials explaining the degree; (5) met with the clinic manager regarding the changes associated with her new title and role; and (6) reassessed the clinic staff's understanding of what a DNP degree is and what it means for practice. DNP graduates can employ these steps, along with the leadership attributes and styles discussed, to institute any change, even change as simple as returning to their clinic one day after graduating with a DNP degree.

■ The Reluctant Leader: Unexpected Leadership

Although the DNP degree curriculum has a strong leadership component, it is evident that not every nurse who earns a DNP degree will want to be in a leadership role. Leadership is not always a role that nurses seek or feel comfortable with (Buonocore, 2004; Joyce, 2001; Philpott & Corrigan, 2006). However, as previously noted in the change discussion, leadership will be expected of DNP graduates in all healthcare settings, regardless of the actual role the DNP graduate assumes.

Leadership versus Management

An explanation of the difference between leadership and management may help to alleviate the anxiety that is sometimes felt by DNP graduates when faced with leadership opportunities. Leadership has previously been defined as "the art and science of influencing a group toward achievement of a goal" (McArthur, 2006, p. 8). Carmen (2002) further defined leadership as "to guide and escort" (p. 133). According to Carmen, leadership implies accompaniment and companionship. Management, on the other hand, implies control through supervision and training. Garrison and McBryde-Foster (2004) define management as controlling resources to accomplish organizational goals. In summary, managers wish the people to have faith in the leader, and leaders wish for faith in the people (Carmen, 2002). Given this clarification, DNP graduates can lessen their anxiety about leadership and realize they have the untapped potential within them to lead.

To augment this point, one may reflect on the literature presented earlier in the chapter, which illustrates that nurses have an instinctive awareness of what attributes are important for effective leadership (Feltner, et al., 2008; Joyce, 2001; O'Connor,

2008). DNP graduates have an opportunity to reflect on these attributes, including the emotional intelligence competencies described, and realize the capacity to lead is within them. Leadership opportunities may be presented in various forms. Self-reflection and honesty will help the DNP graduate to realize his or her true leadership potential when these opportunities are presented.

■ Role Modeling: DNP Graduates Setting the Example

Ralph Waldo Emerson was quoted as saying, "What you do speaks so loudly, I can't hear what you are saying." What a perfect way to sum up the act of role modeling. Although leadership opportunities are presented in various ways, role modeling may be the most subtle form of leadership. Now more than ever, role modeling is an extremely important role for DNP graduates. The DNP degree is still a newer degree for nursing and definitely new to the healthcare setting. It is therefore imperative that DNP graduates act as role models to their nursing colleagues, other healthcare professionals, and patients to demonstrate the potential of a DNP graduate.

Although it may seem like a daunting task, role modeling is something nurses do on a regular basis (Coady, 2003; Davies, 1993; Hicks, 2000; Philpott & Corrigan, 2006). Nurses are role models in every aspect of practice, from providing care at the bedside to leading a research study as a principal investigator. Sister Samantha Philpott (Philpott & Corrigan, 2006) wrote about her experiences as a role model senior nurse. Philpott related the general themes she found to be important as a role model: acting fairly, being honest, and communicating effectively. Acting fairly was described as treating patients and others with respect. Philpott stated that "the perception of unfairness is a major cause of poor staff morale" (p. 11). Being honest extended not only to honesty toward patients but also accepting accountability for one's actions. Communicating effectively included "proactive, honest, and sensitive communication with patients, relatives, and medical staff" (Philpott & Corrigan, 2006, p. 11). Interestingly, Philpott included interpreting body language appropriately as effective communication. Do these themes sound familiar? These themes are reflective of the leadership attributes that were previously discussed.

Although role modeling may seem like an immense responsibility, nursing practice embodies immense responsibility. DNP graduates are building on a foundation already in place. Therefore, many of the leadership styles and characteristics described in this chapter may be familiar to DNP graduates. Self-reflection and evaluation will enable the DNP graduate to promote effective leadership, collaboration, and role modeling in every setting.

■ Case Scenarios Related to the DNP Degree in Leadership and Collaboration

The following case scenarios provide examples of Doctor of Nursing Practice graduates exemplifying roles in leadership.

Case Scenario 1: Leadership in the Clinic Practice Setting

Dr. G. is a women's health nurse practitioner DNP graduate who cares for patients in a suburban outpatient women's health clinic. While seeing a patient who requested an elective termination, she overheard the clinic staff speaking loudly about their opinions regarding elective termination. The patient also overheard these comments and became upset. Dr. G. consoled the patient and offered support as well as a referral for termination. Incidentally, Dr. G. is personally pro-life. After the patient had left the clinic, Dr. G. approached the clinic manager and requested a meeting first alone with the manager and then with the whole clinic staff. In the first meeting with the manager alone, Dr. G. expressed her concerns regarding the incident but requested to handle the situation herself with the staff.

Prior to meeting with the staff, Dr. G. researched sensitivity and diversity training principles and prepared some materials to share with the staff. When she met with the whole staff (providers, staff, and the clinic manager), she introduced the notion that more sensitivity should be expressed when dealing with diverse issues that are often presented in the clinic. She related a similar example to the episode that prompted the meeting. Although those who had been involved knew about the episode, they were not aware that they were overheard. They were also not singled out in this meeting. Remorse was later expressed privately by these individuals, who appreciated the opportunity to express more sensitivity to similar issues in the future.

What is the leadership message in this case? Dr. G. could have used a commanding style and verbally expressed her concerns to the staff members involved either privately or in front of others. Instead, she used self-management skills by maintaining a calm demeanor. She also exhibited relationship management skills and involved the whole group in the shared vision of increased sensitivity to diverse issues. Conflict was also diffused, because Dr. G. avoided singling out the group members who offended the patient. If they had been confronted differently with the situation, the staff may have acted defensively instead of expressing remorse about the incident.

The leadership attributes exhibited by Dr. G. include empathy, trustworthiness, visionary, effective communication, and compassion. Dr. G. also used significant emotional intelligence. A combination of an affiliative and democratic style was employed regarding this issue. Dr. G. approached the whole group and shared a vision openly (affiliative style), but the differing sides as well as consequences were also presented (democratic style) when a specific case involving lack of sensitivity was described. By employing emotional intelligence, the situation was handled effectively, resulting in improved patient care outcomes.

Case Scenario 2: Leadership in the Community

Dr. H. is a clinical nurse specialist (CNS) DNP graduate who works as a CNS at a local hospital and also volunteers at her church as a parish nurse. She began noticing that parish members were not participating in routine health screening events that were sponsored by the parish. Dr. H. approached her parish priest and offered to speak with the congregation after Mass one Sunday. Prior to her presentation, Dr. H. prepared materials for the group that included information regarding the importance of screening and reduced mortality and morbidities resulting from early preventive care. Dr. H. emphasized that health promotion and risk prevention were strongly recommended and that the parish nurses were committed to providing this through health screening to the members of the parish. The parish seemed receptive and appreciative of Dr. H.'s advice and expertise. Further, Dr. H.'s scholarly approach, which included a review of evidence-based practices regarding health promotion and risk reduction, was reflective of her preparation as a DNP graduate.

The leadership attributes that Dr. H. drew from were visionary and motivating in an attempt to inspire the group (the congregation) to buy into a shared vision. Rather than no longer offering the parish health screening, Dr. H. showed compassion and volunteered her time and efforts to educate others and inspire them to take shared responsibility for their healthcare outcomes. Her presentation included evidence from the literature that documented improved outcomes for routine health screening. She also used case studies to explain further the rationale for health screening.

As a result of Dr. H.'s presentation, attendance at the next health screening event nearly tripled, and requests were made for more health education regarding specific topics. Dr. H. started providing educational seminars for her congregation and eventually developed her own consulting health education programs. Her leadership attributes and entrepreneurial skills led her to an additional path in her career that employed the leadership competencies she garnered as a DNP graduate.

Case Scenario 3: Formal Leadership in the Clinical Setting

Dr. C. is a nurse anesthetist DNP graduate who returned to her clinical setting after graduating with a DNP degree. Dr. C. practices at an urban, tertiary care hospital. Prior to graduating from a DNP program, Dr. C. had been the lead nurse anesthetist and performed many managerial duties, such as organizing the schedules, covering when colleagues were off, and generally making sure the anesthesia department provided adequate coverage for all the operating room cases.

Upon graduation from a DNP degree program, Dr. C. had a clearer understanding of leadership and wanted to become more involved as a leader in the anesthesia department. She wanted to develop more programs of research that investigated the impact nurse anesthetists had on patient care and outcomes. Dr. C. also had a vision that included the nurse anesthetists becoming more involved in nursing education for other nursing departments.

Drawing on her new leadership understanding and past experiences in leadership roles, Dr. C. drafted a proposal for her ideas and scheduled a meeting with the service-line director of surgical services. Although they were appreciated, Dr. C.'s ideas were not initially supported by administration due to financial constraints imposed on the hospital. Instead of giving up, Dr. C. consulted and partnered with her mentor from graduate school (a PhD-prepared nurse), submitted a proposal for a research grant, and obtained funding for a research study in her own department. Upon approval from the hospital internal review board (IRB), Dr. C. again approached hospital administration. Now, armed with more resources, Dr. C. eventually was granted approval to conduct the research study. A position was eventually created for Dr. C. within her department (director of research and education for nursing anesthesia), which allowed her to develop more programs of research in the anesthesia department as well as develop educational programs for nursing.

The leadership attributes exhibited by Dr. C. included courage, ability to communicate effectively, collaboration, vision, and clinical competence. The leadership style she employed involved use of an affiliative style. Dr. C. emphasized connections among the anesthesia department, the administration, and a research consultant to bring focus toward a shared goal. Dr. C. also employed a visionary style to motivate those involved to take risks with her and try something new for the anesthesia department. As a result, her leadership skills and abilities allowed Dr. C. to achieve her goals and improve healthcare outcomes.

Interview with a DNP Nurse Leader: Then and Now

Dagmar Raica, DNP, RN, is the chief nursing officer at Marquette General Hospital in Marquette, Michigan. Marquette General is a rural-referral, tertiary care, 350-bed hospital currently attempting to achieve Magnet status. Dr. Raica graduated with a DNP degree in December 2007 from the first DNP program in Michigan at Oakland University, Rochester, Michigan. This program also partnered with Northern Michigan University. Dr. Raica was interviewed for this chapter to share her experiences then and now as a DNP nurse leader. (Interview reprinted with permission.)

Then . . . 2008

Dr. Raica, could you describe your background, including educational and nursing leadership experiences?

I started my nursing career traditionally with a diploma degree and worked as a critical care nurse. I later went on to earn a bachelor's in nursing (BSN) degree, followed by a master's degree in nursing administration. My first leadership position was as an assistant unit manager for 1 year before being promoted to unit manager. I was then promoted to service-line director of cardiac services. After graduating with my DNP degree, Marquette General was going through some structural changes as well as attempting to become a Magnet hospital. I was then approached by my CEO who asked me to assume the role of chief nursing officer. I have been the CNO for approximately 3 months now, and busier than ever! While what I am doing now does not directly affect nursing yet, I am affecting outcomes at the systems level and hope to work on specific nursing projects in the near future.

Dr. Raica, what attracted you to nursing leadership?

My interest in leadership stemmed from a desire to implement positive changes in nursing, which included making nursing better for both patients and nurses. I also wanted to bring nursing's contributions to patient care to the forefront. By being a nurse leader, I am able to highlight to the public what nursing contributes to health care. I also believe that this is what the nursing profession needs: more recognition for what we do as a profession. I feel that as a nurse leader, I am able to focus on this.

Dr. Raica, what prompted your decision to return to graduate school for a DNP degree?

I always returned to school in the past for professional development reasons. I returned for a DNP degree with the same goal in mind. I always knew I wanted to earn the terminal degree in my field. When the opportunity to return for a DNP degree was presented, I was very busy with my career, but I made the time to go back to school. I believe this is reflected back to what I feel the profession needs: nurses who role model and achieve the terminal degree in our field. In turn, we motivate others to strive for further professional development.

Dr. Raica, what did you hope to gain or learn from a DNP degree?

I didn't always realize what I would learn in the past when I returned to school. It was always revealed to me after I pursued the next degree. It was the same way with the DNP degree. I didn't realize what I would gain, but I knew there was always more to learn about my field. I did not expect to be promoted to another level of leadership so quickly, but it worked out perfectly. My hospital setting had a need for more doctoral-prepared nurses, and the timing was right.

Dr. Raica, what did you gain from earning a DNP degree?

I gained more that I ever thought I would. I have a better understanding of the importance of evidence-based practices as well as the implementation of these practices. I also have a better appreciation of the need for nurses to stay involved in research for both the development of the discipline of nursing and the profession. My research project specifically described the improvement of communication between nurses and physicians. By communicating better, we are able to improve collaboration and patient outcomes. I believe that is what it is all about: improving outcomes. Through my DNP degree program, I was able to investigate this further. Now as a DNP leader, I may be able to implement some of these principles to improve communication and overall patient care.

Dr. Raica, what has been the response from your colleagues regarding the DNP degree?

I have been pleasantly surprised by the support and encouragement I have received from completing my DNP degree. Overall, the energy has been congratulatory, supportive, and complementary. One of my nursing PhD colleagues is very excited that another doctoral-prepared nurse is now at Marquette General, and we collaborate on projects regularly. Overall, I believe I set an example to my colleagues that it's never too late to learn more and we never know it all—important concepts for nurse leaders!

Dr. Raica, how has obtaining a DNP degree affected your role as nurse leader?

Nurse leaders in general can influence other nurses. I believe obtaining my DNP degree has elevated the view of the nursing profession. I thought I was a good leader before; however, after returning to school, I realize I have so much more to learn about nursing leadership. I also look at nursing leadership differently since my DNP degree. I always knew evidence-based practice was important, but I now realize how important research is to validate why we do what we do. What I learned about research also made me realize how important it is that we publish what we do and share our findings with the discipline of nursing as well as the profession.

Dr. Raica, how has your responsibility as a role model changed since earning a DNP degree?

I feel even more responsibility to role model effectively. I now have the terminal degree for nursing practice, and therefore my responsibility to elevate the profession is even greater. This degree has broadened my horizons about what leadership and role modeling are. I also feel responsible to be more accountable to my profession and continue to learn how to lead effectively.

Dr. Raica, how has obtaining a DNP degree affected your perceptions of nursing practice?

I look at things more critically, with a more educated eye. I realize the link between theory, research, and practice. I also evaluate research and evidence-based practice literature more critically. I now have the additional knowledge to evaluate what should become practice and what may need more investigation.

Dr. Raica, are you glad you returned to school for a DNP degree?

Yes, absolutely; it was a significant accomplishment with many rewards. I would definitely do it again.

Dr. Raica, would you recommend that others in your role, or in nursing, return for a DNP degree?

Yes, doctoral preparation is so important for the development of nursing as a discipline and as a profession. This degree prepares nurses for the changing environment of health care. Also, earning the terminal degree in our field elevates the profession to higher standards and the recognition nursing deserves.

Dr. Raica, what leadership qualities do you feel are important in a leader?

I think courage, ability to take risks, willingness to grow, listening to others, ability to learn from others, and ability to collaborate with others are all qualities that will enable nurse leaders to take nursing and health care into the future.

Now . . . 2011

Dr. Raica, we discussed your nursing background and education last time we spoke. Could you please describe your current position?

I am the Vice President/Chief Nursing Officer at Marquette General Hospital. We are a regional referral hospital with approximately 600 nurses on staff. I am part of the executive team and attend the monthly hospital board meetings and board quality committee.

Dr. Raica, when we last talked, you had accepted a position as Chief Nursing Officer at Marquette General Hospital in Marquette, Michigan. Could you describe how your role has evolved since then?

It has been a very busy and exciting 3 years! There has never been a time in health care that is as crucial as now to balance safe and effective patient care with quality outcomes and do so in challenging financial and technical times. Finding balance as we remake health care is going to be key. Leading, supporting, communicating, and encouraging change right now is my primary focus not only to the staff nurses but also to nursing leadership. I also see it as my job to educate my fellow executive team with the challenges that nurses face providing care at the bedside as we address system issues that impact the nurse at the bedside. This year we not only implemented an electronic health record, but also automated narcotic dispensing and bar coding medication at the bedside. Supporting nursing staff as well as the nursing leaders through all this change is absolutely essential to success of these projects. At the same time, the Director of Nursing and I are promoting leadership opportunities through shared governance and offering educational opportunities to support evidence-based practice and nursing-led research. Safe, effective patient care in the right environment for both staff and patients is the driving goal.

Dr. Raica, have your reasons for pursuing nursing leadership evolved as your level of responsibility has evolved?

What has evolved is my ability to influence change because of span of control. My focus has always been to look for solutions to issues. Another goal of mine throughout my career has been to promote the role of the nurse on the healthcare team and minimize the concept of hierarchal roles.

Dr. Raica, since being in this role now for approximately 3 years, do you feel the DNP degree prepared you for a high-level leadership position? If so, how?

Yes, I do. The DNP degree enhanced learning on a variety of current issues including healthcare policy, leadership, technology, financial issues, quality, and nursing-led research.

Dr. Raica, are your colleagues now more aware of your degree preparation (DNP) and what that means? If so, could you describe the process of educating your colleagues about the DNP degree?

I think so. Initially I was asked many questions as to what the degree was, but I believe there is a better understanding now with the current literature out there and the increase of DNP programs across the country. Even now when I see articles (and your first book) on DNP-prepared CNOs, I share them with my CEO and the other VPs.

Dr. Raica, would you continue to recommend the DNP degree to your colleagues in nursing leadership roles? Why or why not?

Absolutely, I believe the DNP prepares you with the right focus for nurse leaders in a hospital setting to implement best practices based on nursing-led research, focus on quality outcomes for the hospitalized patient, address the many changes in patient care delivery that we face, and determine the role of nursing in healthcare reform.

Dr. Raica, do you continue to role model in your current setting?

It is something I challenge myself with every day . . . what I say, how I respond . . . everything. For example, to promote staff nurses obtaining certifications in their specialty in our hospital, I decided to take one myself and am now a board certified nurse executive–advanced (NEA-BC).

Dr. Raica, as an experienced DNP-prepared nurse leader, what advice do you have for future nurse leaders?

Continue to challenge yourself and strive to reach new goals. Promote the nursing profession by attaining advanced degrees to give it the credibility and parity it needs and deserves.

SUMMARY

- Leadership and collaboration are included in the curriculum standards provided by the AACN as evidenced by Essential II: Organizational and Systems Leadership for Quality Improvement and Systems Thinking and Essential VI: Interprofessional Collaboration for Improving Patient and Population Health Outcomes.
- Leadership and collaboration are also included in the NONPF *Practice Doctorate Nurse Practitioner Entry-Level Competencies*.
- Research has shown that nurses are able to identify which attributes are important for leadership. These attributes include communication skills, fairness, job knowledge, ability to role model, dependability, participative partnership, confidence, positive attitude, motivation, ability to delegate, flexibility,

compassion, loyalty toward employees, and ability to set objectives (Feltner, et al., 2008).

- Joyce (2001) reported on nurse practitioners' perceptions of leadership attributes and identified four general themes: facilitator, professional, role model, and visionist.

- O'Connor (2008) described several "caring competencies" that were originally adapted from the Center for Nursing Leadership. These competencies describe pertinent and practical leadership attributes that relate to caring.

- Emotional intelligence has been shown to enhance leadership and includes the leadership competencies self-awareness, self-management, social awareness, and relationship management.

- The resonant leadership styles encourage the group to work together in harmony and include visionary, coaching, affiliative, and democratic. The dissonant leadership styles, pacesetting and commanding, should be used sparingly (Goleman, Boyatzis, & McKee, 2002).

- According to Hamric, Spross, and Hanson (2005), successful collaboration can be enhanced by the following characteristics: common purpose, clinical competence, interpersonal competence and communication skills, trust, valuing and respecting diverse, complimentary knowledge, and humor.

- The following team styles have been shown to enhance collaboration: the self-aware team, the self-managed team, and the empathic team (Goleman, Boyatzis, & McKee, 2002).

- DNP graduates can promote change by applying certain steps that include constructing a vision, empowering others throughout the change, providing support, collaborating with others, and evaluating the change after it is in place (Porter-O'Grady, 1998).

- Leadership and management are defined differently with different goals. Leadership implies accompaniment and companionship, and management implies control through supervision (Carmen, 2002).

- Role modeling is an important role for DNP graduates and can be accomplished by nurses who draw on many of the leadership attributes and characteristics they already embody.

REFLECTION QUESTIONS

1. Do you agree that leadership skills/competencies are necessary for most roles that DNP graduates will assume?
2. What leadership attributes do you think are necessary for a DNP graduate to be an effective leader?
3. What leadership attributes do you possess?
4. What leadership style(s) do you think you would most likely adopt, as a DNP graduate, when engaged in a leadership role? Why?
5. Do you confront conflict or avoid it? Why?

6. Do you think collaboration is an important part of leadership? If so, why?
7. What qualities do you think are important for successful collaborating relationships?
8. As a DNP graduate, what pertinent steps do you think are necessary when instituting change?
9. Do you think you are a role model for nursing practice in your healthcare setting? If so, what qualities enable you to role model effectively? If not, what qualities would enhance your ability to role model?

REFERENCES

American Association of Colleges of Nursing (AACN). (2006). *Essentials of doctoral education for advanced nursing practice.* Retrieved from http://www.aacn.nche.edu/publications/position/DNPEssentials.pdf

Bennet, J. (1995). Methodological notes on empathy: Further considerations. *Advances in Nursing Science, 18*(1), 36–50.

Blanchard, K. (1999). *The heart of a leader: Insights on the art of influence.* Colorado Springs, CO: David C. Cook.

Buonocore, D. (2004). Leadership in action: Creating a change in practice. *AACN Clinical Issues, 15*(2), 170–181.

Carmen, T. (2002). *Love em' and lead 'em: Leadership strategies that work for reluctant leaders.* Lanham, MD: Scarecrow Press.

Carroll, T. (2005). Leadership skills and attributes of women and nurse executives: Challenges for the 21st century. *Nursing Administration, 29*(2), 146–153.

Coady, E. (2003). Role models. *Nursing Management, 10*(2), 18–21.

Cook, U., Ingersoll, G. L., & Spitzer, R. (1999). Managed care research, part 1: Defining the domain. *Journal of Nursing Administration, 29*(11), 23–31.

Davies, E. (1993). Clinical role modeling: Uncovering hidden knowledge. *Journal of Advanced Nursing, 18*(4), 627–636.

Emotional intelligence. (n.d.). *Webster's New Millennium Dictionary of English*, Preview Edition (v 0.9.7). Retrieved from http://dictionary.reference.com/browse/emotional%20intelligence

Feltner, A., Mitchell, B., Norris, E., & Wolfle, C. (2008). Nurses' views on the characteristics of an effective leader. *AORN Journal, 87*(2), 363–372.

Garrison, D. R., & McBryde-Foster, M. J. (2004). The baccalaureate nurse as a leader in health care delivery. In L. C. Haynes, H. K. Butcher, & T. A. Boese (Eds.), *Nursing in contemporary society: Issues, trends, and transition to practice* (pp. 504–525). Upper Saddle River, NJ: Pearson/Prentice Hall.

Goleman, D. (1995). *Emotional intelligence: Why it can matter more than IQ.* New York: Bantam Dell.

Goleman, D., Boyatzis, R., & McKee, A. (2002). *Primal leadership: Realizing the power of emotional intelligence.* Boston: Harvard Business School Press.

Greiner, A. C., & Knebel, E. (Eds.). (2003). *Health professions education: A bridge to quality.* Washington, DC: National Academies Press.

Grossman, S., & Valiga, T. (2005). *The new leadership challenge: Creating the future of nursing* (2nd ed.). Philadelphia: F. A. Davis.

Hamric, A., Spross, J., & Hanson, C. (2005). *Advanced practice nursing: An integrative approach* (3rd ed.). St Louis, MO: Elsevier Saunders.

Hicks, D. (2000). Pressure to be a role model. *Nursing Times, 96*(23), 34.

Institute of Medicine (IOM). (2001). *Crossing the quality chasm: A new health system for the 21st century.* Washington, DC: National Academies Press.

Jooste, K. (2004). Leadership: A new perspective. *Journal of Nursing Management, 12*(3), 217–223.

Joyce, E. (2001). Leadership perceptions of nurse practitioners. *Lippincott's Case Management, 6*(1), 24–30.

Kalish, B. (1973). What is empathy? *American Journal of Nursing, 73*(9), 1548–1552.

Kohn, L. T., Corrigan, J. M., & Donaldson, M. S. (Eds). (1999). *To err is human: Building a safer health system.* Committee on Quality of Health Care in America, Institute of Medicine. Washington, DC: National Academies Press.

Lambing, A., Adams, D., Fox, D., & Divine, G. (2004). Nurse practitioners' and physicians' care activities and clinical outcomes with an inpatient geriatric population. *Journal of the American Academy of Nurse Practitioners, 16*(8), 343–352.

LaMonica, E., & Karshmer, J. (1978). Empathy: Educating nurses in professional practice. *Journal of Nursing Education, 17*(2), 3–11.

Lewin, K. (1951). *Field theory in social science: Selected theoretical papers.* New York: Harper & Row.

Mastal, M., Joshi, M., & Schulke, K. (2007). Nursing leadership: Championing quality and patient safety in the boardroom. *Nursing Economic$, 25*(6), 323–330.

McArthur, D. (2006). The nurse practitioner as leader. *Journal of the American Academy of Nurse Practitioners, 18*(1), 8–10.

Merriam-Webster's collegiate dictionary (9th ed.). (1983). Springfield, MA: Merriam-Webster.

National Organization of Nurse Practitioner Faculties (NONPF). (2006). *Practice doctorate nurse practitioner entry-level competencies.* Retrieved from http://www.nonpf.com/associations/10789/files/DNP%20NP%20competenciesApril2006.pdf

O'Connor, M. (2008). The dimensions of leadership: A foundation for the caring competency. *Nursing Administration Quarterly, 32*(1), 21–26.

Philpott, S., & Corrigan, P. (2006). Role modeling. *Nursing Management, 13*(1), 10–12.

Porter-O'Grady, T. (1998). The seven basic rules for successful redesign. In E. C. Hein (Ed.), *Contemporary leadership behavior: Selected readings* (5th ed., pp. 226–235). Philadelphia: Lippincott.

Shelly, J., & Miller, A. (2006). *Called to care: A Christian worldview for nursing* (2nd ed.). Downers Grove, IL: InterVarsity Press.

Smith, T., & Vezina, M. (2004). Mediated roles: Working through other people. In L. A. Joel (Ed.), *Advanced practice nursing: Essentials for role development* (pp. 455–472). Philadelphia: F. A. Davis.

Wong, C., & Cummings, G. (2007). The relationship between nursing leadership and patient outcomes: A systematic review. *Journal of Nursing Management, 15*(5), 508–521.

CHAPTER 3

The DNP Graduate as Expert Clinician

▪ LISA ASTALOS CHISM ▪

"It seems to me shallow and arrogant for any man in these times to claim he is completely self-made, that he owes all his success to his unaided efforts. Many hands and hearts and minds generally contribute to anyone's notable achievements."

—*Walt Disney (1901–1966)*

Many Doctor of Nursing Practice (DNP) graduates will return to various advanced practice nursing or clinician roles in the clinical setting after the completion of their programs. Several years after the development of the DNP degree, one of the most frequently asked questions remains, "How will the clinician's role change or benefit from earning a DNP degree"? This question is often followed by, "If I am in clinical practice, why should I earn a DNP degree"? This question may be addressed, in part, by evaluating the many aspects of clinical practice that are enhanced by the expertise garnered through a DNP degree.

The Institute of Medicine (IOM) has recommended that to meet the changing demands of health care, healthcare professionals should gain increased knowledge in evidence-based practices (EBP), information technologies, and interprofessional collaboration (Greiner & Knebel, 2003). To further meet these changing demands of health care, the American Association of Colleges of Nursing (AACN) and the National Organization of Nurse Practitioner Faculties (NONPF) have developed the curriculum standards for the DNP degree, which include guidelines for course work designed to address the evaluation, integration, translation, and implementation of evidence-based practice, healthcare information systems, and collaboration across healthcare teams and disciplines (AACN, 2006; NONPF, 2006). In addition, clinical practice may also be improved through completion of a DNP degree in more subtle ways. Mentoring and precepting future nurses and other healthcare professionals are also enhanced through the expertise garnered by earning a DNP degree. It should be mentioned that nurses in every setting may frequently be involved in the evaluation and translation of evidence-based practice, information systems, interprofessional collaboration, and mentoring or precepting, but the DNP degree serves to augment these experiences and provide additional expertise to further develop skills in these areas. Hence, the expert clinician's knowledge base in these areas is broadened as a culmination of previous experiences and the knowledge and expertise garnered through a DNP degree.

This chapter reviews the AACN Essentials, the NONPF Competencies, and the National Association of Clinical Nurse Specialists (NACNS) Core Competencies that pertain to specific areas that are likely to improve the delivery of health care and healthcare outcomes in clinical practice. Advanced nursing practice and advanced practice nursing may be confusing terms, and therefore clarification is provided. The newly developed APRN Consensus Model will be reviewed as this model has implications for advanced practice registered nurses (APRNs). Evidence-based practice will be discussed with emphasis on DNP graduates' evaluation and translation of EBP in the clinical setting. Information technology is addressed in relation to how newer technologies can enhance clinical practice from a DNP graduate's perspective. Although nurses frequently collaborate with others in various healthcare settings, interprofessional collaboration, as it relates to DNP graduates' and other healthcare professionals' effect on improved healthcare outcomes in clinical practice, is addressed. Additionally, there is a greater responsibility to mentor and precept others when one earns a terminal degree in his or her field. Therefore, DNP graduates' roles as mentors in the clinical practice setting are discussed. Finally, personal accounts from DNP graduates who are practicing in the clinical setting as well as this author's journey to a DNP degree and beyond are provided.

▪ Curriculum Standards Related to Clinical Practice

The AACN's *Essentials of Doctoral Education for Advanced Nursing Practice* include specific curriculum requirements that pertain to improving nursing practice. Essential III: Clinical Scholarship and Analytical Methods for Evidence-Based Practice addresses the need for increased expertise in the critical evaluation, integration, translation, and implementation of evidence-based practices. This Essential also specifies the need for advanced nursing practice professionals to evaluate practice outcomes, design and evaluate methodologies that improve quality of care, develop practice guidelines based on best practice findings, and work collaboratively with research specialists (AACN, 2006). The NONPF Competency area that addresses the requirement for this area of practice is "Scientific Foundation" (NONPF, 2006). The NACNS also addresses the need for APRNs to evaluate and translate evidence-based practice within the *Core Practice Doctorate CNS Competencies* (NACNS, 2009).

Essential IV: Information Systems/Technology and Patient Care Technology for the Improvement and Transformation of Health Care addresses the need for increased expertise in information technologies that improve overall patient care. Specifically, this Essential requires that DNP graduates garner experience in data mining techniques, the design and implementation of technologies that improve quality of care, and the provision of health consumer information (AACN, 2006). The NONPF Competency area that addresses this area of expertise is "Technology and Information Literacy" (NONPF, 2006). The NACNS also addresses the need for APRNs to "evaluate and improve system-level programs based on the analysis of information from relevant sources such as databases, benchmarks, and epidemiologic data" within the *Core Practice Doctorate CNS Competencies* (NACNS, 2009, p. 13).

Essential VI: Interprofessional Collaboration for Improving Patient and Population Health Outcomes pertains to developing expertise in collaboration across disciplines to improve patient care. Expertise in this area includes analyzing complex practice or organizational issues through participation and leadership of interprofessional teams, acting as a consultant to interprofessional teams, and participating in the development of practice models and policies (AACN, 2006). The NONPF Competency area "Health Delivery System" addresses collaboration and related skills to improve healthcare outcomes (NONPF, 2006). The NACNS emphasizes interprofessional collaboration and the role of APRNs within the *Core Practice Doctorate CNS Competencies* (NACNS, 2009).

Finally, Essential VIII: Advanced Nursing Practice addresses the requirements for practicing as an advanced nursing practitioner in various specialty areas. This Essential includes development of proficiency in comprehensive health assessment, implementation of therapeutic interventions, development of therapeutic relationships with patients and other healthcare professionals, and development of advanced clinical decision-making skills (AACN, 2006). The NONPF Competency area "Independent Practice" requires proficiency in these areas as well (NONPF, 2006). The NACNS includes conducting a "comprehensive assessment of client health care needs, integrating data from multiple sources which include the client and interprofessional team members" within the *Core Practice Doctorate CNS Competencies* (NACNS, 2009, p. 11).

■ Advanced Nursing Practice and Advanced Practice Nursing: Let's Clear This Up

Advanced nursing practice and advanced practice nursing are terms that are often used interchangeably (Brown, 1998; Styles & Lewis, 2000); however, these terms actually have different meanings. Providing a definition of nursing will assist in the clarification of these terms. Nursing was defined by Nightingale (1859) as having "charge of the personal health of somebody and what nursing has to do is to put the patient in the best condition for nature to act upon him." In 1980, the American Nurses Association (ANA) defined nursing as "the diagnosis and treatment of human responses to actual or potential health problems" (ANA, 1995, p. 6). The ANA acknowledges that "nursing philosophy and science have been influenced by a greater elaboration of the science of caring and its integration with the traditional knowledge base for diagnosis and treatment of human responses to health and illness" (ANA, 1995, p. 6). Therefore, contemporary nursing practice is defined as these four essential features (ANA, 1995, p. 6):

1. Attention to the full range of human experiences and responses to health and illness without restriction to a problem-focused orientation;
2. Integration of objective data with knowledge gained from an understanding of the patient's or group's subjective experience;
3. Application of scientific knowledge to the processes of diagnosis and treatment; and
4. Provision of a caring relationship that facilitates health and healing

Nursing practice describes what nurses do when they provide nursing care (Bryant-Lukosius, DiCenso, Browne, & Pinelli, 2004). To further clarify, advanced nursing practice describes what one does in various specialized roles, such as clinical practice, education, research, and leadership. The domain of advanced nursing practice is defined by the type of specialization area one pursues. Put another way, advancement has been defined in nursing as "the integration of theoretical, research-based, and practical knowledge that occurs as part of graduate nursing education" (ANA, 1995, p. 14). Davies and Hughes (1995) expanded on this to further explain that "the term advanced nursing practice extends beyond roles. It is a way of thinking and viewing the world based on clinical knowledge, rather than a composition of roles" (p. 157). Advanced nursing practice is therefore a broad term that describes what nurses do in their various advanced nursing practice roles.

Advanced practice nursing, on the other hand, describes the "whole field of a specific type of advanced nursing practice" (Bryant-Lukosius, DiCenso, Browne, & Pinelli, 2004, p. 522). Advanced practice nursing includes several specialty roles in which nurses function at an advanced level of practice (ANA, 1995; Brown, 1998). The advanced practice registered nurse "acquires specialized knowledge and skills through study and supervised practice at the master's or doctoral level in nursing" (ANA, 1995, p. 14). Advanced practice registered nurses utilize their advanced knowledge and skills within their specialty roles to provide care to individuals, families, and communities.

Hence, the Doctor of Nursing Practice (DNP) degree is the terminal degree for nursing practice, which includes roles in leadership, clinical practice, education, research, and health policy advocacy. Within the domain of advanced nursing practice are the roles defined as advanced practice registered nurses or the clinician roles. These roles include nurse anesthetist, nurse–midwife, clinical nurse specialist, and nurse practitioner. This chapter is primarily focused on the ways in which the DNP degree augments the roles of DNP graduates who are advanced practice registered nurses or in the clinician role.

■ The APRN Consensus Model

The APRN Consensus Model is a regulatory model for advanced practice registered nurses (APRNs). The APRN Consensus Model was developed in 2008 to formally define advanced practice nursing regulation. This regulatory model defines APRN licensure, accreditation, certification, and education (LACE). The electronic platform created to facilitate the implementation and ongoing communication among the regulatory entities is called the LACE network. This model also formally defines advanced practice registered nurse, describes the roles within advanced practice nursing, and defines APRN educational standards and certification standards. The model was developed by the APRN Consensus Workgroup and National Council of State Boards of Nursing APRN Advisory Committee and has been endorsed by many nursing organizations. It has been proposed that all states adopt this model by 2015. The APRN Consensus Model may be accessed at http://www.aacn.nche .edu/education-resources/APRNReport.pdf.

The APRN Consensus Model defines advanced practice roles as nurse anesthetists, nurse–midwives, clinical nurse specialists, and nurse practitioners (Consensus Model, 2008). These roles are related to specific population foci defined as family (across the lifespan), adult/gerontology, neonatal, pediatrics, women's health, and psychiatric/mental health (Consensus Model, 2008). Specialty roles are also addressed within the model and defined as "focus of practice beyond roles and population focus linked to health care needs" (Consensus Model, 2008, p. 10). Examples of specialty roles include (but are not limited to) oncology, palliative care, orthopedics, and nephrology.

The APRN Consensus Model clearly defines APRN education, certification, and licensure requirements as well. Details can be found within the report. Importantly, the implications for DNP graduates are primarily related to the educational requirement of all APRNs. Broad-based APRN education is defined as formal education with a graduate degree (master's or doctorate) or postgraduate certificate awarded by an academic institution and accredited by a nursing or nursing-related accrediting organization (Consensus Model, 2008). The educational requirements for APRNs include preparing the graduate to practice within one of the four delineated APRN roles. Therefore, the APRN Consensus Model will influence the development of DNP degree curricula, particularly the post-BSN DNP curricula for the four APRN roles.

■ Evidence-Based Practice

Evidence-based practice (EBP) "[denotes] disciplines of health care that proceed empirically with regard to the patient and reject more traditional protocols" (Evidence-based, n.d.) Evidence-based practice in nursing has been defined as "integration of the evidence available, nursing expertise, and the values and preferences of the individuals, families, and communities who are served" (Sigma Theta Tau International,

2004, p. 69). Congruent with the aims of the DNP degree, Gibbs (2003) related that evidence-based practitioners adopt a process of lifelong learning that involves continually asking clients questions of practical importance, searching for the current best evidence relative to each question, and taking the appropriate action that is guided by the evidence. The overall goal of evidence-based practice is therefore to promote optimal healthcare outcomes, which are based on critically reviewed clinical evidence, for individual patients, families, and communities.

Although all DNP graduates are expected to evaluate, integrate, and implement evidence-based practices into their particular setting, DNP graduates in the clinician role have a vantage point of evidence-based practice due to their direct impact on care in the clinical setting. Practicing in the clinical setting provides an environment for the DNP graduate clinician to develop and utilize skills pertaining to evaluating, integrating, and implementing evidence-based practice. Further, who better to formulate relevant research questions about practice than the clinicians who provide the care? Jennings and Rogers (1988) recognized that, "While certain aspects of the research process can be shared, it is those nurses in the clinical realm who have the sole opportunity to use research to guide practice" (p. 754).

Barriers to Evidence-Based Practice

It is evident throughout the literature that when evidence-based practices are used to deliver care, the best patient outcomes are achieved (Melnyk, Fineout-Overholt, Feinstein, Sadler, & Green-Hernandez, 2008; Melnyk & Fineout-Overholt, 2005). Despite this, EBP is often met with resistance in the clinical setting. Pravikoff et al. (2005) found that when 1,097 nurses were surveyed, approximately half were not familiar with the term "EBP," and most did not know how to search information databases for literature. This may also be due to the fact that nurses were noted to lack the computer and library training necessary to adequately search the literature for scientific validation (Fink, Thompson, & Bonnes, 2005; Melnyk, 2005; Pravikoff, et al., 2005).

Nurses have also been noted to resist new practice patterns despite evidence that EBP improves patient care outcomes. Nurses regularly practice a certain way because of tradition, past experiences, and intuition rather than utilizing scientific validation (Egerod & Hansen, 2005; Pravikoff, et al., 2005). This may be a function of the lack of knowledge about EBP (Melnyk, et al., 2004) as well as lack of belief regarding the influence of EBP on positive outcomes (Melnyk & Fineout-Overholt, 2005). Please refer to **Table 3-1** for a summary of barriers to EBP. DNP graduates have the opportunity to change these barriers and provide the education to other healthcare professionals regarding the positive outcomes achieved when EBP patterns are employed. Further, DNP graduates may also improve the perceptions about EBP by role modeling and adopting EBP patterns themselves. Mentoring others regarding EBP includes role modeling as well as actively engaging healthcare professionals in activities that promote the use of EBP.

Table 3-1 Barriers to Evidence-Based Practice Summarized

- Lack of computer training
- Lack of library resources and library training
- Resistance to change due to reliance on tradition, past experience, and intuition
- Lack of knowledge about the positive influence of EBP on outcomes
- Lack of belief that EBP will positively influence outcomes
- Poor motivation to investigate EBPs

Reducing Barriers to Evidence-Based Practice

Although employing EBP methods in their own clinical practice is paramount, DNP graduates in clinician roles also have a responsibility to reduce the EBP barriers within their practice settings. Further, DNP graduates' expertise in information systems technology, leadership, clinical decision making, and EBP evaluation, integration, and implementation places them in the perfect position to reduce EBP barriers in the clinical setting. Therefore, the challenge for DNP graduates in the clinician role lies not only in overcoming their own barriers regarding the adoption of EBP patterns but also in providing the leadership and role modeling necessary to promote EBP in the clinical setting.

What interventions will enable DNP graduates to foster the use of EBP in their own practice settings and overcome the barriers to EBP? Research has shown that defining EBP for all who provide care is essential (Hudson, Duke, Haas, & Varnell, 2008). In addition to providing a clear definition of EBP, DNP graduates must provide the knowledge and skills necessary to critically evaluate EBP. Hudson, Duke, Haas, and Varnell (2008) state, "Nurses must have the knowledge and skills to critically question and assist with correcting misguided, inaccurate, or insufficient guidelines in practice" (p. 414). Others in the literature have also agreed that barriers to EBP can be overcome with additional education that strengthens knowledge regarding methods to critically evaluate and integrate EBP (Melnyk, et al., 2004; Melnyk & Fineout-Overholt, 2005; Sheriff, Wallis, & Chaboyer, 2007). Specifically, learning how to navigate information systems databases is a valuable tool to locate and evaluate pertinent EBP information (Melnyk, et al., 2004). DNP graduates gain proficiency in information technologies in their graduate programs and are therefore ideal consultants in this area. Research also suggests that interactive workshops were shown to be effective pedagogical techniques to increase knowledge and understanding of EBP (Sheriff, Wallis, & Chaboyer, 2007). DNP graduates' leadership and collaboration skills facilitate the development and provision of inservice programs and workshops regarding EBP in the clinical setting.

The literature also suggests that it is not enough to have knowledge about EBP; one must believe that EBP actually has a positive effect on outcomes (Melnyk, 2002; Melnyk & Fineout-Overholt, 2005). Hence, DNP graduates in the clinician role may convince others through specific exemplars that adopting EBP patterns is worth the effort. Increasing belief in EBP may also be achieved through mentoring and role modeling the use of EBP. In a study by Melnyk et al. (2004), nurses reported increased use of EBP was directly influenced by "support from faculty, clinical nurse specialists, nurse practitioners, library resources and personnel, administrators, research departments, peer researchers, and specific mentors or clinical experts, as well as time for discussion and use of current research" (p. 191). DNP graduates are often viewed as mentors and role models and therefore are in an ideal position to influence others regarding the use of EBP. **Table 3-2** provides tips for DNPs to reduce barriers to evidence-based practice.

DNP Graduates Evaluating and Translating Evidence-Based Practice

DNP graduates in clinician roles are perfectly positioned to ask questions directly from the clinical setting. Asking questions is the first and most important step toward integrating EBP into clinical practice. Further, asking clinically relevant questions is essential to the development of new knowledge in a field. After the question has been asked, answers may be evaluated in the clinical setting, which allows for direct implementation of EBP. It has been suggested in various dialogues about EBP that it may take up to 18 years to adopt practices based on clinical evidence. Reducing this amount of time to evaluate and translate EBP is essential and well within the domain of DNP graduates. Further, activities such as evaluating research articles in journal clubs, developing inservice programs and workshops that teach evaluation and implementation of research findings, and conducting and reviewing literature searches of the most current evidence will further encourage the adoption of EBP in the clinical setting and foster the improvement of healthcare outcomes. **Table 3-3** provides tips for DNP graduates to evaluate and translate evidence-based practice within their own practices.

Case Scenario of a DNP Graduate Clinician's Experience with Evidence-Based Practice

Dr. C. is a DNP graduate clinician (certified nurse practitioner) working in a hospital-based, internal medicine ambulatory care setting. Dr. C. was a graduate student in a

Table 3-2   Tips for DNPs to Reduce Barriers to Evidence-Based Practice

- Define evidence-based practice to others in the healthcare setting.
- Provide education regarding evidence-based practice that emphasizes positive outcomes through inservice training and workshops.
- Provide consultation regarding information systems, including searching databases for pertinent answers to clinically formulated questions.
- Increase belief in the benefits of EBP by mentoring others in the healthcare setting and providing exemplars through case studies.
- Mentor others in EBP methods, such as searching databases and critically reviewing and evaluating research findings.

Table 3-3 Tips for DNP Graduate Clinicians to Employ Evidence-Based Practices Within Their Own Practices

- Formulate questions when providing care, especially when you don't know if the treatments/recommendations are based on clinical evidence.
- Review/conduct literature reviews regarding treatments or topics you are interested in or question the best practices.
- Start a journal club in your area of clinical practice and meet regularly to discuss pertinent literature.
- If you are in an organization with a library or related resources, ask your reference librarian to conduct searches or automatically alert you regarding pertinent topics you encounter in practice.
- Communicate with other healthcare professionals and ask questions about whether certain practices are based on evidence or simply what has always been done.
- Organize inservice programs for staff and others about how to search for the evidence and find the best answers to questions.

DNP program when she accepted this position. While in school, Dr. C. inquired about resources within the institution that might help her apply the latest research findings to patient care. Dr. C. received assistance from the reference librarian at this institution and began obtaining literature regarding pertinent patient issues.

Initially, sifting through this information was difficult. The myriad results, discussions, and literature reviews made it difficult to decipher what information was accurate and pertinent to best practice recommendations. Through her graduate program, Dr. C. attended a methodology workshop (part of the DNP curriculum) that clarified how to critically review a research article and determine whether the information was indeed valuable. Upon finishing her DNP program, Dr. C. became more proficient at locating and evaluating EBP information. Now, when Dr. C. reviews evidence-based practice articles, she critically evaluates the information for sample sizes, accuracy of statistical analyses, and ability to generalize the results to the given population. As a clinician, Dr. C. is able to apply the EBP patterns she researches and validate effectiveness in her setting.

Taking this knowledge and added expertise a step further, Dr. C. suggested to the physician she practices with that they start a journal club in their setting. Dr. M. was enthusiastic about this and offered to assist with presentation of pertinent topics, even contributing his "Journal Watch" articles for review. Dr. C. also regularly precepts students from various advanced practice nursing programs and now integrates the review of EBP techniques as part of her students' clinical experiences. Dr. C. has found that as she becomes more proficient at reviewing the information, it actually takes her less time to incorporate EBP activities into her day.

■ Information Technology

Following a discussion about EBP, the literature is clear that proficiency in information technology is essential to foster the use of EBP (Carroll, Bradford, Foster, Cato, &

Jones, 2007; Peck, 2005; Zytkowski, 2003). Others refer to the "knowledge explosion" taking place in health care and state that "there has been increasing pressure for health care systems to improve efficiency while standardizing and streamlining organizational processes and maintaining care quality" (Carroll, et al., 2007, p. 39). The amount of information now being accessed to improve quality and healthcare outcomes requires that nurses embrace nursing informatics in every healthcare setting. Curran (2003) relates that "health and knowledge are increasing at a rapid rate. Both the ability to manage information and skilled use of technology are basic tools for practice" (p. 320).

Information technology is also referred to in the nursing literature as nursing informatics. Nursing informatics is defined as "a combination of computer science, information science, and nursing science designed to assist in the management and processing of nursing data, information, and knowledge to support the practice of nursing and the delivery of nursing care" (Graves & Corcoran, 1989, p. 227). The International Medical Informatics Association's Special Interest Group on Nursing Informatics (IMIA-NI) offers a similar definition that includes the "integration of nursing, its information, and information management with information processing and communication technology, to support the health of people worldwide" (IMIA-NI, 1998). From these definitions, it may be extrapolated that the purpose of nursing informatics is to develop systems that manage, organize, and process health information (Zytkowski, 2003) in an effort to improve quality of care and healthcare outcomes. Nursing informatics has become so essential to improving quality and healthcare outcomes that in 1992 the American Nurses Association (ANA) designated nursing informatics as an approved nursing specialty (Zytkowski, 2003). The ANA (2001) refers to nursing informatics as "a specialty that integrates nursing science, computer science, and information science to manage community data, information, and knowledge in nursing practice" (p. vii). For the purpose of this discussion, the broader term "information technology," which includes nursing informatics, is used.

Is Nursing Overcoming Technophobia? Embracing Information Technology

Traditionally, nursing has been somewhat reluctant to embrace information technology (Gaumer, Koeniger-Donohue, Friel, & Sudbay, 2007; Peck, 2005; Simpson, 2004). However, due to the need for improvement in quality and healthcare outcomes, nursing has begun the challenge of integrating information technologies into patient care. Further, the Institute of Medicine's call for improvement in quality and healthcare outcomes specifically designates proficiency in information systems as a requirement for healthcare professionals (IOM, 2001). The IOM's report *To Err Is Human* (Kohn, Corrigan, & Donaldson, 2000) was the initial call for a decrease in medical errors. *Crossing the Quality Chasm* (IOM, 2001) followed this report and specifically called for an emphasis on information technology to improve healthcare outcomes and reduce errors. In 2003, the IOM published a report outlining the requirements for healthcare professionals' education and recommended that information technologies be included as a core competency for all healthcare professionals (Greiner & Knebel, 2003). These reports, as well as nursing's desire to improve patient care outcomes, has contributed to nursing's increasing acceptance of information technology.

Consequently, recent research has shown that nursing noted improved care through the adoption of information technology. A study by Gaumer, Koeniger-Donohue, Friel, and Sudbay (2007) described the use of information technologies by APRNs. Seventy percent of the APRNs surveyed reported that they were able to perform their job better due to information technologies. Nearly all (87%) of the APRNs stated that their time was more efficiently spent because of information technology. Further, 81% perceived that patient safety was improved through information technologies. Overall, 75% responded that their caregiving was improved by the use of information technologies.

Simpson (2004) also stated that information technology improves nursing practice by "counteracting human error, by improving human behavior, and by putting nurses where they need to be to be more effective" (p. 303). Further, information technology has the potential to improve more specific aspects of nursing. Recruitment and retention are improved due to improvement of job satisfaction through information technologies, such as electronic charting, electronic mobile devices, and innovative devices such as smart intravenous pumps (Simpson, 2005). Patient care is improved by information technologies that facilitate the "data-to-information-to-knowledge continuum" (Simpson, 2005, p. 346). Evidence-based practices are more accessible via information technologies and are therefore more quickly adopted by nursing. Overall, the use of information technology to evaluate and implement EBP improves quality and patient care outcomes.

Specific to advanced nursing practice, Zytkowski (2003) relates that information technology has an impact on nurse practitioners' practices by influencing "access to individual health information, reimbursement, and practice based on evidence from research" (p. 278). Further, nurse practitioners are responsible for improving patient care while adhering to organizational standards for scope of practice. These demands are dependent on access to real-time resources and information (Zytkowski, 2003). Information technology provides this information in the most up-to-date fashion through Internet resources.

More Than Just Nuts and Bolts: Technology Used to Improve Clinical Practice

Information technology is used by nurses in many specialty areas related to nursing practice, such as leadership roles (computer software for management of health information), education roles (distance education technologies), and clinician roles (personal digital assistants or PDAs). The employment of information technology in nursing practice is becoming commonplace. Further, many nurses, especially in the clinical environment, are using various information technologies and do not realize they are doing so.

Nursing leaders may be found using information technology to perform data mining. This technique enables the sorting of data from large populations to reveal healthcare-related patterns that may improve the quality of care and healthcare outcomes. Nursing leaders may also use software that organizes large amounts of systems information to streamline the management of systems issues. Information technology may also be used by nurse leaders to communicate information to large groups of people who are not in the same location through Internet technology.

Nursing educators may also be found using information technologies to share information with students. Online course work, e-mail, and interactive live meetings are now integral aspects of distance education. These technologies allow the sharing of information to those previously not able to attend courses on campus.

Nurses in the clinical setting are inundated with data related to patient care and frequently use very innovative types of information technologies. Personal digital assistants are often found in the pocket of many nurses in the clinical setting. They may be loaded with software such as Epocrates, 5-Minute Clinical Consult (5MCC), and various other programs that are available on the Internet and are designed to provide information in the palm of one's hand. Some of these programs are free and may be downloaded immediately. Clinical pharmacists endorse the use of PDAs by nurses in the clinical setting and find that PDAs provide general management and data collection, drug referencing for side effects, adverse reactions, compatibility, dose-specific reactions, and clinical references relating to diagnoses, disease management, and laboratory referencing (Shneyder, 2002). Software programs such as Epocrates offer pharmacology, diagnostic, and symptom information. Epocrates also offers a medical dictionary and an International Classification of Diseases/Current Procedural Terminology (ICD/CPT) billing code feature to allow for accurate terminology and billing for diagnoses and procedures.

Another example of nurses in the clinical setting employing nursing informatics is the use of "telehealth" technologies. Telehealth is defined as "the use of electronic information and telecommunication technologies to support long-distance clinical health care, patient and professional health-related education, public health, and health administration" (Sharp, 1998, pp. 68–69). Nursing tends to prefer telehealth because of the emphasis on patients' long-term wellness, self-management, and health (Peck, 2005). Telehealth can be used as an interactive technique or as a method to track patient data. As access to patient care data improves, patient care improves as well (Peck, 2005). Telehealth also includes care that is provided despite distance. Collaboration between physicians and advanced practice registered nurses (APRNs) frequently takes place from one location to another. Nursing home care companies are also employing telehealth by providing nurses in the field with PDAs that can take photos of wounds, upload the photos to a web-based site, and allow an APRN to view the photos through an online portal. The patient's status is evaluated and care is provided without the APRN leaving his or her clinical setting.

Advanced practice registered nurses may also integrate information technology into patient education. Internet resources can provide patient information quickly and easily. However, patients are often intimidated by the Internet and are not sure how to accurately search for information. Advanced practice registered nurses can access this information for patients quickly and print patient education resources that are frequently available on various health-related websites. Further, APRNs can decipher accurate information for patients while advising them what information is accurate and appropriate for patient education. Knowing what information is appropriate and deciphering this information for patients is a form of information technology (Curran, 2003).

DNP Graduates Navigating the Information Highway

As information technology specialists, how do DNP graduates in clinician roles utilize nursing informatics to improve quality and healthcare outcomes? Many of the answers are reviewed in this chapter. It should also be mentioned that nurses in all clinical settings frequently engage in the use of information technology. However, of the information technologies reviewed, some are essential proficiencies for DNP graduates who are most directly involved in patient care.

The use of PDAs is vital for the provision of up-to-date, efficient, and accurate information to DNP graduates in the clinician role. The use of this technology improves access to information regarding medications, treatment regimens, and billing and coding information. This information improves quality of care, safety, and cost.

Techniques to provide patient information accessed on the Internet are also essential for DNP graduates in the clinician role. Advising patients on accurate health-related websites is a skill that is appreciated by patients who do not feel comfortable looking for this information themselves. Simply utilizing a search engine to print information for patients, in their language, is a nursing informatics skill that is often overlooked as information technology. However, this skill improves patient education, and therefore quality and patient care outcomes are improved.

The use of telehealth is also a valuable tool to improve nursing practice by allowing care to be more accessible. APRNs can utilize Internet portals to view patient data and modify care as the data change to allow for seamless, efficient, and improved care. Telehealth as a means to share information is also essential for DNP graduates in clinician roles. Physician–DNP graduate collaboration may be improved through telehealth technologies by providing consultation in rural areas.

Partnering with nursing administration to perform data mining techniques also allows DNP graduates in clinician roles to observe patterns in large amounts of patient data. This information provides insights about patient patterns regarding their health status and facilitates solutions to improve patient care. Data mining also facilitates the development of evidence-based practice patterns.

Finally, exhibiting an overall comfort with the utilization of information technology will enable DNP graduates in clinician roles to influence others' comfort with technology. Teaching others how to access information on the Internet, sharing information obtained on PDAs, and participating in the development of inservice training regarding nursing informatics will encourage others to become involved in learning about and using these technologies. It is widely known that participation in the design, development, and use of information technology will increase the likelihood that it is accepted (Carroll, et al., 2007; Courtney, Demiris, & Alexander, 2005).

Please refer to **Tables 3-4** and **3-5** for lists of ways that DNP graduates can use information technology and websites regarding information technology.

Case Scenario of a DNP Graduate Clinician's Experiences with Information Technology

As one can see, information technology can be integrated into the clinical setting in various ways to improve quality and patient outcomes. Dr. A. is a DNP graduate nurse practitioner who works in an off-site hospital outpatient setting. Dr. A. utilizes various information technologies throughout his day while seeing patients.

Dr. A. frequently utilizes his hospital reference librarian to obtain new information technologies that are available within his system as well as in any healthcare setting.

Additionally, when caring for patients, Dr. A. frequently uses a search engine to obtain patient information while patients are in the clinic. Dr. A. believes that this empowers patients and provides much-needed information at a time when patients are vulnerable.

Dr. A. also uses a PDA loaded with Epocrates software. He uses Epocrates regularly to check for medication interaction and obtain information about specific diagnoses. In addition, Dr. A. recently upgraded his Epocrates software and is able to obtain ICD/CPT codes to ensure accurate billing.

Recently, Dr. A. became aware of a local home care company that equips its nurses with PDAs to document patient care while at the bedside. These home care nurses also have the capability to photograph wounds, download the photos on the

Table 3-4 Utilization of Information Technology for DNP Graduates in Clinician Roles

- Use PDAs to access up-to-date information regarding medications, diagnostics, and symptoms.
- Use Internet search engines to access patient information materials.
- Review websites for patients to determine if the most accurate and appropriate information is being relayed.
- Utilize reference librarians at your institution or locally to obtain information technology resources and assist with literature searches.
- Partner with administration to become involved in data mining to evaluate patterns in patient data.
- Provide inservice training to other healthcare professionals regarding information technology.
- Role model and utilize information technologies in your clinical setting and share what technologies improve your clinical practice.

Table 3-5 Websites for Information Technology in Nursing

www.himss.org/ASP/topics_nursinginformatics.asp
This website provides information from the Healthcare Information and Management Systems Society Nursing Informatics Task Force.

www.cinjournal.com
This is the website for the *Computers, Informatics, Nursing* journal.

www.ojni.org
This is the website for the *Online Journal of Nursing Informatics.*

www.informaticsnurse.com
This website lists informatics nursing jobs and miscellaneous nursing informatics information.

www.nursinginformatics.com
This website provides information regarding education and continuing education courses about nursing informatics.

www.ania.org
This is the website for the American Nursing Informatics Association.

---

home care secure site, and provide a portal for healthcare professionals to view these photos from the clinical setting. Interestingly, Dr. K., the physician who works with Dr. A., was not interested in sampling this website with the home care agency until Dr. A. convinced him to view the wound photos on the site. Both Dr. A. and Dr. K. now regularly consult this home care company and are able to update the plan of care while still in their clinical setting.

Because of the expertise in information technology Dr. A. garnered while in a DNP program, he is comfortable discovering and utilizing new information technologies within his clinical setting. Prior to his DNP program, Dr. A. shared some of the same reluctance many others express with regard to information technologies. However, Dr. A.'s awareness of the IOM's call for improved health care through the utilization of information technologies and the importance of obtaining up-to-date information that is available through information technologies confirmed for him that it is necessary to become comfortable with these technologies.

■ Interprofessional Collaboration in the Clinical Setting: More Than Just Getting Along

Interprofessional collaboration was discussed previously as it relates to DNP graduates in leadership or potential leadership roles. The current discussion regarding interprofessional collaboration relates specifically to DNP graduates in clinician roles. The recognition that one caregiver alone is unable to support the complexity of current healthcare delivery led to the IOM's recommendation that interprofessional collaboration be included in the educational standards of healthcare professionals in the future (Greiner & Knebel, 2003). Given the additional preparation in this area garnered through a DNP program, the DNP graduate in a clinician role is in a perfect position to influence and exemplify interprofessional collaboration.

Interprofessional collaboration from the clinician's perspective involves more than just getting along with your collaborating physician. The word "collaborate" is derived from the Latin word *collaborare*, which means "to work with one another" (Webster, 2004). The American Nurses Association (ANA, 1995) has defined collaboration as a partnership with shared power, recognition and acceptance of separate and combined practice spheres of activity and responsibility, mutual safeguarding of the legitimate interests of each party, and a commonality of goals.

Interprofessional collaboration has repeatedly been shown to decrease health-care costs and improve both quality of care and healthcare outcomes. Cowan et al. (2006) found that collaborative relationships between physicians and nurse practitioners reduced hospital length of stay without altering readmissions or mortality. McKay and Crippen (2008) also found that instituting a collaborative practice model decreased length of hospital stay and overall healthcare costs. Schmalenberg et al. (2005) also noted that interdisciplinary collaborative relationships between nurses and physicians were linked to improved quality of care. Finally, Knaus, Draper, Wagner, and Zimmerman (1986) reported that when collaborative relationships were present in hospitals, 41% lower mortality occurred than the predicted number of deaths.

Although evidence clearly supports interprofessional collaboration, others have reported barriers. Stein-Parbury and Liaschenko (2007) reported that interprofessional collaboration was hindered when physicians dismissed nurses' knowledge, clinical assessment skills, and concerns about patients. Another frequently noted barrier was lack of recognition regarding other healthcare professionals' roles or knowledge base (Yeager, 2005). The overwhelming solution presented in the literature regarding these barriers was improved communication between healthcare professionals (Gerardi & Fontaine, 2007; McKay & Crippen, 2008; Rossen, Bartlett, & Herrick, 2008; Stein-Parbury & Liaschenko, 2007). Other antecedents to interprofessional collaboration included shared vision between healthcare professionals (Hallas, Butz, & Gitterman, 2004; Yeager, 2005) and trust and respect regarding fellow healthcare professionals' knowledge and expertise (Stein-Parbury & Liaschenko, 2007).

Creating the Bridge: The Challenge for DNP Graduate Clinicians

What does this all mean to the DNP graduate clinician? Although fostering collaboration was discussed in the previous chapter in relation to leadership, one may begin to see how the roles of DNP graduates are truly integrated. The DNP graduate in a clinician role may not be in a formal leadership position; however, the same set of skills is required to promote interdisciplinary collaboration in the clinical setting. These skills will enable DNP graduates in a clinician role to create a bridge between all members of the healthcare team.

Gerardi and Fontaine (2007) described collaboration in relation to the American Association of Critical-Care Nurses' (AACN) *Standards for Establishing and Sustaining Healthy Work Environments* (2005). Six key components were found to be essential for a healthy work environment and "true collaboration" was included.

Gerardi and Fontaine state that "true collaboration is a way of being and a way of working" (2007, p. 10). These are words for DNP graduates to live by. Gerardi and Fontaine also related that true collaboration is a "continuum of engagement" that involves "self-reflection, information sharing, negotiation, feedback, conflict, engagement, conflict resolution, and finally forgiveness and reconciliation" (2007, p. 10).

DNP graduates in clinician roles engage in balancing acts daily when collaborating with other healthcare professionals. Communication techniques that include open listening, understanding multiple perspectives, and developing patient-oriented solutions negotiated together within a team have been noted repeatedly to foster interdisciplinary collaboration (Goleman, Boyatzis, & McKee, 2002; Hamric, Spross, & Hanson, 2005).

Apker, Propp, Zabava Ford, and Hofmeister (2006) explored how nurses communicate professionalism while collaborating with other healthcare team members. These authors noted that displaying professionalism can lead to beneficial outcomes for patients, nurses, and organizations (Apker, Propp, Zabava Ford, & Hofmeister, 2006). Moreover, this study found that four specific types of communication fostered collaboration as well as enabled nurses to display professionalism. These were named the "Four C's of Professional Nurse Communication in Health Care Team Interactions" and included collaboration, credibility, compassion, and coordination (Apker, Propp, Zabava Ford, & Hofmeister, 2006, p. 183).

Collaboration was further elaborated on as updating team members regularly and preparing appropriately before presenting the information. Nurses who "had their ducks in a row" when collaborating were viewed as being professional as well. Further, nurses who engaged in dialogue with physicians to identify solutions for problems and shared in the decision making also displayed professionalism as well as effective collaboration.

Credibility was further described as how nurses display their proficiency while collaborating with other healthcare team members. Establishing credibility when collaborating may also reduce barriers to collaboration associated with lack of recognition of team members' knowledge and expertise. Interestingly, nurses who effectively displayed credibility while adjusting their communication style depending on the varied roles, personalities, and situations were viewed as effectively collaborating with other healthcare team members. Terms such as "sensing the environment" and "adapting to the situation" were used to describe nurses who displayed credibility while collaborating (Apker, Propp, Zabava Ford, & Hofmeister, 2006, p. 184). These terms are similar to the emotional intelligence competencies that were noted to improve communication and leadership in the previous chapter.

Compassion was described as showing consideration for all team members, especially those who were considered to be novices (Apker, Propp, Zabava Ford, & Hofmeister, 2006). Mentoring and demonstrating social support to newer team members were considered key to displaying professionalism and compassion. Advocacy was another behavior noted to be associated with compassion. Respondents stated that when other team members were advocated for, compassion was displayed. Finally, communication that included an optimistic, supportive, and positive attitude was noted to display compassion (Apker, Propp, Zabava Ford, & Hofmeister, 2006).

The final communication skill set included coordination. The manner in which nurses coordinate healthcare delivery speaks to nurses being in the center of the "hub" of the healthcare team (Apker, Propp, Zabava Ford, & Hofmeister, 2006, p. 185). This communication skill demonstrates the leadership nurses must assume every day when providing care. The ability to coordinate care while collaborating with the healthcare team demonstrates nursing professionalism as well.

With regard to DNP graduates, Apker, Propp, Zabava Ford, and Hofmeister's (2006) work describes valuable insights for collaboration and professionalism in nursing. DNP graduates have earned the terminal degree in their field. Therefore, demonstrating professionalism through effective collaboration is vital to their success in every role they may assume.

Realizing that "true collaboration is a way of being" (Gerardi & Fontaine, 2007, p. 10) will also enable DNP graduates to successfully build bridges among all healthcare disciplines. Knowing how to effectively communicate while collaborating will enable DNP graduates to effectively collaborate and build bridges among healthcare disciplines. Building these bridges will facilitate interprofessional collaboration and enable DNP graduates to continually improve quality and healthcare outcomes in an ever-changing, complex healthcare environment. Please refer to **Table 3-6** for bridge-building tips.

Case Scenarios of Interprofessional Collaboration

The following case scenarios describe two types of interprofessional collaboration: one in which the DNP graduate is unsuccessful in building a collaborative relationship and one in which the DNP graduate experiences interprofessional collaboration.

Table 3-6 Tips for Building Bridges Among Healthcare Disciplines

- Respect the knowledge and expertise of other members of the healthcare team in the clinical setting.
- Frequently seek out input and feedback from other members of the healthcare team, especially members in other disciplines.
- Provide accurate and complete information when discussing patients or patient care issues with members of the healthcare team.
- Organize team meetings with members of the healthcare team to focus on new treatment guidelines and evidence-based practices.
- Communicate effectively by utilizing active listening, compassion, and empathy.
- Use emotional intelligence competencies to accurately assess the needs of the healthcare team and feel the room's emotional environment.
- Mentor new team members and provide social support through compassion and empathy.

Case Scenario 1: An Attempt to Build a Bridge

Dr. L. is a new graduate from a BSN-to-DNP program. His experience with collaboration involves working with physicians in a small, rural emergency room setting. His specialization in his DNP program prepared him to become certified as an acute care clinical nurse specialist. Upon graduating, Dr. L. took a position as an emergency room nurse practitioner and began working with the same healthcare team he previously worked with.

Early on, Dr. L. attempted to develop a grand rounds program in the emergency room that would include case presentations with input from all disciplines in the ER setting, including pharmacy, nursing, and medicine. Unfortunately, this idea was met with much resistance from the ER staff physicians. Additionally, when attempting to collaborate with the physicians regarding patient care, Dr. L. was treated poorly and frequently questioned in an accusatory fashion when he suggested different evidence-based treatments. Dr. L. overheard staff physicians making statements such as, "Who does he think he is recommending this treatment?" The medical staff treated him disrespectfully in front of other staff members and patients. As a result, the nursing staff did not exhibit any trust in his abilities.

Dr. L. approached the nurse manager of the ER and was again met with resistance regarding additional educational programs for the staff. Instead of the physicians and nurse manager providing mentoring, Dr. L. was left to fend for himself. Hospital administration offered no assistance and did not have previous experience dealing with the issues related to advanced nursing practice. Eventually, Dr. L. left the hospital he worked at and relocated to work in a large university setting with other advanced practice registered nurses. Dr. L. felt he would get the support and mentoring he needed to grow as an advanced practice registered nurse and a valued member of the healthcare team. Sadly, the small, rural hospital lost a DNP graduate who attempted to improve quality of care and patient outcomes through collaboration.

Case Scenario 2: A Bridge Built

Dr. N. is a DNP graduate working as a nurse–midwife in a university-affiliated outpatient clinic. Dr. N. began to notice that she has been caring for an increasing number of patients who had previously undergone bariatric surgery and are now pregnant. Upon doing a literature search to obtain information regarding caring for this unique population, Dr. N. noted that there was a paucity of evidence-based practice guidelines available pertaining to pregnant postbariatric surgery patients.

Dr. N. took the first step to integrating evidence-based practice and asked a question: What are the increased risks to both mother and baby when the mother has had bariatric surgery? Dr. N. requested a grand rounds meeting with the departments of obstetrics, surgery, and dietary. She contacted her reference librarian, who provided her with literature regarding bariatric surgery and postsurgical complications, including risks that persist well after surgery. Dr. N. also contacted the information technology department, and with their assistance she was able to arrange a satellite meeting with another teaching institution that had recently begun a clinical trial involving pregnant patients who had previously undergone bariatric surgery.

The grand rounds meeting was well attended by nursing, medicine, obstetrics, surgery, and dietary. Many questions were raised regarding how to care for this population, including how to address their unique nutritional needs. The team initiated steps to develop a research program in their institution, and Dr. N. was able to actively participate in this endeavor. Dr. N. used the knowledge she had garnered in her DNP program to integrate evidence-based practice, utilize information technologies, and build a bridge between disciplines. This process had started with her simply asking a question while caring for her patient.

■ Mentoring: DNP Graduates Shaping the Future of Clinician Roles

"Mentor" has been defined as a trusted counselor or guide (McKinley, 2004; Webster, 2004). The term "mentor" originated in Greek mythology and refers to Odysseus's trusted counselor, who became his son Telemachus's teacher (Webster, 2004). Odysseus entrusted the care of his son to Mentor while he went to fight in the Trojan War. Mentor's job was not just to teach Telemachus but to help him develop as a man and prepare him for the responsibilities he would assume (McKinley, 2004). In the professional realm, mentoring involves helping others achieve goals as well as offering support in a nonthreatening way. Hence, the clinical setting is an ideal place for DNP graduates to mentor and shape the future of nursing.

DNP Graduates: From Experts to Novices and Back to Experts

Mentoring involves the mentor having a certain level of expertise. A discussion about expertise and mentoring would not be complete without mentioning Patricia Benner's (1984) work *From Novice to Expert*. Dr. Benner's work is derived from The Dreyfus Model of Skill Acquisition. This model posits that while developing a set of skills, one progresses through five levels of proficiency: novice, advanced beginner, competent, proficient, and expert (Benner, 1982; Dreyfus & Dreyfus, 1980). Dr. Benner has purported that these levels of skill development may be used to describe how nurses develop proficiency as experts. Dr. Benner's premise was that experience results in expertise. Nurses begin their careers as novices and move through the levels by gaining experience in the clinical setting. Expertise has been characterized as knowing the vision of what is possible (Benner, 1982). In other words, knowing the goals and possible outcomes from an expert's interventions is what allows a nurse to move from proficiency to expertise.

By definition, DNP graduates are in a position of expertise. DNP graduates are acutely aware of the goals of healthcare delivery as well as various interventions to improve these goals. However, many of the new skills introduced (or reinforced) to

DNP graduates place them in the position of novice after spending perhaps years in the position of expert. Concepts such as evidence-based practice, information technologies, leadership skills, interprofessional collaboration, and research methodology may be less familiar to many DNP graduates who may be functioning at high levels of expertise in the clinical setting. Therefore, garnering newer, sophisticated skills in a DNP program may make many DNP graduates feel less like experts and more like novices.

Despite this, many DNP graduates will find themselves in the role of mentor. However, the wealth of clinical expertise many DNP graduates possess may allow them to move from novice to expert quite easily. The new skills DNP graduates garner in their programs are integrated into their nursing practice. Further, the skills acquired in a DNP program enable graduates to develop an enlarged view of healthcare delivery and design ways to improve healthcare outcomes, which will foster expertise in nursing practice. Dracup and Bryan-Brown (2004) relate that "the expert has gone beyond the tasks and responds to the whole picture" (p. 449). DNP graduates are well beyond the tasks of nursing and are able to envision the whole picture.

The Robert Wood Johnson Executive Nurse Fellows Program (2009) has identified five competencies that are essential for mentoring. These competencies may be related to ways in which DNP graduates may increase their level of expertise and eventually provide mentoring. The first competency is the ability to translate a strategic vision into a motivating message. Each time a DNP graduate expresses why he or she returned to school for a DNP degree, a strategic vision is shared, which serves to motivate others. This author is often told that she has inspired others to return to school either for nursing or for a graduate degree in nursing. The second competency is risk taking and creativity. Again, earning a new, innovative degree demonstrates risk taking and creativity. Further, the ability to complete a research project that is grounded in clinical practice also displays creativity. The third competency is the ability to understand and develop the self with regard to self-knowledge and individual motivation. DNP graduates are challenged through their DNP programs to know themselves and their individual motivation, as well as their own personal leadership styles. The choice to earn a DNP degree illustrates awareness of the need for additional knowledge to meet the changing demands of health care. Further, the additional leadership skills they garner enable DNP graduates to develop awareness regarding their own strengths and weaknesses. DNP graduates are experts at knowing what they do not know and discovering ways to enrich their knowledge base. The fourth competency includes inspiring and leading change. DNP graduates will be leaders regardless of their area of expertise. They will be called on to inspire and guide others in times of change. The final competency is effective communication and interpersonal effectiveness. DNP graduates will mentor through their ability to engage in mutual and equal relationships. Many DNP graduates will have had previous experiences that involved hierarchical relationships with other healthcare professionals. These experiences will serve to remind DNP graduates that successful mentoring relationships are built on empathy, compassion, respect, and nurturing behaviors. Therefore, DNP graduates will have sensitivity regarding what type of mentoring relationship is mutual and equal.

Precepting: The Ideal Opportunity to Mentor

For the DNP graduate in the clinical setting, precepting is often integrated into the clinical role. Precepting is a time-limited commitment that evolves into a teaching–learning relationship between student and preceptor. However, "mentoring is more than just training or precepting" (McKinley, 2004, p. 207). Mentoring has been described as a way to assist in human development, where one invests time, energy, and personal knowledge to enable another to grow and develop (McKinley, 2004). Although precepting differs from mentoring, precepting presents the perfect opportunity for DNP graduates in the clinical setting to become mentors.

Hayes (1998) studied the stories of students who felt they had experienced a mentoring relationship with their clinical preceptor. Specific descriptors were cited by the students related to their experiences. These specific descriptors included the following: a vested interest in the student, a love for teaching, openness, friendship, trust, acting as a life jacket, patience, sharing job advice, and role modeling kind, empathetic, competent patient care (Hayes, 1998). These characteristics mirror many of the leadership attributes previously discussed. Further, when thinking of a teacher/preceptor/clinical instructor who inspired, led, and truly made a difference in their lives, many DNP graduates will be able to recall similar experiences. Hence, self-reflection, previous experiences, and the skills garnered in a DNP program will enable DNP graduates to seize the opportunity to build mentoring relationships in the clinical setting.

McKinley (2004) wrote about mentoring in nursing and related three steps to the mentoring process that may foster successful mentoring relationships both in and out of the clinical setting: reflecting, reframing, and resolving. Reflecting involves the creation of the relationship (McKinley, 2004). This includes sharing personal information to build a common ground as well as discussing the goals of the relationship. DNP graduates in the preceptor role may share their personal journeys in nursing as a way to inspire and guide. Also, DNP graduates may ask students what their expectations are for the semester as well as share what they hope to accomplish while teaching. This author often advises students she precepts to ask all the silly questions, not just questions about clinical scenarios. Frequently, questions about certification, relationships with staff, and how to interview for a job are cited among the most valuable pointers students think they received during a clinical rotation. Reframing encourages connecting and allows the mentor to challenge the student (McKinley, 2004). DNP graduates may use their broadened knowledge base about information technologies to encourage students to look outside the box for information. This may also be done by challenging students to integrate evidence-based practice when developing a plan of care. At this time, the DNP graduate may demonstrate these skills to the student and reinforce learning in an ongoing process. Melnyk et al. (2004) found that evidence-based practice (EBP) increased with mentorship from others utilizing EBP. These behaviors strengthen the relationship between mentor and student and allow the student to grow (McKinley, 2004). Resolving involves the mentor empowering the student to develop solutions (McKinley, 2004). This is when the foundation built by reflection and reframing is put into action. The DNP graduate allows the student to examine the options and consequences of the options. Previously it was mentioned that expertise means knowing the vision of what is possible (Benner, 1982). DNP graduates may have experienced this type of learning from mentors while acquiring new skills in their DNP programs. These experiences will allow DNP graduates to let the students own their solutions. This process is similar to DNP graduates developing and owning their solutions through their own evidence-based research projects—a process that came to fruition through the mentoring they once received.

■ Conclusion

The ways in which DNP graduates may shape the future of nursing through mentoring are numerous (please refer to **Table 3-7**). In the clinical setting DNP graduates are in the forefront of health care and therefore in a position to improve quality and healthcare outcomes. Mentoring new nurses, advanced practice registered nurses, and other healthcare professionals will ensure that the DNP graduates' focus on improved healthcare delivery will be a priority of the future of nursing practice.

Table 3-7   Tips for DNP Graduates Mentoring in the Clinical Setting

- Express an interest in students personally.
- Share personal experiences, especially personal setbacks or failures.
- Express a love for teaching.
- Stay open to ideas, input, and suggestions.
- Be willing to give advice about jobs, interviewing, and creating good staff relations.
- Role model empathetic and compassionate patient care.
- Motivate students to have a vision, especially a vision of themselves when they complete their degree.
- Challenge students to come up with their own solutions and empower them to own their solutions.
- Allow students to be wrong, and give constructive, noncritical feedback when they are wrong.
- Create opportunities to be creative and utilize evidence-based practice or information technology to develop solutions.
- Role model effective interdisciplinary collaboration by demonstrating or role playing the discussion of care with other disciplines.

Interviews with DNP Clinicians: Then and Now

The following interviews with Doctor of Nursing Practice (DNP) graduates provide invaluable insight from practicing clinicians with DNP degrees.

Interview with Dr. Kathleen A. Payson

Kathleen A. Payson, DNP, APRN, BC is a faculty member at Wayne State University School of Nursing in Detroit, Michigan. She is also a private practice women's health and internal medicine adult nurse practitioner.

Then . . . 2008

Dr. Payson, could you please describe your current position?

I am a contracted services nurse practitioner in a women's health and internal medicine private practice as well as part-time faculty at Wayne State University in Detroit, Michigan. I plan to continue my clinical practice with an emphasis on pursuing a joint role in academia and nursing research. In addition, I plan on completing my Osteoporosis Prevention Research Project—Phase 2 with a goal to publish the final outcomes.

Dr. Payson, what motivated you to return to school for a DNP degree?

Overall, I liked the concept of the DNP role because it focused more on the clinical aspect of nursing at the doctorate level. First and foremost, the motivation for me to advance my education was due to our country's critical nursing shortage—a shortage that will worsen when our men and women return from war and one that has already been significantly impacted by the aging population in America. The realization and impact of the nursing shortage became more evident when I started my academic role as a WSU nursing educator. There are not enough professors to handle the demand for nurses entering the nursing/healthcare arena. Secondly, being a nurse is a motivating force alone.

I would also like to mention that the accelerated pace of the DNP program at Oakland University (OU) in Rochester, Michigan was an attraction to apply for the DNP program. OU has a stellar reputation for higher education along with being the first DNP program in the state of Michigan. Education is the power and the highway to make a difference within the discipline of nursing! Having the opportunity for advancement in nursing to better serve my patient population was the utmost priority. In addition, a Doctor of Nursing Practice degree can facilitate the growing need to keep pace towards clinical and technological skills required for the future of health care.

Dr. Payson, could you describe your experience in a DNP program?

The DNP experience at OU prepared me to be in the forefront and to become a leader in nursing whether it is in the academic, clinical, or research environment. The nurse leaders who were part of the DNP program encouraged us to be strong, flexible, and to excel within the discipline of nursing. This advanced preparation in leadership responsibilities has influenced my involvement in healthcare policy, thereby enabling significant changes toward health promotion/education. For example, new experiences and educational opportunities include, and are not limited to, writing a grant to support my research project towards osteoporosis prevention among postmenopausal women utilizing a nurse-led educational intervention. These educational opportunities created excitement to further explore various avenues in nursing research, thus enhancing health care for all.

Dr. Payson, how has your practice changed since earning a DNP degree?

As an APRN with a DNP degree, I am better prepared to become an expert in managing the complex balance between quality of care, access to care, and fiscal responsibilities. A difficult task to accomplish without an advanced degree! Ultimately, health care is a business, and we are all entrepreneurs! I feel that the DNP degree is the stepping stone for the future of nursing, allowing improved quality and continuity of health care. Additionally, there has been great respect shown among my colleagues, staff, and patients with earning the Doctor of Nursing Practice degree.

Dr. Payson, how has your view of nursing and nursing practice changed since earning a DNP degree?

It has changed considerably and with a great deal of confidence. My understanding of nursing has evolved by realizing the influence that we have among ourselves and with knowing that power in numbers can make significant changes. We must take a stance and support one another by promoting our profession and learn to overcome obstacles in order for enormous changes in health care to occur. Nursing must continually promote further education in our profession, ensuring enough leaders and educators for our next generation of nurses.

The afforded privilege of acceptance and completion of the DNP degree has also given me the perseverance to go forth and continue to strive and commit myself to excellence in the nursing discipline. I also feel it is imperative for nursing to have nursing leaders prepared at the doctorate level as many other nonhealthcare professions require. The demand for nurses continues to escalate, and leaders in nursing are in the forefront to make the public aware of both the art and science of nursing.

Dr. Payson, how have others reacted to you earning a DNP degree?

Favorably and with great respect, especially from those who know what a nurse practitioner role is. I have found that this new role has required a huge educational component. I now make a concerted effort and spend a great deal of time educating my colleagues, patients, family, and friends about the DNP degree and our evolving roles.

Dr. Payson, have your responsibilities in the clinical setting changed since earning a DNP degree?

Yes, the DNP degree has prepared me to take on leadership positions in research and clinical care delivery, thereby allowing improved patient outcomes and enhanced system management among my patient population I serve.

Dr. Payson, would you encourage other advanced practice registered nurses to return to school for a DNP degree?

Yes, because of the emerging clinical doctoral focus emphasizing clinical practice-oriented leadership development. The goal of the DNP degree is to prepare the APRN as a nurse scientist encompassing investigative skills of a researcher as well as the clinical and leadership skills that are required in this ever-changing healthcare system. Health outcomes measurement, healthcare economics, statistical analysis, and informatics are common focus areas and a major trend for the future. Furthermore, these areas were incorporated and a main focus in Oakland University's first DNP program.

Dr. Payson, if given the opportunity, would you return to school to earn a DNP degree again?

Absolutely, without a doubt. Since the program, my level of maturity, motivation, self-confidence, and strength of commitment to provide leadership for the nursing role have been greatly enhanced. Knowledgeable clinicians are required to navigate healthcare systems. The discipline of nursing must continually strive to synthesize and integrate various bodies of knowledge, thereby allowing enhanced quality care in an interdisciplinary evidence-based healthcare environment.

Now . . . 2011

Dr. Payson, we discussed your nursing background and education last time we spoke. Could you please describe your current position?

My current position is an adult nurse practitioner, with a Doctor of Nursing Practice degree, within an urban women's health care setting. My role within the practice is an administrator and provider of direct patient care.

Dr. Payson, has your position evolved at all over the last 4 years since earning a DNP degree? If so, how?

Yes, my position has evolved since earning my DNP degree. The advanced training and education have permitted me to function to the fullest capacity as a healthcare provider toward health promotion and disease prevention in the OB/GYN setting. This role has given me additional respect from my peers and has allowed me the opportunity to partner with physicians in redesigning women's health care, therefore leading to improved health outcomes.

Dr. Payson, has your clinical/academic practice evolved at all since earning a DNP degree?

Yes, my clinical/academic practice has evolved since the DNP degree. I became more involved in actively participating toward the advancement of nursing by serving as adjunct faculty, nurse educator/lecturer, and as a student preceptor for the adult nurse practitioner program at Wayne State University in Detroit, Michigan.

Dr. Payson, have you experienced a salary or responsibility increase since earning your DNP degree?

Yes, in reviewing the current DNP salary averages, I am at the top of the salary range for the DNP profession. Since earning a DNP degree, my scope of practice has been enhanced, resulting in an increase in my hourly rate, an annual bonus based on profitability, and 2 additional weeks of vacation.

Dr. Payson, have your patients/students adapted to your degree preparation? How did you educate your patients/students about your degree preparation?

Yes, my staff, patients, and students have adapted to my degree preparation. The transition took a great deal of time in explaining the role of a DNP-prepared nurse practitioner, but perseverance has paid off. Repetition is the "key." It was critical to first educate my staff to appropriately explain my role and appropriately address my title to patients, family members, ancillary departments, or to any healthcare provider whether communicated in person, by phone, or documentation. My credentials are listed on the building directory, door, and our phone. The office phone message clearly informs callers of my title, stating "Dr. Payson, our nurse practitioner." This change in credentials from NP to DNP was a learning curve for all. Having to explain or defend my role is now limited to new patients who are unfamiliar with the DNP title.

Dr. Payson, do you use the title "Dr." in your clinical or academic setting? If so, how do you introduce yourself?

Yes, how I introduce myself is as follows: "Good morning or afternoon, I am Dr. Payson, the nurse practitioner."

Dr. Payson, would you continue to encourage others to return to school for a DNP degree? Why or why not?

Absolutely! I will always encourage others to further their education from a NP to DNP degree. Attaining a doctoral degree in nursing advances and shapes the nurse practitioner role and the entire future of nursing. Advanced education facilitates utilization of evidence-based healthcare practice and the implementation of relevant research into practice. These higher standards of patient care ultimately enhance beneficial changes toward advancing health outcomes.

Dr. Payson, do you agree with the AACN's recommended target date of 2015 for the DNP degree as entry into practice for advanced practice registered nurses? If so, how do you recommend we continue to strive toward this goal?

I agree with the AACN's recommendation for the DNP degree as entry into practice for APRNs but I do not agree with the targeted date of 2015. We are only 4 years out and with the current shortage of nurses and nurse educators, this will be a difficult task to attain and ultimately may compromise patient health care. It is imperative to continually promote the purpose and goal of the DNP degree as entry into practice for APRNs. This can be effectively achieved by our colleagues within the nursing profession since we are the largest segment of the nation's healthcare workforce. Continued efforts in educating all healthcare professionals, staff, students, and most importantly our patient population, is the ultimate driving force to accomplish the AACN's future goal. "Word of mouth" can either promote or harm our profession. Therefore, it is ultimately our responsibility to provide the "best" care so that our patients are willing to promote and support our advanced role. Other avenues are to utilize available health information systems, participate in healthcare forums and research studies, become published, and be actively involved in the public healthcare policy arena.

Interview with Dr. Sheila Behler

Sheila Behler, DNP, APRN, BC is a nurse practitioner at John D. Dingell VA Medical Center in Detroit, Michigan.

Then . . . 2008

Dr. Behler, could you please describe your practice setting?

I am certified as a family practice nurse practitioner. I work full time in primary care at John D. Dingell VA in Detroit, Michigan. I have a caseload of 1,400 to 1,500 patients. Most have an element of mental health issues and substance dependence issues. Most also have chronic diseases like diabetes and hypertension. We are frequently overbooked for several appointments due to the government mandate that all veterans must be seen within 30 days. My clinic runs from 0800 until 1600, but I am always there by 0700 to review labs, X-rays, consultation reports, fill out forms, and a variety of other issues that need follow-up.

Dr. Behler, what motivated you to return to school for a DNP degree?

I decided to return to school for my DNP degree because of the appeal that this was the last step I could take towards validating my profession. I already had a master's degree in nursing and two post-master's certificates. I felt this would be the final frontier, so to speak. Additionally, I have always enjoyed learning and challenging myself to learn.

Dr. Behler, could you describe your experience in the DNP program?

The rigor of the program enabled me to enhance my organizational skills and increase my focus. The distance education aspects of the program were unique but also very challenging. I learned to prioritize due to the fact that I worked full time while attending school. Also, I am very proud to have been part of the first DNP program in Michigan.

Dr. Behler, how has your practice changed since earning a DNP degree?

I am very much more focused on research-based standards for care. I am not swayed by new medications unless I have seen the articles in my journals and read that they are indeed more beneficial then other less costly ones. The knowledge I gained in the DNP program validated for me the importance of evidence-based practice.

Dr. Behler, how has your view of nursing and nursing practice changed since earning a DNP degree?

As DNP graduates I feel we have a professional obligation to provide leadership to fellow NPs. I also feel the need to further educate the public regarding what advanced practice registered nurses are, including what a DNP degree is. We also have an obligation to incorporate evidence-based research into our practice. In this area in particular, others look to us for leadership, even though we are in a clinical role.

Dr. Behler, how have others reacted to the knowledge and skills you garnered in the DNP program?

People are proud, both my coworkers and especially my patients. I presented a PowerPoint presentation of my research to others in my practice setting, and they were delighted to see my research as well as the outcomes. After the presentation, one of the physicians in our group asked me about hypertension medications for his personal use in managing his health. He is using the medication I suggested to control his hypertension that was based on my research with evidence-based practice. This reinforces our role in educating others about evidence-based practice and how we can mentor others to change their practice patterns.

Dr. Behler, have your responsibilities changed in your clinical setting since earning a DNP degree?

Yes, I am being asked to be on more committees like the credentialing committee for all primary care providers to bring a higher standard of care. Also, I have been more involved in research projects, including applying for a grant related to my work in hypertension. I plan to continue to pursue research, and I also believe it is important to publish our work and contribute to nursing's body of knowledge. New opportunities have also been presented for me in my practice setting, such as initiating an educational program for registered nurses to finish their bachelor's degree. Finally,

I should also mention the constant need to educate patients regarding nursing and this newer terminal degree. Many of my patients say, "Oh, you're a doctor now, are you leaving?" I constantly provide reassurance and education regarding my DNP degree. This is part of having a practice-focused doctorate.

Dr. Behler, would you encourage other advanced practice registered nurses to pursue a DNP degree?

Yes, I would. I feel the more we push ourselves professionally, the better the health outcomes will be for our patients. I also feel it is important to grow as a nurse.

Dr. Behler, if given the opportunity, would you earn a DNP degree again?

Yes, I would. It was without a doubt one of the hardest things I have done in my life, and I am still, after 6 months out, amazed I did so much and learned so much. I know I give better patient care because of the DNP degree.

Now . . . 2011

Dr. Behler, we discussed your nursing background and education last time we spoke. Could you please describe your current position?

I am still employed in the same position, providing primary health care to veterans whom I enjoy.

Dr. Behler, has your position evolved at all over the last 4 years since earning a DNP degree? If so, how?

The position itself has not evolved into anything different only because I have chosen to have it remain the way it is. My preference is to provide direct patient care based on the latest evidence-based research. I have been fortunate to be able to precept nurse practitioner students, which is also very gratifying as we need to replace ourselves as some of us prepare to retire.

Dr. Behler, has your clinical practice evolved at all since earning a DNP degree?

Without a doubt it has. I read research articles with more understanding and critique as to which ones have merit that influences my clinical practice.

Dr. Behler, have you experienced a salary or responsibility increase since earning your DNP degree?

Yes, I am very happy to say I have and I have also published my original research, which merited a small bonus and acknowledgement.

Dr. Behler, have your patients adapted to your degree preparation? How did you educate your patients/students about your degree preparation?

My patients love it that I am a doctor nurse! I explain that a doctoral-prepared nurse does extra study and rigorous research to assist in providing the best care for them.

Dr. Behler, do you use the title "Dr." in your clinical or academic setting? If so, how do you introduce yourself?

Always and I am very clear; I state I am Dr. Behler, a nurse practitioner. Sometimes this leads to further discussions, sometimes not.

Dr. Behler, would you continue to encourage others to return to school for a DNP degree? Why or why not?

Yes, keeping in mind this is a clinical degree and you may or may not change careers, it is about one's own self-growth, the growth of our profession to establish standards, and for our patients.

Dr. Behler, do you agree with the AACN's recommended target date of 2015 for the DNP degree as entry into practice for advanced practice registered nurses? If so, how do you recommend we continue to strive toward this goal?

I do because currently when you become a nurse practitioner there are several avenues to do this, which I find confusing for myself as well as my patients. You could have a women's health practitioner working in urology; I know someone who does this and is an expert but with the doctoral degree you are confident that person has looked at research and standards with a critical eye and is not influenced by some studies that may not have merit. It sets a standard across the board.

Interview with Dr. Andrea Kwasky

Andrea Kwasky, DNP, APRN, BC is a family psychiatric/ mental health nurse practitioner

Then . . . 2008

Dr. Kwasky, could you please describe your practice setting?

I work in a residential treatment center for children and adolescents who live with severe mental health issues. I started this position shortly before entering the program, which made the choice to also return to school particularly interesting. The residents that I care for range in age from 9 to 19. They have all had multiple treatment failures within the acute care inpatient setting and have had great difficulties at home, school, and within the community. Residents generally reside within the program from 6 months to several years until they can be reintegrated back into the community at a less intense level of treatment. My role is to improve the quality of care for vulnerable youth who have not been able to be successful in previous treatment. I collaborate with a treatment team to provide staff education, milieu management, crisis intervention, and medication management.

Dr. Kwasky, what motivated you to return to school for a DNP degree?

A fellow nurse practitioner introduced me to the DNP degree. I became aware that Oakland University was planning to start the first program in Michigan. After further investigation of the degree and various universities that offered this type of program, I decided to apply for the first and only program in existence in Michigan. I was excited to once again feel like a pioneer blazing a new nursing trail within the state of Michigan as my bachelor of science degree with a major in nursing was a community-based program and the first of its kind in Michigan (Western Michigan University). I knew that the DNP program would be challenging, but with that came the great reward of being on the forefront of furthering the nursing profession.

Dr. Kwasky, were there any additional factors that motivated you to return to school for a DNP degree?

Yes, at the time I was accepted to the program I was 29 years old. It was in a time of self-reflection and transition in my life. I had recently lost my mother, and she had always been a very supportive force behind the various goals that I had set for myself. The DNP program presented an opportunity to enhance my knowledge base in my field and allow me to refocus my goals. I am a believer that education and knowledge are with you everywhere you go. I am not a career student, and I have worked full time most of my nursing career. However, I love to learn, and I feel that anything I can do to enhance my nursing practice is essential to improve the care of my patients.

Also, I would like to add that I was the youngest DNP student in my class. I add this to emphasize the point that despite nursing's unwritten rule that one must obtain experience before pursuing higher education, I feel that one can gain experience along the way while enhancing their education. I want to encourage others like myself to not feel intimidated about returning to school early in your nursing career. You can increase your experience as you increase your knowledge base!

Dr. Kwasky, could you please describe your experience in the DNP program?

Challenging, exhausting, rewarding, excruciating, and well worth every moment. Not only did I gain valuable skills and knowledge related to research, theory, as well as how to navigate the political process, but also I was able to cultivate relationships with a cohort of visionary nursing leaders.

Dr. Kwasky, how has your practice changed since earning a DNP degree?

The primary way that my practice has changed is in the way that I conceptualize nursing. Additionally, I now feel more of a responsibility to mentor and cultivate relationships with individuals who are interested in becoming nurses or individuals who have just entered a nursing program. Several of the residential care specialists that I work with have just entered nursing school. I feel an obligation to discuss my experiences within the profession of nursing and to expose them to all of the possibilities that await them. In fact, I will be teaching a mental health clinical rotation with a group of second-degree students this fall.

I also have had the pleasure to act in the role of public relations and marketing for the "Doctor Nurse" within my community. Educating the public about [the] role of the DNP has certainly been interesting.

Dr. Kwasky, how has your view of nursing and nursing practice changed since earning your DNP degree?

I am better able to articulate the difference between discipline and the profession of nursing. I have a more intimate understanding of the theoretical and historical background of my chosen field.

Dr. Kwasky, how have others reacted to your DNP degree and the skills/knowledge you garnered in the program?

With questions, many questions. For example, "Why didn't you just go to medical school?" People are curious, and the general public especially does not understand the DNP degree. I more fully realize the obligation I have to educate patients, families, other healthcare professionals, and the public about my field and my degree. Also, I feel an obligation to become involved in public policy and impact the future of nursing educational standards. The DNP degree is now the terminal practice degree. I feel that policy protecting our right to use the title "doctor" and represent our field as doctoral-prepared nurse[s] is important. Policies that would prevent this are rapidly coming to the forefront, perhaps sparked by our higher educational standards. I feel DNP graduates as well as the nursing profession as a whole need to unite and become involved in policies that affect nursing and health care in general.

Dr. Kwasky, have your responsibilities changed in your clinical setting since earning a DNP degree?

The responsibilities outlined in my job description have not changed as a result of earning the DNP degree. However, the accountability that I have to myself, the patients that I care for, and the nursing profession have dramatically shifted. I have learned to think about what I do in a more global way. What I mean by this is that the methodology by which I practice has changed. I am always seeking to identify the evidence and rational[e] behind my interventions.

Dr. Kwasky, would you encourage other advanced practice registered nurses to return to school for a DNP degree?

Yes! However, I would caution others that with great knowledge comes great responsibilities. The educational process does not end with the DNP degree. Prospective students should also know that the way they practice will never be the same. Instead of perhaps feeling frustrated by this, they need to feel a renewed sense of responsibility to educate others about their degree and using their new knowledge and skills to continually improve the quality of health care they provide.

Dr. Kwasky, if given the opportunity, would you earn a DNP degree again?

This is an interesting question. Am I glad that I have obtained the degree? Absolutely! However, being on the forefront of something that the public has never been exposed to is not for everyone. Every conversation with a new patient or family starts out with, "Hello, I am Dr. Kwasky. The children I work with call me Dr. Andrea. I am a family psychiatric/mental health nurse practitioner, and I also have a doctorate in nursing practice. I work in collaboration with the physician." This relates back to the challenge for DNP graduates to educate others about our profession, our degree, and our role in healthcare delivery. As DNP graduates, we know who we are, we know where we have been, and we know we are different. The challenge lies in using this knowledge every day to improve healthcare delivery.

Now . . . 2011

Dr. Kwasky, we discussed your nursing background and education last time we spoke. Could you please describe your current position?

Currently, I hold a full-time assistant professor faculty position with the University of Detroit Mercy, McAuley School of Nursing. In addition to teaching I remain clinically immersed in the area of mental health through my advanced practice role with children and adolescents at a long-term residential treatment center for children/adolescents who have significant mental health issues.

Dr. Kwasky, has your position evolved at all over the last 4 years since earning a DNP degree? If so, how?

Yes, after obtaining my DNP degree from Oakland University I continued my full-time employment at the residential treatment center that I previously referenced. I remained there while I contemplated my career path and how I could best utilize the knowledge and skills gained from my recent educational endeavor. After thoughtful consideration I decided to challenge myself by pursuing a career educating future nurses. As I look back on my own academic career, I can specifically identify nursing mentors and role models that influenced my path. I wanted to share my passion for nursing and commitment to vulnerable populations with students in an effort to engage them in the important work that we do as professional nurses. While working with students in their mental health clinical rotation I tell them that the only thing that I can think of that is better than working with the children and adolescents at the treatment center is hopefully igniting the spark in one of them to want to do something similar for the members of our population that have been marginalized and stigmatized.

Dr. Kwasky, has your clinical/academic practice evolved at all since earning a DNP degree?

In both realms of academia and practice I find that I am able to more effectively evaluate systems issues and understand the multiple layers (individual, systemic, programmatic, and political) that can contribute to both a problem or solution.

Dr. Kwasky, have you experienced a salary or responsibility increase since earning your DNP degree?

I have not experienced a salary increase as a result of earning my DNP. One of the goals of DNP preparation is to assist with education of future nurses. This is certainly not as financially lucrative as being clinically immersed full time; however, the rewards are great. Therefore, I think that being an educator must be something that one is passionate about. With regard to an increase in responsibility, I have not been formally given more responsibility. However, with advanced education comes a responsibility to act on that knowledge. Since completing my DNP I have published and have several articles in process, written and obtained grant funding for a study related to vitamin D and depression in young women, established a relationship with a PhD mentor who has been instrumental in partnering to conduct research, I attend conferences to disseminate information related to my specialty area, and I continue to grow in my newest role as an educator.

Dr. Kwasky, have your patients/students adapted to your degree preparation? How did you educate your patients/students about your degree preparation?

I teach an introductory nursing course titled Self-Awareness for Nurses in the Interdisciplinary Environment. The focus of the course is to develop a better understanding of what it means to be a professional nurse. Part of my responsibility as an educator is to help the students understand the various ways in which nurses are educated. This includes teaching the students about the DNP degree. I also have the opportunity to work with nursing students who are nearing graduation. They generally have misconceptions about the degree and frequently have very good questions about academic preparation and the AACN's recommended target date of 2015 for the DNP degree as entry into practice for advanced practice registered nurses. When I explain to the students that the DNP is a degree, not a role, they seem to have a better understanding. Students and patients seem to have adapted well as long as they are educated appropriately. However, in my opinion, some controversy still exists regarding the belief that the DNP is a terminal degree for those that may not value practice as scholarship, which seems ludicrous in a practice-driven profession. Additionally, I still think that our physician counterparts require education regarding this degree and how we can partner with them in the healthcare environment.

Dr. Kwasky, do you use the title "Dr." in your clinical or academic setting? If so, how do you introduce yourself?

Yes, I use my title as "Dr." in both my clinical and academic setting. In the clinical setting when I am working with children, I am Dr. Andrea, and in the academic setting I am Dr. Kwasky. I use the same explanation that I did when I first earned my degree. I educate the children, adolescents, families, students, and other healthcare providers that I am a family psychiatric mental health nurse practitioner who also has earned a doctoral degree in nursing practice.

Dr. Kwasky, would you continue to encourage others to return to school for a DNP degree? Why or why not?

Yes. For those individuals who are clinically immersed and would like to pursue advanced education in nursing I think that the DNP is a great option.

Dr. Kwasky, do you agree with the AACN's recommended target date of 2015 for the DNP degree as entry into practice for advanced practice registered nurses? If so, how do you recommend we continue to strive toward this goal?

I think that it is an interesting idea. With so many entry levels into practice, I can see why this goal has been established. I hear many senior nursing students who are seeking a BSN to DNP program to attend as soon as they have completed their undergraduate degree. I think that students should be cautious about this and that universities should be cognizant that the DNP teaches higher level concepts and thinking. Therefore, students should be required to have a minimum number of practice hours completed prior to admission. Otherwise, some concepts can be lost in translation as students are trying to assimilate concepts that they only know in theory and have not been exposed to in practice.

■ A DNP Graduate's Personal Journey: Who, Me?

I always knew I would go back to school after earning a master's degree in nursing. I was impatiently waiting for a true practice doctorate to become a reality. I intended to stay involved in nursing practice as an advanced practice registered nurse. Therefore, when the opportunity to earn a DNP degree in the first program in Michigan presented itself, I was the first student to apply. In graduate school I wasn't quite sure what the result would be upon completing my degree; I just knew I needed to learn more. Now, as a DNP graduate clinician, I am beginning to understand how a DNP degree enhances my ability to deliver and improve health care. I am more aware of the needs of my patients as individuals as well as members of communities, and I have developed more complex skills to meet their needs. Moreover, I have a more acute awareness of the needs of my profession and the increasing complexities in health care today.

The skills I developed through the DNP program are reflected in how I care for my patients. I regularly evaluate and translate evidence-based practice for my patients and seek new ways to integrate this information into the plan of care. When patient care is not optimal due to systems or organizational issues, I use my leadership and collaboration skills to develop solutions to improve care. I mentor others in nursing who wish to pursue a DNP degree and have developed a specialty preceptor program within my clinical setting. Finally, I am committed to promoting nursing, the nurse practitioner role, and the DNP degree through pedagogical methods that will increase others' understanding.

I believe I knew a great deal about nursing when I was prepared at the master's degree level. Earning a DNP degree not only broadened this knowledge base but also made me more aware of my role in nursing practice and healthcare delivery. I am also more aware of where nursing—as a practice profession—has been, where we are going, and where we need to be. Now, almost 5 years since graduating with a DNP degree, I have begun to realize the impact this degree will have on health care. As leaders and practice experts, DNP graduates are beginning to shape the future of health care by influencing healthcare policy and the evaluation and translation of evidence-based practice. I am very proud to be a DNP graduate and am more fully committed to promoting the DNP degree.

■ Why a DNP for Clinicians?

In the beginning of the chapter, the question was posed, How will the clinician's role change or benefit from earning a DNP degree? After a discussion regarding the many aspects of the DNP graduates' role as clinician, it is this author's anticipation that a broader understanding has developed. Many readers will turn to this section to look for the answer to, Why a DNP for clinicians? As a DNP graduate who finished her degree almost 5 years ago, this author has realized the answer to this question is somewhat complex. Healthcare delivery is improved through expertise in evaluating, translating, and implementing evidence-based practice, information technology, interprofessional collaboration, and mentoring. However, one may not fully appreciate the benefits of the DNP degree until some time after graduation. The experience of doctoral study also shapes and defines how clinicians' roles are actualized after graduation. Clinicians should understand that realizing the benefits of a DNP degree is a process that will continue to unfold years after graduation. Be assured, however, that this process is worthwhile, rewarding, and exciting. Nursing is uniquely positioned to improve health care through increased knowledge and education. As Dr. Kathleen Payson so accurately stated, "Education is power and the highway to make a difference."

SUMMARY

- Advanced practice nursing and advanced nursing practice are often used interchangeably but actually have different meanings. Advanced nursing practice describes what nurses do when they provide nursing care. Advanced practice nursing describes the whole field of specific types of nursing practice (Bryant-Lukosius, et al., 2004).
- The APRN Consensus Model defines advanced practice nursing as well as regulation for licensure, accreditation, certification, and education (LACE) of APRNs.
- Evidence-based practice (EBP) serves to promote optimal healthcare outcomes, which are based on critically reviewed clinical evidence for individual patients, families, and communities.

- Although all DNP graduates are expected to evaluate, translate, and implement EBP into their particular settings, DNP graduates in clinician roles have a vantage point of EBP due to their direct impact on care in the clinical setting.
- Barriers to EBP exist and include resistance to change, lack of preparation regarding EBP, lack of resources for EBP, lack of belief in EBP, and poor motivation to investigate EBPs.
- DNP graduates in the clinical setting, as well as other settings, can reduce barriers to EBP by defining EBP to others, providing education regarding EBP, providing consultation in researching EBP, and mentoring others regarding EBP outcomes.
- DNP graduates can evaluate and translate EBP by asking relevant questions in the clinical setting, reading literature reviews regarding pertinent topics, starting a journal club in their practice setting, communicating to others regarding EBP, and organizing educational programs to increase the knowledge of other healthcare professionals in their setting.
- Information technologies serve to manage, organize, and process health information (Zytkowski, 2003) in an effort to improve the quality of care and healthcare outcomes.
- The IOM reports in 2000, 2001, and 2003 all express an increased need for healthcare professionals to increase proficiency in information technologies to meet the complex demands of health care.
- Nursing uses information technologies to improve care, improve care delivery, and provide accurate, up-to-date information to patients. This is done through the use of PDAs, telehealth technologies, and reference librarians for consultation regarding information technology resources.
- Interprofessional collaboration is more than just getting along. DNP graduates are perfectly positioned to influence and exemplify interprofessional collaboration.
- Improved communication has been shown to be the most effective avenue to decrease barriers to interprofessional collaboration.
- DNP graduates will be looked to as mentors in health care. This involves DNP graduates in clinician roles displaying expertise, even when they may feel like novices regarding the new skills they have garnered in their DNP programs.
- Precepting students presents the ideal opportunity for DNP graduates in the clinical setting to act as mentors.
- DNP graduates may shape the future of nursing and influence the improvement of healthcare outcomes by mentoring others in the healthcare arena.

REFLECTION QUESTIONS

1. Do you think you understand the importance of evidence-based practice in nursing and in health care?
2. Do you think you evaluate and translate EBP into your nursing practice?

3. What ways can you think of to further evaluate and translate EBP into your nursing practice?
4. Do you think nursing has embraced information technologies?
5. In what ways do you think you could utilize information technologies in your nursing practice?
6. Do you think interprofessional collaboration is important to meet the demands of a complex healthcare system?
7. In what ways can you improve interprofessional collaboration in your setting?
8. Do you think you have, or have had, a mentor? If so, how can your experience with a mentor improve your ability to mentor others?
9. In what ways do you think DNP graduates in clinician roles, as well as other roles, have the opportunity to shape the future of nursing?

REFERENCES

American Association of Colleges of Nursing (AACN). (2006). *Essentials of doctoral education for advanced nursing practice.* Retrieved from http://www.aacn.nche.edu/publications/position/DNPEssentials.pdf

American Association of Critical-Care Nurses (AACN). (2005). *AACN standards for establishing and sustaining healthy work environments: A journey to excellence.* Retrieved from http://www.aacn.org:88/WD/HWE/Docs/HWEStandards.pdf

American Nurses Association (ANA). (1995). *Nursing's social policy statement.* Washington, DC: Author.

American Nurses Association (ANA). (2001). *Scope and standards of nursing informatics practice.* Washington, DC: Author.

Apker, J., Propp, K., Zabava Ford, W., & Hofmeister, N. (2006). Collaboration, credibility, compassion, and coordination: Professional nurse communication skill sets in health care team interactions. *Journal of Professional Nursing, 22*(3), 180–189.

Benner, P. (1982, March). From novice to expert. *American Journal of Nursing, 82*(3), 402–407.

Benner, P. (1984). *From novice to expert: Excellence and power in clinical nursing practice.* Menlo Park, CA: Addison-Wesley.

Brown, S. J. (1998). A framework for advanced practice nursing. *Journal of Professional Nursing, 14*(3), 157–164.

Bryant-Lukosius, D., DiCenso, A., Browne, G., & Pinelli, J. (2004). Advanced practice nursing roles: Development, implementation, and evaluation. *Nursing and Health Care Management and Policy, 48*(5), 519–529.

Carroll, K., Bradford, A., Foster, M., Cato, J., & Jones, J. (2007). An emerging giant: Nursing informatics. *Journal of Nursing Management, 38*(3), 38–42.

Consensus model for APRN regulation: Licensure, accreditation, certification & education. (2008). Retrieved from http://www.aacn.nche.edu/education-resources/APRNReport.pdf

Courtney, K., Demiris, G., & Alexander, G. (2005). Information technology: Changing nursing processes at the point-of-care. *Nursing Administration Quarterly, 29*(4), 315–322.

Cowan, M., Shapiro, M., Hays, R., Abdelmonem, A., Vazitani, S., Ward, C., et al. (2006). The effect of a multidisciplinary hospitalist/physician and advanced practice nurse collaboration on hospital costs. *Journal of Nursing Administration, 36*(2), 79–85.

Curran, C. (2003). Informatics competencies for nurse practitioners. *AACN Clinical Issues, 14*(3), 320–330.

Davies, B., & Hughes, A. M. (1995). Clarification of advanced nursing practice: Characteristics and competencies. *Clinical Nurse Specialist, 9*(3), 156–160.

Dracup, K., & Bryan-Brown, C. (2004). From novice to expert to mentor: Shaping the future. *American Journal of Critical Care, 13*(6), 448–450.

Dreyfus, S., & Dreyfus, H. (1980). *A five stage model of the mental activities involved in directed skill acquisition.* Unpublished doctoral study supported by the Air Force Office of Scientific Research, USAF (contract F49620-79-C0063), University of California, Berkeley.

Egerod, I., & Hansen, G. M. (2005). Evidence-based practice among Danish cardiac nurses: A national survey. *Journal of Advanced Practice, 51*(5), 465–473.

Evidence-based. In E. McKean (Ed.), *New Oxford American Dictionary* (2nd ed.) [Computer software]. New York: Oxford University Press.

Fink, R., Thompson, C. J., & Bonnes, D. (2005). Overcoming barriers and promoting the use of research in practice. *Journal of Nursing Administration, 35*(3), 121–129.

Gaumer, G., Koeniger-Donohue, R., Friel, C., & Sudbay, M. (2007). Use of information technology by advanced practice nurses. *Computers, Informatics, Nursing, 25*(6), 344–352.

Gerardi, D., & Fontaine, D. (2007). True collaboration: Envisioning new ways of working together. *AACN Advanced Critical Care, 18*(1), 10–14.

Gibbs, L. (2003). *Evidence-based practice for the helping professions: A practical guide with integrated multimedia.* Pacific Grove, CA: Brooks/Cole-Thompson Learning.

Goleman, D., Boyatzis, R., & McKee, A. (2002). *Primal leadership: Realizing the power of emotional intelligence.* Boston: Harvard Business School Press.

Graves, J., & Corcoran, S. (1989). The study of nursing informatics. *Image: Journal of Nursing Scholarship, 21*(4), 227–231.

Greiner, A. C., & Knebel, E. (Eds.). (2003). *Health professions education: A bridge to quality.* Washington, DC: National Academies Press.

Hallas, D., Butz, A., & Gitterman, B. (2004). Attitudes and beliefs for effective pediatric nurse practitioner and physician collaboration. *Journal of Pediatric Health Care, 18*(2), 77–86.

Hamric, A., Spross, J., & Hanson, C. (2005). *Advanced practice nursing: An integrative approach* (3rd ed.). St Louis, MO: Elsevier Saunders.

Hayes, E. (1998). Mentoring and self-efficacy for advanced practice nursing practice: A philosophical approach for nurse practitioner preceptors. *Journal of American Academy of Nurse Practitioners, 10*(2), 53–57.

Hudson, K., Duke, G., Haas, B., & Varnell, G. (2008). Navigating the evidence-based practice maze. *Journal of Nursing Management, 16*(4), 409–416.

IMIA-NI: The Nursing Informatics Special Interest Group. (1998). *Nursing informatics definition.* Retrieved from http://www.imiani.org

Institute of Medicine (IOM). (2001). *Crossing the quality chasm: A new health system for the 21st century.* Washington, DC: National Academies Press.

Jennings, B. M., & Rogers, S. (1988). Merging nursing research and practice: A case of multiple identities. *Journal of Advanced Nursing, 13*(6), 752–758.

Knaus, W., Draper, E., Wagner, D., & Zimmerman, J. (1986). An evaluation of outcome from intensive care in major medical centers. *Annals of Internal Medicine, 104*(3), 410–418.

Kohn, L. T., Corrigan, J. M., & Donaldson, M. S. (Eds.) (1999). *To err is human: Building a safer health system.* Committee on Quality of Health Care in America, Institute of Medicine. Washington, DC: National Academies Press.

McKay, C., & Crippen, L. (2008). Collaboration through clinical integration. *Nursing Administration Quarterly, 32*(2), 109–116.

McKinley, M. (2004). Mentoring matters: Creating, connecting, empowering. *AACN Clinical Issues, 15*(2), 205–214.

Melnyk, B. (2002). Strategies for overcoming barriers in implementing evidence-based practice. *Pediatric Nursing, 28*(2), 159–161.

Melnyk, B. (2005). Advanced evidence-based practice in clinical and academic settings. *Worldviews on Evidence-Based Nursing, 2*(3), 161–165.

Melnyk, B., & Fineout-Overholt, E. (2005). *Evidence-based practice in nursing and healthcare: A guide to best practice.* Philadelphia: Lippincott Williams & Wilkins.

Melnyk, B., Fineout-Overholt, E., Feinstein, N., Li, H., Small, L., Wilcox, L., et al. (2004). Nurses' perceived knowledge, beliefs, skills, and needs regarding evidence-based practice: Implications for accelerating the paradigm shift. *Worldviews on Evidence-Based Nursing, 1*(3), 185–193.

Melnyk, B., Fineout-Overholt, E., Feinstein, N., Sadler, L., & Green-Hernandez, C. (2008). Nurse practitioner educators' perceived knowledge, beliefs, and teaching strategies regarding evidence-based practice: Implications for accelerating the integration of evidence-based practice into graduate programs. *Journal of Professional Nursing, 24*(1), 7–13.

National Association of Clinical Nurse Specialists (NACNS). (2009). *Core practice doctorate clinical nurse specialist (CNS) competencies.* Retrieved from http://www.nacns.org/docs/CorePracticeDoctorate.pdf

National Organization of Nurse Practitioner Faculties (NONPF). (2006). *Practice doctorate nurse practitioner entry-level competencies.* Retrieved from http://www.nonpf.com/associations/10789/files /DNP%20NP%20competenciesApril2006.pdf

Nightingale, F. (1859). *Notes on nursing: What it is and what it is not.* London: Harrison and Sons.

Peck, A. (2005). Changing the face of standard nursing practice through telehealth and telenursing. *Nursing Administration, 29*(4), 339–343.

Pravikoff, D., Pierce, S., Tanner, A., Bakken, S., Feetham, S., Foster, R., et al. (2005). Evidence-based practice readiness study supported by academy nursing informatics expert panel. *Nursing Outlook, 53*(1), 49–50.

Robert Wood Johnson Executive Nurse Fellows Program. (2009). Retrieved from http://www.executivenurse fellows.org

Rossen, K., Bartlett, R., & Herrick, C. (2008). Interdisciplinary collaboration: The need to revisit. *Issues in Mental Health Nursing, 29*(4), 387–396.

Schmalenberg, C., Kramer, M., King, C., Krugman, M., Lund, C., Poduska, D., et al. (2005). Excellence through evidence: Securing collegial/collaboration nurse–physician relationships, part 1. *Journal of Nursing Administration, 35*(10), 450–458.

Sharp, N. (1998). From "incident to" to telehealth: New federal rules and regulations affect NPs. *Nurse Practitioner, 23*(8), 68–69.

Sheriff, K., Wallis, M., & Chaboyer, W. (2007). Nurses' attitudes to and perceptions of knowledge and skills regarding evidence-based practice. *International Journal of Nursing Practice, 13*(6), 363–369.

Shneyder, Y. (2002). Personal digital assistants (PDAs) for the nurse practitioner. *Journal of Pediatric Health Care, 16*(6), 317–320.

Sigma Theta Tau International Evidence-Based Practice Task Force. (2004). Evidence-based nursing: Rationale and resources. *Worldviews on Evidence-Based Nursing, 1*(1), 69–75.

Simpson, R. (2004). The softer side of technology: How IT helps nursing care. *Nursing Administration Quarterly, 28*(4), 302–305.

Simpson, R. (2005). From tele-ed to telehealth: The need for IT ubiquity in nursing. *Nursing Administration Quarterly, 29*(4), 344–348.

Stein-Parbury, J., & Liaschenko, J. (2007). Understanding collaboration between nurses and physicians as knowledge at work. *American Journal of Critical Care, 16*(5), 470–477.

Styles, M., & Lewis, C. (2000). Conceptualizations of advanced nursing practice. In A. Hamric, J. Spross, & C. Hanson (Eds.), *Advanced nursing practice: An integrative approach* (pp. 33–51). Philadelphia: W. B. Saunders.

Webster's concise English dictionary. (2004). New Lenark, Scotland: David Dale House.

Yeager, S. (2005). Interdisciplinary collaboration: The heart and soul of health care. *Critical Care Nursing Clinics of North America, 17*(2), 143–148.

Zytkowski, M. (2003). Nursing informatics: The key to unlocking contemporary nursing practice. *AACN Clinical Issues, 14*(3), 271–281.

CHAPTER 4

The DNP: Expectations for Theory, Research, and Scholarship

■ MORRIS A. MAGNAN ■

"Gather in your resources, rally all your faculties, marshal all your energies, focus all your capacities upon mastery of at least one field of endeavor."

—John Haggai

The words "theory," "research," and "scholarship" are inextricably linked to the notion of doctoral study. Of these three, "theory" and "research" seem to be the most troublesome for DNP hopefuls. For some reason these two words tend to stimulate affective responses ranging from ennui to mild anxiety to panic, but rarely exhilaration. Undoubtedly, some DNP hopefuls have skipped over this chapter or decided to read it last simply because the words "research" and "theory" appear in the title. It is for this group, especially, that the chapter is written. It is hoped that the information provided will serve as a resource that increases the reader's capacity to succeed in being and becoming a Doctor of Nursing Practice.

The chapter is divided into two major sections to provide information that might be helpful to DNP hopefuls: (1) during doctoral study, and (2) beyond graduation. The first major section of the chapter begins with a brief discussion of theory and highlights the importance of learning how to work with middle-range theory to guide observation and plan interventions. Then, research expectations are discussed, with particular attention given to discussing what is needed to support evidence-based practice. A section on scholarship follows, which provides detailed information about skills of scholarship that must be developed to succeed in doctoral study. In addition, the scholarship section includes information about the DNP final project: what it is, how to choose a topic, and how to choose a committee. This first major section of the chapter ends by providing tips on getting the

DNP final project published. The second major section of the chapter focuses on scholarship and research beyond graduation. This section opens with a discussion of scholarship expectations and barriers to scholarship that DNPs who work in academic or clinical service settings may encounter. The discussion then turns to mentorship and the role it might play in achieving scholarship and research goals. The chapter ends by providing some pointers on building a network of support for research and scholarship.

■ The DNP and Theory

Human beings invest a great deal of time and effort in trying to understand how the world works. When this effort is characterized by systematic, rigorous, and reproducible modes of inquiry, it is referred to as science. Scientists in a field strive to provide systematic and responsibly supported descriptions and explanations about phenomena (objects and events) in the world of human experience. The overall goal is to advance these descriptions and explanations to the level of theoretical formulations. Thus, theory is a valued product of scientific inquiry. Some authors have even taken the position that the aim of science is theory (Kerlinger, 1973) and that the aim of nursing science is to produce practice-relevant nursing theory (Jacobs & Huether, 1978). Doctoral programs in nursing prepare PhD students to develop theory for nursing practice, whereas DNP students are prepared to use theory in practice.

The complexities of doctoral-level practice require that DNP students have a broad base of knowledge gleaned from a number of sciences, not just nursing. To be adequately prepared to address current and emerging practice issues, the DNP Essentials (AACN, 2006) recommends a foundation in biology, genomics, the science of therapeutics, the psychosocial sciences, and the science of complex organizational structures. In addition, there is a clear expectation that DNP graduates will have some facility in using theory from nursing and other sciences to, for example: (1) determine the nature and significance of health-related phenomena, (2) describe strategies to ameliorate health-related phenomena, (3) address problems related to the delivery of health care, and (4) develop and evaluate new approaches to practice (AACN, 2006). The implications of these expectations seem clear: DNP graduates need to be proficient in applying theory to diverse practice situations. The application of theory to practice may extend along a number of lines, such as using relevant theories to address patient-centered clinical problems, conceptualize quality improvement initiatives, or address organizational problems related to the uptake and diffusion of well-tested, innovative approaches to clinical practice.

There are many definitions of theory. One useful definition of theory comes from Kerlinger, who defined theory as "a set of interrelated constructs (concepts), definitions, and propositions that present a systematic view of phenomena by specifying relations among variables, with the purpose of explaining and predicting the phenomena" (1973, p. 9). The utility of a theory comes from the organization it provides for (1) thinking, (2) observing, and (3) interpreting what is observed (Fawcett, 2005).

Historically, nursing theory has provided both a guide for practice and a basis for research. Nursing theory consists of concepts connected by relational statements that describe, predict, or explain phenomena that are consistent with nursing's perspective (Donaldson & Crowley, 1978). Attempts have been made to classify nursing's theoretical formulations into a hierarchy consisting of conceptual models, grand theories, and middle-range theories (Fawcett, 2005). Conceptual models often have as their purpose to communicate knowledge that is useful to the whole discipline of nursing. Grand theories are more delimited in their scope than conceptual models and tend to focus on developing one aspect of a conceptual model, such as health or self-care. In contrast, middle-range theory describes, explains, or predicts concrete and specific phenomena (Fawcett, 2005). Thus, middle-range theory, unlike grand theory, is narrower in scope, more amenable to validation through empirical testing (Lenz, Suppe, Gift, Pugh, & Milligan, 1995), and more immediately applicable to clinical practice (Fawcett, 2005; Lenz, 1998a, 1998b).

Over the last 2 decades, a burgeoning interest in middle-range theory has led to the publication of several books on middle-range theory. Some of these books provide a compendium of middle-range nursing theories, and others present middle-range theories from nursing as well as middle-range theories from other disciplines that have had some utility in addressing problems encountered in clinical practice. DNP students might want to consider adding to their library one or both of the following resources: *Middle Range Theories: Application to Nursing Research* (Peterson & Bredow, 2004); and *Handbook of Stress, Coping, and Health: Implications for Nursing Research, Theory, and Practice* (Rice, 2000). These and other compendia should be viewed as introductory, secondary sources of information about the theories discussed. If a decision is taken to use a particular middle-range theory as the conceptual framework for a scholarly project (e.g., the DNP capstone project), it is always best to access and have a thorough understanding of the theorist's original work rather than relying on interpretations of the theorist's work offered by other authors.

In a book chapter titled "Nursing Science for Nursing Practice," Donaldson (1995) discusses the importance of taking a pragmatic approach to using theory in practice. From Donaldson's perspective, the "pragmatist nurse" will use knowledge from nursing, nursing science, and other disciplines only if it has utility for achieving the desired clinical outcomes. Extending Donaldson's views to the application of middle-range theory in practice, it could be argued that middle-range theories that facilitate a straightforward approach to the conceptualization of clinical problems and patient outcomes, delineate effective interventions, and point to appropriate modes of measuring patient outcomes are likely to be more useful in addressing clinical problems encountered in doctoral-level practice than conceptual models and grand theories (Donaldson, 1995).

Nursing science can generate some, but not all, of the theory needed to inform nursing practice (Donaldson & Crowley, 1978). Therefore, introducing DNP students to middle-range theories from nursing as well as from other health-related disciplines will help them build an armamentarium of theory from which they can draw upon. Some theories (not all are middle range) that DNP students have found to be immediately applicable to problems encountered in the clinical setting can be found in **Table 4-1**.

In a very practical sense, exposing DNP students to a large number of middle-range theories may be of lesser importance than helping them acquire skills needed to apply middle-range theory to practice. The ability to apply middle-range theory to practice should be viewed as an important, learned, transferable skill. In other words, acquiring skill at applying one middle-range theory to a practice situation should transfer to the application of other middle-range theories to practice situations. To acquire this skill, DNP graduates will need to: (1) have a foundation in the language of theory (e.g., concepts, relational statements), (2) learn how to distinguish modifiable from nonmodifiable predictors and understand the meaning this has for planning theory-based interventions, and (3) understand how to interpret the research literature to determine the level of empirical support for relationships between theoretical concepts. In addition, DNP graduates need to understand thoroughly how to frame a health-related phenomenon (e.g., a clinical problem) within a theoretical perspective and then use the selected theory as a guide: (1) for theory-driven assessment, (2) to select theory-based intervention(s), and (3) to develop theoretically congruent measures for predicted outcomes.

According to the DNP Essentials, the DNP program should prepare the graduate to "develop and evaluate new practice approaches based on nursing theories and theories from other disciplines" (AACN, 2006, p. 9). The importance of having DNPs prepared to develop and evaluate theory-driven interventions cannot be overstated. In *Nursing's Social Policy Statement* (ANA, 2003), society is promised nursing interventions that are based on theoretical and evidence-based knowledge. Thus, society's confidence in the profession depends, in part, on nursing's ability to deliver on this promise. DNP graduates are functioning at the highest level of professional practice. Moreover, their education prepares them to bridge the gap between theory and practice. Therefore, DNP graduates are well positioned to help nursing fulfill its promise.

Table 4-1   **Theories DNP Students Have Found to Be Applicable to the Clinical Setting**

- The Health Belief Model (Rosenstock, 1990)
- Theory of Planned Behavior (Ajzen & Madden, 1986)
- Self-Efficacy (Bandura, 1977, 1997)
- Transtheoretical Model of Behavioral Change (Prochaska & DiClemente, 1983)
- Interaction Model of Client Health Behavior (Cox, 1982)
- Theory of Unpleasant Symptoms (Lenz, Pugh, Milligan, Gift, & Suppe, 1997)
- Uncertainty in Illness (Mishel, 1990)
- Middle-Range Theory of Empathy (Olson & Hanchett, 1997)

■ The DNP and Research

The DNP is not a research degree. The DNP Essentials (AACN, 2006) clearly states that practice-focused doctoral programs leading to the DNP place "less emphasis . . . on research methodology and statistics than is apparent in research-focused programs" (AACN, 2006, p. 3). However, it is important that DNP hopefuls understand that less emphasis on research methodology and statistics does not mean no emphasis. In fact, it is expected that DNP graduates will play a pivotal role in nursing's research enterprise, particularly at the juncture of providing leadership for evidence-based practice (AACN, 2006; Lenz, 2005). In addition, it is expected that DNP graduates will have a foundation in research sufficient to support participation in translational research, initiate practice inquiry, and collaborate effectively in knowledge-generating research (AACN, 2006).

Curriculum standards for research and statistics are not stated explicitly in the DNP Essentials document (AACN, 2006). However, the DNP Essentials does make it clear that "DNP curricula are designed so that all students attain DNP end-of-program competencies" (AACN, 2006, p. 7). The term "curriculum" can be understood broadly as all the learning that is planned and guided by a school. Designing DNP curricula and making decisions about what courses and learning activities should be included in a DNP program are the responsibility of the academic unit that offers the DNP program. Therefore, each school develops its own DNP curriculum and includes courses in research and statistics based on the faculty's understanding of what is needed to achieve competencies outlined in the DNP Essentials. A careful review of the entire DNP Essentials document suggests that a foundation in research ethics, the fundamentals of research methodology, core statistical principles, and the critical appraisal of research literature is needed to achieve some of the DNP competencies listed under Essentials I, II, IV, V, VII, and VIII and all of the DNP competencies listed under Essential III. The extent to which DNP curricula—planned learning activities—facilitate the creation of a solid foundation in research ethics, research methods, core statistical procedures, and the critical appraisal of literature will vary from school to school. Given the newness of DNP programs, there are, understandably, no data available to compare the research capabilities of DNP graduates across programs. This absence of comparative information places a greater responsibility on DNP hopefuls to shop carefully for a DNP program that will help them meet competencies that require a foundation in research. A thorough understanding of the research foundations specified or implied in the DNP Essentials document can facilitate making a wise choice. In addition, DNP hopefuls may find Magyar, Whitney, and Brown's (2006) article on the research foundations of the practice doctorate particularly helpful as they strive to understand more fully the research expectations of DNPs.

Research Capabilities for Evidence-Based Practice

In nursing, there is a general consensus that practitioners can no longer rely solely on experience, pathophysiologic rationale, or opinion-based processes to achieve high-quality, contextually relevant patient outcomes. Dramatic changes in healthcare delivery with an increased focus on containing costs while promoting patient safety and achieving high-quality outcomes have intensified the demand for evidence-based health care. Evidence-based medicine (EBM) is widely understood as "the conscientious, explicit, and judicious use of current best evidence in making decisions about the care of patients," whereas the practice of evidence-based medicine means "integrating individual clinical expertise with the best available external clinical evidence from systematic research" (Sackett, Rosenberg, Gray, Haynes, & Richardson, 1996, p. 71). Evidence-based nursing practice (EBNP) differs from EBM. In the medical model, evidence from randomized clinical trials (RCTs) is weighted more heavily than all other forms of evidence (Sackett, et al., 1996). In nursing, practitioners take into account evidence from RCTs but cast a much wider net to inform their clinical decision making by taking into account evidence from both qualitative and quantitative research, clinician expertise, the patient's clinical state, the clinical setting and circumstances, and patient values, preferences, and beliefs (DiCenso, Guyatt, & Ciliska, 2005; Melnyk & Fineout-Overholt, 2005). One useful definition describes EBNP as "the conscientious integration of best research evidence with clinical expertise and patient values and needs in the delivery of quality, cost-effective health care" (Burns & Grove, 2005, p. 736).

Essential III of the DNP Essentials (AACN, 2006) states explicitly that curricula should prepare DNP graduates to "use analytic methods to critically appraise existing literature and other evidence to determine and implement the best evidence for practice" (AACN, 2006, p. 12). In the current healthcare climate, adequate preparation in the area of evidence-based practice is likely to carry more weight with DNP prospective employers than capabilities related to participating in translational research, initiating practice inquiry, or collaborating effectively in knowledge-generating research. Moreover, research has shown that employers expect advanced practice registered nurses to be aware of the most current practice information so they can serve as a resource for others (McDiarmid, 1998; Stetler & DiMaggio, 1991). Thus, DNP hopefuls may want to pay particular attention to developing knowledge, skills, and habits of inquiry needed to build competencies for evidence-based practice.

The critical appraisal of research literature is particularly relevant to evidence-based practice. In nursing, the research literature is broadly divided into two dominant paradigms: quantitative research and qualitative research (Weaver & Olson, 2006). Quantitative research is characterized by objectivity and the use of numerical data to obtain information about the world (Burns & Grove, 2005). Qualitative research is characterized by the use of subjective, interactive approaches to describe life experiences and give meaning to them (Burns & Grove, 2005). Both approaches employ systematic modes of inquiry, and both require rigor in implementation. Criteria have been established for evaluating the rigor of quantitative and qualitative research (Burns & Grove, 2005). To critically appraise the research literature emanating from these two paradigms, DNP graduates need to know about and understand the paradigm-specific criteria used to evaluate quantitative and qualitative studies. Then, analytic methods, such as comparison, can be used to critically evaluate whether and to what extent attributes of rigor are evident within a particular study. Greater confidence can be placed in decisions to change practice patterns when evidence to support the decision comes from more rigorous studies.

Decisions about how best to prepare DNP students for evidence-based practice are the curricular concerns of schools that offer DNP programs. However, the level of competency attained at end of program and beyond will depend largely on the DNP student. The DNP student's commitment to developing learning skills for the immediate future, the ability to adapt these skills to meet the requirements of changing circumstances, and, above all, the ability and will to apply learning to action will likely play a critical role (Titmus, 1999). With respect to evidence-based practice, one learning skill that must be mastered by all DNP students is the ability to access relevant information using computer information technology (CIT). Getting connected to the right web-based resources is critical. Popular search engines, such as Google and Yahoo!, are a starting point, but learning how to navigate these search engines is no substitute for developing the skills needed to use library computer information technology (CIT) efficiently to glean information from electronic sources and bibliographic databases, such as CINAHL, ProQuest Nursing Journals, MEDLINE, PsycINFO, and others.

University students now learn how to search computerized bibliographic databases as part of their undergraduate education. Thus, library literacy is an a priori expectation for all graduate-level students. DNP hopefuls who have not yet learned how to search electronic bibliographic databases need to do so quickly. University librarians often provide traditional, face-to-face library workshops as well as online tutorials to help students become proficient in using library services and in conducting bibliographic searches. DNP students, especially those who have been away from the academic setting for some time, should think seriously about participating in these learning activities to ensure that their level of library literacy is equal to the demands of doctoral study. Although research consistently has shown that nursing students tend to use learning resources that are easily accessible and familiar to them (Barnett-Ellis & Restauri, 2006; Dee & Stanley, 2005), DNP students need to move beyond what is easy and familiar to locate the cross-disciplinary information that informs their practice and scholarship.

The DNP's involvement in evidence-based nursing practice is likely to proceed along two distinct dimensions. One dimension relates to the requirement to continuously update one's own practice. Nurturing the habit of regularly conducting keyword searches in one's area of expertise, getting linked to relevant RSS (Rich Site Summary) feeds, and serving as a sentinel reader of research in one's area of expertise are strategies DNPs can employ to ensure timely access to evidence pertinent to their areas of practice. McMaster University's Health Information Research Unit (accessible at http://plus.mcmaster.ca/np) provides access to current best evidence to support evidence-based decision making for nursing practice. To become a sentinel reviewer for McMaster University's evidence-based nursing initiative, contact them directly by e-mail at MOREebn@mcmaster.ca. A second dimension for DNP involvement in evidence-based practice has more to do with promoting and facilitating its use within healthcare organizations.

The movement toward evidence-based nursing practice within an organization is more likely to occur in organizations that value the use of knowledge and provide resources to access that knowledge (Rosswurm & Larrabee, 1999). Although evidence-based practice is rapidly becoming an expectation for nurses at all levels of practice, this expectation may be an unrealistic one. Research has shown that staff nurses tend to undervalue research, rely heavily on informal sources to inform practice-related decisions, and are poorly equipped to access and critically appraise research literature (Pavikoff, Tanner, & Pierce, 2005; Spenceley, O'Leary, Chizawsky, Ross, & Estabrooks, 2008). Moreover, staff nurses who know about evidence that supports a change in practice are not at liberty to implement practice changes that supersede institutional policies. In contrast, DNPs are well equipped for evidence-based practice. Moreover, DNPs with clinical concentrations that prepare them to work in clinical nurse specialist (CNS) and administrative roles are likely to be hired into positions of authority where they can build human capital and bring about changes in policy to promote the use of evidence-based practice within an organization.

▪ The DNP and Scholarship

Scholarship is a way of thinking and being in the world. The term "scholarship" is used to refer to the character, qualities, activities, and attainments of a scholar; a learned person (Merriam-Webster, 1993). Doctoral education in nursing, whether research or practice focused, prepares graduates for a scholarly approach to the discipline of nursing (AACN, 2006). However, it is important to recognize that scholarship is developed, not awarded. Earning the DNP or PhD degree is a noteworthy accomplishment; it is not a mark of scholarship. Ideally, the work of earning a doctoral degree as well as the exposure to and close interaction with scholars from nursing and other fields will set into motion certain habits of thought, a questioning attitude, and a disciplined approach to work that might eventually lead to the full bloom of scholarship. As budding scholars, DNP hopefuls might want to think carefully about scholarship, what it means, how it might be developed over the course of one's career, and most important, what skills of scholarship are required to succeed in doctoral study and beyond.

There is no agreed-upon definition of scholarship. However, the literature consistently points to three recurring themes: (1) breadth and depth of knowledge within a defined area, (2) innovation and creativity, and (3) exposure of the scholarly product(s) to public scrutiny and peer review (AACN, 1999; Kitson, 2006; Morahan

& Fleetwood, 2008). The American Association of Colleges of Nursing defines scholarship in nursing as:

> Those activities that systematically advance the teaching, research, and practice of nursing through rigorous inquiry that (1) is significant to the profession, (2) is creative, (3) can be documented, (4) can be replicated or elaborated, and (5) can be peer reviewed through various methods. (AACN, 1999, p. 3)

Developing one's self as a scholar takes time and dedication. Typically, it takes decades of scholarly productivity before one is recognized as a scholar in one's field. Acquiring the skills of scholarship often begins, unavoidably, during doctoral study. Kitson (2006) has identified four skills of scholarship deemed to be relevant for nursing research and practice that seem to coalesce around:

1. being able to find and understand what has gone before (literature searching, comprehension, critical appraisal, interpretation);
2. reviewing the published literature in a fair and unbiased way, accurately reflecting the state of the field, showing judgment and the ability to integrate and synthesize a diverse body of knowledge;
3. the ability to communicate ideas effectively, cogently, coherently, and concisely through the written word (using proper grammar, syntax, punctuation and spelling) and orally;
4. the ability to think logically and clearly and knowing how to present the pros and cons of an argument in a balanced way. (2006, p. 541)

The first skill listed was already discussed in this chapter under the section titled "Research Capabilities for Evidence-Based Practice." The fourth skill seems to be somewhat self-explanatory and probably learned best within the context of participating in doctoral-level seminars. The second and third skills seem worthy of some additional comments because doctoral students seem to have difficulty getting a good start on developing these skills.

Developing scholarship in the area of "reviewing the published literature in a fair and unbiased way, accurately reflecting the state of the field, showing judgment and the ability to integrate and synthesize a diverse body of work" (Kitson, 2006, p. 541) can be particularly difficult to master if the mind is not open to alternative views. In other words, the problem of introducing bias is one that novice readers must overcome when reading scholarly publications. The challenge in reading scholarly publications is to first try to understand what the author is trying to say from the author's point of view rather than disputing what the author says in an off-handed way because it does not concur with one's own point of view. A second problem that must be overcome is the problem of believing everything in print. Doctoral students may feel reluctant to dispute what is written, especially if the author has a recognized, famous name. However, it is important to recognize that doctoral faculty often assign specific readings for the very reason that the author's ideas, as presented, are indefensible. This is one way faculty help students learn how to critically appraise the literature.

In reviewing the published literature, it is important to recognize that it is reviewed one manuscript at time. Thus, learning how to read articles published in professional journals is a foundational skill that must be mastered before taking on the challenge of integrating and synthesizing a diverse body of literature. Given the vast amount of reading required of doctoral students, it would seem that some rules of engagement should be in place beyond the old standby of just "reading for ideas." One thing that must be understood is that articles published in professional journals are basically of two types, research and nonresearch, and each requires a distinct approach. **Table 4-2** lists some tips for reading nonresearch articles.

Research reports generally follow a standard format with relatively standard subheadings, such as an introduction, review of literature, methods (including sample, setting, instrumentation, measurement, etc.), results, discussion, and conclusion.

Reading research reports is not the same as critiquing research. When reading research, it helps to understand thoroughly what should be included in each major section of the research report. For example, the introduction section should identify a knowledge gap and a statement of purpose. The knowledge gap is, as it implies, an area of knowledge that is missing or only partially understood. The knowledge gap is usually identifiable by statements such as, "little is known about," or "the extent to which . . . something occurs . . . is poorly understood." The purpose statement often is identified by the words "the purpose of this study is." Also, there should be a logical relationship between the knowledge gap and the purpose such that if the purpose of the research is fulfilled, the knowledge gap will be closed or narrowed. A full discussion of the details of reading research reports is beyond the scope of this chapter. However, Macnee and McCabe (2008) have published an excellent book on research utilization that states explicitly what readers should expect to find in each section of a research report. Although the book was designed for undergraduate students, I found it to be a useful starting point when teaching DNP students how to read and interpret research reports.

Kitson (2006) notes that one skill of scholarship (the third skill previously listed) is "the ability to communicate ideas effectively, cogently, coherently, and concisely through the written word (using proper grammar, syntax, punctuation, and spelling)" (p. 541). In acquiring this skill of scholarship, smart DNP students learn quickly that academic success depends upon mastering the parenthetical elements first. Doctoral-level faculty tend to be highly critical of poor punctuation and grammar, get unnerved when referenced works are cited improperly, and some go absolutely bonkers when a reference list is incomplete or poorly punctuated. To achieve some consistency in the production of scholarly papers (which, in this case means every paper written for a class), many schools of nursing endorse following guidelines set forth in the *Publication Manual of the American Psychological Association* (APA, 2001). Every doctoral student should posses a current copy of the APA manual. Abridged and online versions of the APA manual are available but should be avoided because they often do not provide full or correct rules for referencing materials (especially electronic sources), and they are definitely not the rules being used by the faculty.

After purchasing the APA manual (or whichever style manual is endorsed by your school), it is important to learn how to work with the manual. Buying lunch for a colleague who knows the APA manual well in exchange for some APA pointers is money well spent. Trying to figure out how to use the APA manual the night before a paper is due is a recipe for disaster.

Table 4-2   Tips for Reading Nonresearch Articles

1. Read with a pen and highlighter in hand. There are some important seminal works in the nursing literature, but there are no sacred documents. Highlighting key points and writing in the margins is not sinful, and it can help with retention of information.
2. Avoid the sickness of highlighter mania. Highlight sparingly so that important ideas and key points can be found easily when the document is revisited, for example, during class discussion or when writing a literature review.
3. Inspect the article critically before reading. This critical inspection should include looking at the title and the subheadings in the body of the article. The title should give a general idea of the topic being addressed, and the subheadings should relate to the title and provide some early insight into how the author is approaching the topic or building an argument. Then, look at the credentials and affiliation of the author(s) to determine whether the author is likely to be an authoritative source of information.
4. Read the abstract. Abstracts of nonresearch articles vary in length and degree of helpfulness. Some may actually state the purpose of the article and provide a conclusion or summary statement.
5. Read the introductory paragraphs to locate the purpose or thesis of the article. The purpose will jump off the page when it is stated as "the purpose of this article is." More subtle statements of purpose might be written, such as "to more fully understand." A thesis is an argument that the author wants to challenge or defend. Theses often are prefaced by the words "but" and "however." When located, it helps to write in the margin "purpose" or "thesis" then look again at the subheadings in the article. The subheadings should provide insight and anticipation about the approach the author is taking to achieve the purpose or defend the thesis.
6. In reading the remainder of the article, use a highlighter or preferably an ink pen to number and comment on key points that relate directly to the purpose or thesis.
7. Finally, read the conclusion critically. Try to determine to what extent the author's conclusion is supported by key points made in the article. It is equally important to determine whether the conclusion goes beyond what can be supported by the key points made in the body of the article.
8. Conclude your reading by writing a brief synopsis (I put this on the front page of the article) using bullet points and sentence fragments. This final step, while tedious, should not take more than 5 minutes, and it really helps lock into memory what was read. Generally, the synopsis uses a format such as:
   - The author proposes/argues that . . . [state purpose or thesis].
   - The author's position is supported by . . . [bullet point two to three strong key points].
   - Weak and contradictory points of support include . . . [bullet point two to three points].
   - The author's conclusion is reasonable [supported by the key points] or unreasonable [goes beyond what has been reported].
   - Sometimes an additional note is added if it is immediately apparent that current work agrees or disagrees with the work of another author. In this case, I make a note, such as "compare to Smith, 2004."

Learning to communicate ideas effectively, cogently, and concisely in writing is a skill that comes with practice. However, even the most practiced and highly skilled authors ask colleagues to review their manuscripts before submitting them for publication in peer-reviewed journals. Doctoral students are well advised to follow this lead. Having a colleague, such as another doctoral student, read a scholarly paper for grammar, punctuation, APA format, clarity of thought, and conciseness before turning it in for grading can save embarrassment and grade points. The choice of colleague is important. It is best to choose a trusted colleague with writing skills that are equal to or greater than your own. A friend or family member who is unwilling to provide honest critique, including negative feedback, is never a good choice.

Some DNP students, especially those with poor writing skills, become bitter about the amount of scholarly writing required. Typically, the argument hinges on the notion that the DNP is, after all, a clinical degree and/or the faculty expectations are too high. Unfortunately, curriculum standards are not going to change to accommodate students who do not produce doctoral-level work. Fortunately, most universities have a writing center where tutors are available to help students learn how to develop their ideas and express them in writing. Students with weak writing skills but a strong commitment to completing their doctoral studies should avail themselves of these services.

One additional challenge that DNP students must learn to deal with is the experience of feeling marginalized—socially and professionally. Doctoral study is demanding and transformative. Involvement in doctoral study as well as the effort invested in acquiring the skills of scholarship will change one's habits of thought, introduce new language into one's vocabulary, and stimulate the acquisition of new behaviors. These changes inevitably find their way into the students' personal and professional lives. Family and spouses, no matter how supportive, will grow tired of hearing about what's happening at school and may become frustrated when the demands of school and scholarship seem to constantly interfere with family time. Professional colleagues may question the student's motives for pursuing the DNP. Even long-standing colleagues may choose to distance themselves when the DNP student starts to act and talk differently. As a result, the DNP student may start to feel marginalized, misunderstood, and cut off from valued sources of support at a time when support is needed most. That is the time to turn to fellow doctoral students for support. Collateral support from fellow doctoral students often is the only source of support that seems to genuinely ease the discomfort that comes from feeling marginalized and misunderstood.

The DNP Scholarly Project

Students can gain entry into a DNP program without knowing in advance what will be the focus of their final DNP project, but nobody graduates without completing a final scholarly project. Although academicians tend to agree that all students must complete a final project, there is disagreement about what it should be called. In the DNP Essentials document (AACN, 2006) it is referred to as the "final DNP project," and others refer to it as a "capstone project" (Lenz, 2005). By whatever name, DNP students need to appreciate that the final project is not just one more paper. Instead, it is a scholarly project that demonstrates synthesis of course content, including research and theory.

The focus of the final DNP project will depend, in part, on the candidate's point of entry into the doctoral program of study. Students with master's degrees already functioning as advanced practice registered nurses may choose to focus on a practice or policy issue pertinent to their area of specialization. Postbaccalaureate students will be required to complete a clinical residency. In this case, the capstone project is likely to be an end product emerging from and completed during the course of the clinical residency. It has been suggested that projects emanating from the clinical residency might focus on such things as "the development of a program of intervention, or an analysis of health care policy, or a discussion of patient care provided" (Lenz, 2005, p. 4). In the final analysis, the focus of the final project may be of lesser importance than the rigor of the project. The final project should be of sufficient rigor that it meets program requirements and warrants recognition as doctoral-level work.

Success in completing the final DNP project depends, in part, on knowing exactly what is required. Universities routinely establish guidelines for the completion of scholarly projects. Guidelines for scholarly projects may vary across academic units (e.g., psychology versus nursing) and within departments depending upon the degree being sought: bachelor's, master's, PhD, or DNP. Typically, a doctoral student handbook provides detailed information about departmental expectations regarding the final project, approvals needed to initiate and complete the project, as well as important information about style, formatting, and deadlines. DNP students need to get their hands on this important document early, study it thoroughly, and refer to it often through the course of their program.

Choosing a Topic

Choosing a topic for the final DNP project can be difficult. It is best to choose something that captures one's intellectual interests in a sustainable way. Passion for a topic seems to be important. However, do not worry if absolute passion and motivation for the topic seem to be insufficient. Passion and motivation tend to be somewhat fickle. Expect both to wax and wane then gain momentum once again as the project nears completion. Do worry if passion for the subject matter seems to be driven by strong emotions (e.g., anger, frustration) or value conflicts (e.g., social injustice) rather than intellectual curiosity. The quest for knowledge and understanding requires some degree of impartiality and scientific objectivity. The prospects of maintaining objectivity and finishing the capstone project on time are dismal if encounters with the literature, the study subjects, or the data trigger strong emotions. Although it is possible to acknowledge, clarify, and bracket strongly held feelings and beliefs to achieve an impartial, balanced view of one's subject matter, this often requires special guidance and instruction, which may not be available or sufficient. Therefore, DNP students are well advised to discuss with their chairpersons any concerns they have about their ability to maintain an objective, impartial view of their topic.

An early decision regarding the topic for the final DNP project is better than a later decision—maybe! Students who enter the DNP program with a topic in mind or latch onto a topic early in the program have the distinct advantage of using course work efficiently to enlarge and refine their understanding of the subject matter. On the other hand, there is a risk of cutting one's self off from exciting, new ideas encountered as one proceeds through the program.

Whether the choice of topic for the final project is made early or late, the student's original view of the final project, undoubtedly, will get modified along the way. Often, refinements are needed to clarify what question(s) are being raised, to set boundaries on the scope of the project, and to ensure that the data collected will yield valid and reliable information pertinent to the question(s) being asked. Typically, the student's committee will recommend modifications and refinements before the student launches the project. These recommendations often mean more work for the student, but they also mean that the committee is doing its job.

DNP students should never commit to a final project that is too large to finish within a reasonable time frame. Committee members, especially the chairperson, should help the student determine what is a reasonable time frame. In more structured settings, for example when the capstone project is completed during the course of the clinical residency, specific indicators of semester-to-semester progress are likely to be identified in advance and detailed in writing in the doctoral student handbook.

Securing approval for capstone projects that require review by an internal review board (IRB) can be a time-consuming process. IRBs and human subjects committees are known for their thoroughness, not their speed. Often, proposed projects need to be reviewed by several IRBs, for example, the university-level IRB as well as the human subjects committee of the hospital(s) or institution(s) where data will be collected. Typically, it is best to proceed in an orderly fashion by first getting approval from the university-level IRB before submitting the project proposal to a hospital or outside institution. During my own doctoral-level study, I was advised to allot one full semester (4 months) to the IRB approval process. This proved to be sound advice.

Choosing a Committee

Typically, a committee of faculty collaborators is assembled to mentor the student through the final DNP project. Bringing together the right group of people is important to the success of the project. Getting the right person to chair the committee is absolutely critical. It is nice if the chairperson of the committee likes the student. It is more important that the chairperson has, at least, a passable interest in the student's topic; better if he or she has theoretical, methodological, or content expertise; but absolutely essential that he or she knows how to get the student through the final project on time.

Students should choose their chairperson first. When the chairperson understands the nature of the student's project and agrees to chair the project, he or she can provide direction and facilitate decision making about additional areas of expertise needed to ensure a well-rounded committee. The committee should be configured so that it lends strength to the project. If, for example, the planned project focuses on conducting a depth analysis of healthcare policy related to access to health care, then at least one committee member should have expertise in the area of healthcare policy. Students need to establish and maintain productive working relationships with committee members. Similarly, committee members need to establish and maintain productive working relationships with one another. If the chairperson suggests that a certain faculty member may not be a good choice for committee membership, the wise student will accept this suggestion at face value and widen the search until a more suitable, mutually agreed upon, committee candidate is found. It is always good practice to check with the committee chairperson first before inviting someone to join the committee.

Getting the DNP Scholarly Project Published

There are many reasons to write for publication. One well-recognized reason to write for publication is to advance nursing knowledge by disseminating the results of nursing research. Other reasons include advancing professional practice and the quality of nursing care by publishing exemplars of excellence in nursing care or the results of quality improvement initiatives. In addition, reporting new and interesting observations in the literature is one way of influencing professional opinion by drawing attention to, stimulating dialogue about, and shifting perspectives on pesky clinical problems or troublesome professional issues. More personal reasons for publishing include establishing one's self as an expert within a specialized area of practice or building a portfolio of scholarship that includes publication in peer-reviewed journals, a requirement for nursing academicians living under the publish or perish edict of university tenure systems. Whatever reason motivates one to write for publication, rest assured that the work of writing will stimulate brain activity (Johnson, 2008). Good writing brings the added benefits of cultivating clear thinking, discipline, analytical ability, the emergence of logically coherent arguments, and a deep sense of accomplishment (Fahy, 2008; Johnson, 2008).

In this chapter, the DNP final project is referred to as a scholarly project. Scholarship is open to public scrutiny, debatable, adaptable, and subject to improvement. Conferences and peer-reviewed journals are the venues most commonly used to showcase one's scholarship. Disseminating findings from the DNP scholarly project at conferences and in peer-reviewed journals is a mark of good scholarship. DNP students should think seriously about using both venues to showcase their scholarly work. Presenting at professional conferences brings with it the distinct advantage of meeting and networking with professional colleagues who share similar interests. Publishing in peer-reviewed journals has the advantage of reaching a wider audience.

Getting a manuscript published in a peer-reviewed journal requires good writing, but journal choice and following author guidelines are equally important. The focus of a manuscript submitted for publication in a refereed journal must match the mission of the journal. Also, the presentation and style of the manuscript must match exactly the journal's guidelines for authors. Nothing is more aggravating for journal editors than disregard for journal format or mission or both (Froman, 2008).

By the time DNP students come to the end of their program of study, they should have a good idea about which professional peer-reviewed journals publish work similar to their own. These are the journals that should be targeted for publication. The manuscript can be submitted to only one journal at a time. It is recommended that the would-be author choose from among two or three of these journals, then review the journal mission, access the journal's author guidelines, and decide which journal seems to be most appropriate. Author guidelines should be kept close at hand throughout the production of the manuscript, but don't start writing yet! Although most journals accept unsolicited manuscripts, a query letter to the editor can be extremely beneficial because it (1) helps the editor decide whether a proposed manuscript is in keeping with the mission of the journal, (2) avoids problems of having a manuscript rejected because the journal has recently accepted a manuscript of similar content and focus, and (3) helps the author synthesize manuscript ideas within one or two short paragraphs. Well-written query letters are difficult to produce, but they are well worth the effort. A number of online resources are available to guide new writers through the do's and don'ts of crafting an effective query letter. See, for example, recommendations made by John Hewitt at http://www.poewar.com /how-to-write-a-query-letter.

Human Subjects Concerns

Federal guidelines define research as "a systematic investigation, including research development, testing and evaluation, designed to develop or contribute to generalizable knowledge" and go on to note that "some demonstration and service programs may include research activities" (National Institutes of Health, 2005, p. 6). The Belmont Report specifically states that "if there is any element of research in an activity, that activity should undergo review for protection of human subjects" (U.S. Department of Health and Human Services, 1979, p. 4). The interpretation of these guidelines continues to evolve. It has been argued, for example, that data collected outside the confines of standard practice and presented at a public meeting or in a publication should require the same IRB approval and informed consent as data collected for research purposes (Glatstein, 2001). Thus, data-based quality improvement initiatives that involve human subjects may be subjected to the same level of scrutiny as research that involves human subjects (Newhouse, Pettit, Poe, & Rocco, 2006).

DNP students who are interested in publishing the results of data-based projects that involve human subjects should anticipate that journal editors will ask them to explicitly disclose whether IRB approval was obtained. Also, journal editors will ask whether an informed investigational consent explaining, in clear language, the purpose, possible risks, and benefits of the study was signed by all participating subjects. Often this information must be included within the body of the manuscript.

Any attempt to deceive the journal on these points would be considered evidence of ethical misconduct.

Whose Work Is Getting Published?

Decisions about authorship may seem straightforward but can become complex very quickly. This is especially true when generating publications from the final DNP project. At first blush it seems reasonable to think about the capstone project as the student's work alone. However, it is important to remember that doctoral projects, whether a dissertation or final DNP project, are mentored, collaborative projects. Typically, the collaborators—faculty chairperson and committee members—provide guidance and input into the conceptualization and design of the project as well as considerable time and effort in directing/redirecting the project, facilitating interpretation of results, and editing the final report. Thus, each collaborator may have a substantial claim to some of the intellectual property reflected in the final DNP project. To avoid contention, it is wise to discuss the topic of authorship early in the development of a project (King, McGuire, Longman, & Carroll-Johnson, 1997). This discussion should address important issues such as who will be included as authors, the order of authorship, who will be acknowledged, and an agreement to revisit these points of concern as publication draws near. A final agreement on author inclusion should be stated in writing to dispel erroneous assumptions that could lead to embarrassment and erosion of professional relationships down the road (King, et al., 1997).

Relying on standards or guidelines to direct decision making about authorship is highly recommended (King, et al., 1997). A dependable and frequently cited formal statement of criteria for authorship comes from the International Committee of Medical Journal Editors (ICMJE, 2008):

> Authorship credit should be based on 1) substantial contributions to conception and design, acquisition of data, or analysis and interpretation of data; 2) drafting the article or revising it critically for important intellectual content; and 3) final approval of the version to be published. Authors should meet conditions 1, 2, and 3.

The preceding statement helps clarify what is meant by "substantial contribution." To further avoid problems of loose authorship and questions regarding order of authorship, journals routinely ask for written certification from all authors whose names appear on the byline of an article. In addition, journals increasingly require each author to specify the nature of their contribution to the published product. In some journals a brief description of the functional role of each author is appended to the end of the published piece (for example, see recent publications from the *Journal of Advanced Nursing*). In the final analysis, "all persons designated as authors should qualify for authorship, and all those who qualify should be listed" (ICMJE, 2008).

The faculty member who chairs the student's committee often will initiate discussions about authorship and help negotiate finer points, such as what constitutes a substantial contribution worthy of authorship versus minor contributions worthy of acknowledgment. However, if the chairperson does not take the lead, it is in the student's own best interest to launch the discussion. Moving to publication as sole author on a manuscript without consulting one's collaborators is bad form at best and scientific misconduct at worst, especially if the intellectual work of collaborators is presented as though it were the student's own work (Grinnell, 1997). On the other hand, DNP graduates should not naïvely weight the contributions of collaborators more heavily than their own by giving away first authorship. Students have a right to list their name as first author when they publish major findings of their final DNP project. Moreover, the American Psychological Association explicitly endorses listing the student "as principal author on any multiple-authored article that is substantially based on the student's dissertation or thesis" (APA, 2001, p. 396).

New authors may find it especially helpful to read Baggs's (2008) excellent editorial, which speaks clearly and succinctly to issues of authorship, acknowledgement, duplicate publication, self-plagiarism, and salami slicing (i.e., trying to slice too many publications out of one piece of research).

Peer Review

Peer review is one way of ensuring that what is being printed in the literature is relevant, innovative, and nonredundant. Double-blind peer review is a long-standing tradition in nursing. When double blinded, the manuscript under review moves, through the editor, from an unidentified writer to a similarly unidentified reviewer (hence, double blind) (Walker, 2004). The peer-review process can be highly politicized and may even squelch creativity. However, it is unlikely that peer-review processes will change between now and the time that current DNP students submit their manuscripts for publication, so it is probably best for students to adopt a healthy attitude toward peer review. To begin with, it helps if new authors try to think about reviewers as colleagues.

Rarely is a manuscript accepted as is, without revision. Authors may not like what reviewers say about their manuscripts, but constructive criticism from objective reviewers with relevant expertise can be used to clarify thinking and sharpen writing skills (Fahy, 2008). Therefore, recommendations for revision with resubmission should be viewed optimistically, especially if the reviewers have provided substantive feedback. Reviewer feedback almost always tells the author exactly what needs to be done to the manuscript to increase the chances of getting it published. All reviewer comments must be addressed. Addressing reviewer comments does not mean the author agrees with every critique or recommendation. It does mean that the author should provide rationale for reviewer recommendations that have not been followed. Editors do not look favorably upon authors who ignore reviewer comments (Froman, 2008). Multiple revisions and resubmissions may be needed before a manuscript is finally accepted for publication. Enduring what might seem like an overabundance of help from peer-review colleagues requires a special kind of perseverance, but don't give up! If the reviewers were not interested in seeing the manuscript in print, they would not persist in providing collegial feedback.

Dealing with Rejection

Outright rejection is a hard blow to the ego, but rejection should not lead to dejection. It is important to remember that it is the work that is being rejected, not the author. One of the leading causes for rejection of a manuscript is a mismatch between the journal's mission and the focus of the manuscript (Froman, 2008). Also, the choice of journal can influence the likelihood of rejection. Highly competitive, top-tier journals, such as *Advances in Nursing Science, Nursing Research*, and *Research in Nursing and Health*, tend to have higher rejection rates than specialty journals, such as *Clinical Nurse Specialist, Journal of Advanced Nursing, Heart & Lung*, and *Dimensions in Critical Care Nursing*.

■ Scholarship and Research Beyond Graduation

Scholarship and scholarly productivity are work-related expectations of university faculty. New DNP graduates who interview for faculty appointments at university schools of nursing need to come away from those interviews with a full understanding of the scholarship expectations of their potential employers. It is important, for example, to know what counts as scholarship, expectations regarding scholarly productivity, and the level of support provided for faculty scholarship. Historically, publication of research findings in peer-reviewed journals has been the gold standard of faculty scholarship. However, since the publication of Boyer's (1990) seminal work, *Scholarship Reconsidered: Priorities of the Professoriate*, many schools of nursing have broadened the definition of scholarship, especially as it relates to the scholarship of clinical faculty (see, for example, Jones & Van Ort, 2001). Boyer's (1990) conceptualization of scholarship includes four categories: discovery, integration, application, and teaching. The scholarship of discovery generates new and unique knowledge. The scholarship of integration refers to the synthesis of knowledge across fields. The scholarship of application focuses on using new knowledge to solve social problems. Finally, the scholarship of teaching takes into account the relationship between teaching and learning and upholds the importance of using creative approaches to bridge the gap between what the teacher knows and what the student learns.

Job security at universities as well as decisions about tenure and promotion are based upon scholarly productivity. Therefore, it is important for DNP graduates to know whether potential employers define scholarship exclusively as research publications or along a number of categories, such as those described by Boyer (1990). In university settings, expectations for scholarly productivity are typically stated in quantifiable terms; for example, one to two publications per year or two to four paper presentations at local, regional, or national professional conferences. It is important that DNP graduates who are seeking faculty appointments understand that a continuous, identifiable, year-to-year record of scholarly productivity is expected. The volume of scholarly work produced may fluctuate from year to year, but long dry spells should be avoided. Partnering with other faculty to coauthor a publication, copresent at a conference, or redesign a course can help carry new faculty members through dry spells.

Partnering often brings with it the unexpected benefits of stimulating creativity and reinvigorating interest and excitement about one's own area of scholarship.

Making time for scholarship is a huge problem. University faculty carry heavy workloads that include course preparation and evaluation, teaching, service to the school and university, as well as student advisement and counseling. Learning to make time for scholarship can be very challenging, especially for new faculty members. Often, workload documents specify that a percentage of time (for example, 10% or 20%) is allotted for faculty scholarship. However, it is up to the faculty member to protect this time. In other words, if 4 hours per week are allotted for scholarship, then a 4-hour block of time should be scheduled in one's personal calendar as time protected for scholarship. Self-discipline is required to ensure that the time protected for scholarship is, in fact, used for the intended purpose and not frittered away on other activities. Creating a protected work space for scholarship is equally important. It is difficult to be productive when one's work space is constantly invaded by phone calls and drop-in visits from faculty and students. Posting an office schedule, closing the office door, and turning the phone off are some strategies that can be used to protect the work space from these distractions.

DNP graduates who take positions in clinical service settings may find that their employers have no clearly stipulated expectations for scholarship and scholarly productivity. In these situations, the DNP needs be highly self-directed when it comes to: (1) clarifying his or her value orientations toward scholarship, (2) choosing an area(s) for scholarship that will advance the profession, (3) determining how his or her scholarship will be developed, (4) negotiating release time for scholarship, and (5) garnering recognition for scholarly productivity in annual performance evaluations. Currently, there are no widely recognized models of scholarship for clinical practice. In medicine, Morahan and Fleetwood (2008) have proposed a conceptual model of scholarship in which practice activities, such as teaching students, teaching patients, providing services, and conducting research, are linked to scholarship activities, such as teaching others how to teach students; teaching procedures to other clinicians; informing others how to design, implement, and evaluate programs; and informing others of research findings by presenting results at conferences and publishing papers. DNP graduates might use a similar strategy to conceptualize linkages between their own practice-related activities and areas of scholarship. Alternatively, DNPs who work in clinical service settings might consider adapting Boyer's (1990) four dimensions of scholarship—discovery, integration, application, and teaching—to organize their thinking about scholarship in practice. For example, advanced practice registered nurses who work at the Detroit Medical Center demonstrated the scholarship of teaching when they developed, tested, and disseminated a teaching program designed specifically for the purpose of helping staff nurses learn how to use the Braden Scale correctly to assess a patient's level of risk for developing pressure ulcers (Maklebust, et al., 2005).

Getting caught in the practice trap is a barrier to scholarship for all practitioners. DNPs will know they are caught in the practice trap if all their work time is dedicated to clinical practice. To advance the profession, it is imperative that DNPs make time in their work schedules (and time at home) for scholarship. Dialogue and up-front negotiation with potential employers may be needed to ensure adequate release time and financial support for involvement in scholarly activities. In exchange for release time and financial support, DNP employers should expect to see tangible results, such as presentations (not merely attendance) at conferences and/or publications in professional peer-reviewed journals.

Mentored Scholarship

There is an assumption in nursing that mentoring is critical to career success, especially if one chooses to develop one's self as a productive scholar after earning the doctoral degree (Morse, 2006; Roy & Linendoll, 2006). Mentors typically are defined as individuals with advanced experience and knowledge who are committed to providing support—career building and psychosocial—to less experienced, more junior individuals, who are referred to as protégés or mentees (Maas et al., 2006; Yonge, Billay, Myrick, & Luhanga, 2007). A number of mentoring models are portrayed in the literature. One model of mentoring depicts mentoring as a long-standing, dyadic relationship between a mentor and a protégé that begins during doctoral study and proceeds throughout the span of one's career. Another model of mentoring depicts mentoring as an activity orchestrated within the hierarchical structure of an organization, for example, when a senior faculty member is assigned to mentor a junior faculty member. Other, more contemporary, models suggest that mentoring may come from multiple sources and that the exchange between the mentor and the protégé emerges from what is needed at some point in time (Broome, 2003; de Janasz & Sullivan, 2004). Parse (2002), for example, speaks of mentoring moments that emerge as individuals engage in a dialogue about a scholarly project or career development. From Parse's (2002) perspective, mentoring moments are characterized by choice rather than a long-standing relationship. Accordingly, the mentor chooses to offer wise counsel for the moment and the project, whereas the protégé chooses to accept mentoring from someone who espouses value orientations similar to his or her own. Higgins (2000) has suggested that the amount and type of help provided (i.e., career versus psychosocial) can be used to conceptualize mentoring and that mentors can range from acting merely as an ally (someone who helps only if and when help is needed) to friend (someone who provides high amounts of psychosocial support) to sponsor (someone who provides high amounts of career support) to true mentor (someone who provides high amounts of both career and psychosocial support).

The literature on mentoring consistently identifies the mentor as the helper and the protégé as the one being helped; however, it has been suggested that "the best mentoring relationships include mutual benefits and positive attitudes between the mentor who enjoys guiding and supporting the protégé and the protégé who seeks to model the behaviors and achievements of the mentor" (Maas, et al., 2006, p. 184). The chairperson of the DNP student's capstone project may be the first person to take an active interest in guiding the DNP's scholarly development. The relationship between the capstone advisor and the DNP student often resembles what Higgins (2000) describes as a sponsored mentorship in which the mentor (advisor) provides a high amount of project mentoring to ensure that the protégé (doctoral student) succeeds in meeting curriculum requirements for the capstone project. Thus, the relationship between the chairperson and the doctoral student might be more appropriately understood as a time-limited, project-specific, advisor–advisee relationship. There is no way of predicting whether this type of sponsored mentorship will transition to a true mentoring relationship that extends beyond the duration of the capstone project. There is always the risk that expectations of either the mentor or protégé will not be met, especially when one considers how extensive these expectations can be. Maas et al. (2006) have noted that:

> Protégés expect mentors to be role models and to have the expertise, interest, and demeanor needed to guide and support protégés in seizing and using opportunities to develop a successful career. Mentors seek protégés who are motivated for success and leadership, and are a good match with the mentor in terms of career interests and a mutually beneficial relationship. (Maas et al., 2006, pp. 183–184)

After graduation, finding a mentor—whether a true mentor, an ally, a sponsor, or a cadre of mentors—to guide, support, and inspire the development of one's scholarship can be challenging. The DNP graduate may long for a true mentor, but until one is found it might be best to make good use of whatever qualified help is available. As Dave Thomas, the founder of Wendy's, has stated, "Instead of waiting for someone to take you under his [sic] wing, go out and find a good wing to climb under" (Phillips-Jones, 2001, p. 1). This may require learning how to network effectively in the hallways, at meetings, by e-mail, and at professional conferences.

The search for a mentor(s) and mentoring can be made easier if the DNP graduate (protégé) proactively identifies areas where mentoring is wanted and needed. This search should be guided by a clear understanding that mentoring often occurs in phases (Broome, 2003). What is needed in the early part of one's DNP career will not be equal to what is needed in the later part of one's DNP career. New DNP graduates, for example, may find that situation-specific mentoring from multiple mentors is sufficient to help them negotiate job interviews, get their scholarly project published, overcome self-doubt, redefine their professional identity, and become comfortable using their new title. Often it is within the context of engaging in mentoring moments that relationships take shape; values, ideas, and aspirations are exchanged; and the ground is made fertile for developing an enduring relationship between the mentor and the protégé.

Mentored Research

It has been established that the DNP is not a research-focused degree. Nevertheless, results from a survey of DNP students (N = 69) have shown that nearly one-third of the students surveyed anticipated being involved in research after graduation (Loomis, Willard, & Cohen, 2006). It is unclear from the survey report whether the anticipated postgraduation research involvement is limited to evidence-based practice or extends to actual involvement in knowledge-generating research. Although it is recognized that the DNP is not a research degree, no universal law prohibits DNPs from conducting knowledge-generating research. However, DNP graduates who are interested in conducting research may find it helpful to work with a PhD-prepared nurse who can bring research and statistical expertise to the project. If the DNP is interested in serving as the sole principal investigator on the project, then a research consultant or mentor might be brought on board. Research consultants and mentors can provide "advice regarding research-related questions and issues, proposal development, funding sources, and manuscript development" (Whittemore, 2007, p. 235). Typically, a consultant is paid whereas a mentor is not. Alternatively, the DNP may choose to work more collaboratively with a PhD-prepared nurse as a coinvestigator on a project. In a collaborative effort there is shared accountability for the outcome. My own experience collaborating with advanced practice registered nurses (APRNs) on research projects has been personally and professionally enriching and has led to a number of coauthored publications in peer-reviewed journals (see, for example, Magnan & Maklebust, 2008a, 2008b, 2009a, 2009b; Magnan & Reynolds, 2006; Magnan, Reynolds, & Galvin, 2005; Reynolds & Magnan, 2005). These authors identified trust as the most important feature of a collaborative relationship. The APRNs needed to trust that their important research ideas would not be stolen by the PhD-prepared nurse. In addition, it seemed to be very important to the APRNs that the PhD-prepared nurse understood nursing practice and respected the clinical expertise of the APRNs. DNP graduates might recognize from this personal account that effective, productive collaborations with a PhD-prepared nurse need to be based on trust and mutual respect.

■ Building a Network for Research and Scholarship

A network is a circuit through which things flow: ideas, energy, dialogue, information, favors, and so on. Networking involves proactive involvement in activities to develop and maintain personal and professional relationships with others for the purpose of mutual benefit in their work or career (Forret & Dougherty, 2001). Thus, one common purpose of networking is career advancement, which may extend from finding a first job to finding a new job with higher pay and status. Networking also plays an important role in building professional identity and reputation (Rojas-Guyler, Murnan, & Cottrell, 2007). The more extensive the network, the more people there are who know about your skills, initiative, areas of interest, scholarly pursuits, and reputation. Other purposes of networking include identifying and cultivating mentoring relationships and meeting research collaborators (de Janasz & Forret, 2008).

Opportunities for networking are almost limitless. Networking can be done in person, over the phone, via the Internet, and through professional organizations. Professional conferences are great venues for networking. However, it is important to use conference time wisely; planning ahead helps. Plan to attend conference symposia and breakout sessions where the topic being presented is likely to attract an audience with interests similar to your own. Little networking occurs during the actual presentation, so plan to linger afterwards to meet the presenter(s), especially if the presenter is a known expert in your area of interest. Traveling to the next session with a newly found colleague is a good way of extending your network. If you are the presenter, be prepared to graciously engage members of the audience who stay afterwards to talk about your presentation.

For networking purposes, wise use of conference time must include taking full advantage of all conference-hosted social events, especially if food is being served! Nonfood events may include guided tours of historical sites or morning walks. Food events usually include a continental breakfast, a box lunch, and, at some conferences, a posh evening event complete with chamber music, a shrimp bar, a cash bar, and several serpentine tables stacked with hors d'oeuvres and desserts. These food events provide opportunities to network in a relaxed social setting while sharing a bite to eat. The conference-hosted evening event is a must attend for all serious networkers. Often, more formal evening wear is required and, because these are usually stand-up events (no seating available), sensible shoes are a must. It is extremely difficult to work a room and network effectively if your feet are killing you. Do not carry a handbag to an evening event. The hands must be kept free to handle tiny food plates, but more important, the hands must be free to shake hands. Do take business cards but keep them in a pocket or an over-the-shoulder bag so that they are accessible but out of the way.

Networking often begins with a succinct introductory icebreaker followed by an introduction. Painfully shy people may want to rehearse responses to questions such as, "Where do you work?", "What are your areas of interest?", and "Are you working on any exciting projects?" However, learning how to lead a conversation by asking questions of others is more important to networking than reporting on one's own accomplishments (Puetz, 2007).

The biggest barrier to networking is avoiding it altogether. Introverted individuals with low self-esteem may find it especially difficult to engage in networking activities (Forret & Dougherty, 2001). However, training with opportunities for practice and feedback can help individuals increase their confidence and comfort with networking skills (de Janasz & Forret, 2008). Setting a goal to make at least two or three new contacts at a conference can help motivate one in the right direction. Other mistakes in networking include leaving business cards at home, asking others for too much too soon, failing to follow-up with new contacts, and not having clearly identified career-related goals (Agre, 2002; Puetz, 2007; Nickleston, 2008).

Building a network of support to advance scholarship and research requires some up-front self-reflection. It is important to come to terms with what you are about and what your scholarship and research interests are. The following advice seems especially relevant: "Don't follow fashion. Don't imagine that the world compels you to work on certain topics or talk a certain way. First things first: once you can explain what you care about, then you can build a community of people who also care about that. That's what networking is for" (Agre, 2002, p. 4). It is important that DNP graduates recognize that they are pioneering a new role in the profession. The frontiers for DNP scholarship and involvement in research that will advance the discipline and the profession of nursing are wide open, so find out what you really care about then gather in your resources, rally all your faculties, marshal all your energies, and focus all your capacities upon mastery in your chosen area of scholarship and research.

Summary

- The utility of a theory comes from the organization it provides for (1) thinking, (2) observing, and (3) interpreting what is observed.
- Acquire skills needed to apply middle-range theory to practice.
- A foundation in research ethics, the fundamentals of research methodology, core statistical principles, and the critical appraisal of research literature is needed to achieve some of the DNP competencies.
- DNP graduates will play a pivotal role in nursing's research enterprise, particularly at the juncture of providing leadership for evidence-based practice.
- Doctoral study provides opportunities to start developing skills of scholarship, especially skills related to reviewing the literature and writing cogently, clearly, and concisely.
- Publishing findings from the final DNP project is a mark of good scholarship. Acknowledging contributions of collaborators is a mark of ethical conduct.
- Make good use of mentors and mentoring moments to advance career, scholarship, and research goals.
- Build a network of support to advance scholarship and research goals beyond graduation.

Reflection Questions

1. Does theory add anything to daily practice? In what ways might you use theory in practice?
2. Should DNP graduates avoid engaging in research undertaken to generate new knowledge?
3. How important is it to foster a mentoring relationship(s) to advance your scholarship and/or research?
4. What qualities would you find most helpful in a mentor?
5. Do you think networking will help you grow as a scholar? If so, have you started networking with others who have similar interests?

REFERENCES

Agre, P. (2002). *Networking on the network: A guide to professional skills for PhD students.* Retrieved from http://vlsicad.ucsd.edu/Research/Advice/network.html

Ajzen, I., & Madden, T. J. (1986). Prediction of goal-directed behavior: Attitudes, intentions, and perceived behavioral control. *Journal of Experimental Social Psychology, 22*, 453–474.

American Association of Colleges of Nursing (AACN). (1999). *Defining scholarship for the discipline of nursing.* Washington, DC: Author.

American Association of Colleges of Nursing (AACN). (2006). *Essentials of doctoral education for advanced nursing practice.* Retrieved from www.aacn.nche.edu/publications/position/DNPEssentials.pdf

American Nurses Association (ANA). (2003). *Nursing's social policy statement* (2nd ed.). Silver Spring, MD: Author.

American Psychological Association. (2001). *Publication manual of the American Psychological Association* (5th ed.). Washington, DC: Author.

Baggs, J. G. (2008). Issues and rules for authors concerning authorship versus acknowledgements, dual publication, self plagiarism, and salami publishing. *Research in Nursing & Health, 31*(4), 295–297.

Bandura, A. (1977). Self-efficacy: Toward a unifying theory of behavioral change. *Psychological Review, 84*(2), 191–215.

Bandura, A. (1997). *Self-efficacy: The exercise of control.* New York: W. H. Freeman.

Barnett-Ellis, P., & Restauri, S. (2006). Nursing student library usage patterns in online courses: Findings and recommendations. *Internet Reference Services Quarterly, 11*(4), 117–138.

Boyer, E. L. (1990). *Scholarship reconsidered: Priorities of the professoriate.* Princeton, NJ: Carnegie Foundation for the Advancement of Teaching.

Broome, M. E. (2003). Mentoring: To everything a season. *Nursing Outlook, 51*(6), 249–250.

Burns, N., & Grove, S. K. (2005). *The practice of nursing research: Conduct, critique, and utilization* (5th ed.). St. Louis, MO: Elsevier Saunders.

Cox, C. L. (1982). An interaction model of client health behavior: Theoretical prescription for nursing. *Advances in Nursing Science, 5*(1), 41–56.

Dee, C., & Stanley, E. E. (2005). Information-seeking behavior of nursing students and clinical nurses: Implications for health sciences librarians. *Journal of Medical Librarians Association, 93*(2), 213–222.

de Janasz, S. C., & Forret, M. L. (2008). Learning the art of networking: A critical skill for enhancing social capital and career success. *Journal of Management Education, 32*(5), 629–650.

de Janasz, S. C., & Sullivan, S. E. (2004). Multiple mentoring in academe: Developing the professorial network. *Journal of Vocational Behavior, 64*(2), 263–283.

DiCenso, A., Guyatt, G., & Ciliska, D. (2005). *Evidence-based nursing: A guide to clinical practice.* St. Louis, MO: Elsevier Mosby.

Donaldson, S. K. (1995). Nursing science for nursing practice. In A. Omery, C. E. Kasper, & G. G. Page (Eds.), *In search of nursing science* (pp. 3–12). Thousand Oaks, CA: Sage.

Donaldson, S. K., & Crowley, D. M. (1978). The discipline of nursing. *Nursing Outlook, 26*(2), 113–120.

Fahy, K. (2008). Writing for publication: The basics. *Women and Birth, 21*(2), 86–91.

Fawcett, J. (2005). *Contemporary nursing knowledge: Analysis and evaluation of nursing models and theories.* Philadelphia: F. A. Davis.

Forret, M. L., & Dougherty, T. W. (2001). Correlates of networking behavior for managerial and professional employees. *Group & Organizational Management, 26*(3), 283–311.

Froman, R. D. (2008). Hitting the bull's eye rather than shooting yourself between the eyes. *Research in Nursing & Health, 31*(5), 399–401.

Glatstein, E. (2001). What is research? *International Journal of Radiation Oncology, Biology, & Physics, 5*(2), 288–290.

Grinnell, F. (1997). Truth, fairness, and the definition of scientific misconduct. *Journal of Laboratory and Clinical Medicine, 129*(2), 189–192.

Higgins, M. (2000). The more, the merrier? Multiple developmental relationships and work satisfaction. *Journal of Management Development, 19*(4), 277–296.

International Committee of Medical Journal Editors (ICMJE). (2008). *Uniform requirements for manuscripts submitted to biomedical journals: Writing and editing for biomedical publications.* Retrieved from http://www.icmje.org/index.html

Jacobs, M. K., & Huether, S. E. (1978). Nursing science: The theory-practice linkage. *Advances in Nursing Science, 1*(1), 63–73.

Johnson, T. M. (2008). Tips on how to write a paper. *Journal of the American Academy of Dermatology, 59*(6), 1064–1069.

Jones, E. G., & Van Ort, S. (2001). Facilitating scholarship among clinical faculty. *Journal of Professional Nursing, 17*(3), 141–146.

Kerlinger, F. N. (1973). *Foundations of behavioral research* (2nd ed.). New York: Holt, Rinehart, & Winston.

King, C. R., McGuire, D., Longman, A., & Carroll-Johnson, R. M. (1997). Peer review, authorship, ethics, and conflict of interest. *Image, 29*(2), 163–167.

Kitson, A. (2006). The relevance of scholarship for nursing research and practice. *Journal of Advanced Nursing, 55*(5), 541–545. [Reprinted from Kitson, A. (1999). The relevance of scholarship for nursing research and practice. *Journal of Advanced Nursing, 29*(4), 773–775.]

Lenz, E. R. (1998a). The role of middle-range theory for nursing research and practice: Part 1. Nursing research. *Nursing Leadership Forum, 3*(1), 24–33.

Lenz, E. R. (1998b). The role of middle-range theory for nursing research and practice: Part 2. Nursing practice. *Nursing Leadership Forum, 3*(2), 62–66.

Lenz, E. R. (2005). The practice doctorate in nursing: An idea whose time has come. *Online Journal of Issues in Nursing, 10*(3), Manuscript 1. Retrieved from www.nursingworld.org/MainMenuCategories/ANAMarketplace/ANAPeriodicals/OJIN/TableofContents/Volume102005/No3Sept05.aspx

Lenz, E. R., Pugh, L. C., Milligan, R. A., Gift, A., & Suppe, F. (1997). The middle-range theory of unpleasant symptoms: An update. *Advances in Nursing Science, 19*(3), 14–27.

Lenz, E. R., Suppe, F., Gift, A. G., Pugh, L. C., & Milligan, R. A. (1995). Collaborative development of middle-range theory: Toward a theory of unpleasant symptoms. *Advances in Nursing Science, 17*(3), 1–13.

Loomis, J. A., Willard, B., & Cohen, J. (2006, December). Difficult professional choices: Deciding between the PhD and DNP in nursing. *OJIN: The Online Journal of Issues in Nursing, 12.* Retrieved from http://www.doctorsofnursingpractice.org/UserFiles/File/Loomis2006.pdf

Maas, M. L., Strumpf, N. E., Beck, C., Jennings, D., Messecar, D., & Swanson, E. (2006). Mentoring geriatric nurse scientists, educators, clinicians, and leaders in the John A. Hartford Foundation Centers for Geriatric Nursing Excellence. *Nursing Outlook, 54*(4), 183–188.

Macnee, C. L., & McCabe, S. (2008). *Understanding nursing research: Using research in evidence-based practice* (2nd ed.). Philadelphia: Lippincott Williams & Wilkins.

Magnan, M. A., & Maklebust, J. (2008a). The effect of web-based Braden Scale training on the reliability and precision of Braden Scale pressure ulcer risk assessments. *Journal of Wound, Ostomy and Continence Nursing, 35*(2), 199–208.

Magnan, M. A., & Maklebust, J. (2008b). Multi-site web-based training in use of the Braden Scale for predicting pressure sore risk. *Advances in Skin & Wound Care, 21*(3), 124–133.

Magnan, M. A., & Maklebust, J. (2009a). The effect of web-based Braden Scale training on the reliability of Braden subscale ratings. *Journal of Wound, Ostomy and Continence Nursing, 36*(1), 51–59.

Magnan, M. A., & Maklebust, J. (2009b). The nursing process and pressure ulcer prevention: Making the connection. *Advances in Skin & Wound Care, 22*(2), 83–92.

Magnan, M. A., & Reynolds, K. E. (2006). Barriers to addressing sexuality across five areas of specialization. *Clinical Nurse Specialist, 20*(6), 285–292.

Magnan, M. A., Reynolds, K., & Galvin, L. (2005). Barriers to addressing patient sexuality in nursing practice. *Medical-Surgical Nursing, 14*(5), 282–289.

Magyar, D., Whitney, J. D., & Brown, M. A. (2006). Advancing practice inquiry: Research foundations of the practice doctorate in nursing. *Nursing Outlook, 54*(3), 139–151.

Maklebust, J., Sieggreen, M. Y., Sidor, D., Gerlach, M. A., Bauer, C., & Anderson, C. (2005). Computer-based testing of the Braden Scale for predicting pressure sore risk. *Ostomy Wound Management, 51*(4), 40–42, 44, 46.

McDiarmid, S. (1998). Continuing nursing education: What resources do bedside nurses use? *Journal of Continuing Education in Nursing, 29*(6), 267–273.

Melnyk, B., & Fineout-Overholt, E. (2005). *Evidence-based practice in nursing and healthcare: A guide to best practice*. Philadelphia: Lippincott Williams & Wilkins.

Merriam-Webster's collegiate dictionary (10th ed.). (1993). Springfield, MA: Merriam-Webster.

Mishel, M. H. (1990). Reconceptualization of the Uncertainty in Illness theory. *Image: Journal of Nursing Scholarship, 22*(4), 256–262.

Morahan, P. S., & Fleetwood, J. (2008). The double helix of activity and scholarship: Building a medical education career with limited resources. *Medical Education, 42*(1), 34–44.

Morse, J. M. (2006). Deconstructing the mantra of mentorship in conversation with Phyllis Noerager Stern. *Health Care for Women International, 27*(6), 548–558.

National Institute of Health (NIH). (2005). *45 CFR Part 46 § 46.102 definitions*. Retrieved from http ://ohsr.od.nih.gov/guidelines/45cfr46.html

Newhouse, R. P., Pettit, J. C., Poe, S., & Rocco, L. (2006). The slippery slope: Differentiating between quality improvement and research. *Journal of Nursing Administration, 36*(4), 211–219.

Nickleston, P. (2008, April). 7 networking mistakes to avoid. *Dynamic Chiropractic, 29*(19). Retrieved from http://www.dynamicchiropractic.com/mpacms/dc/article.php?id=53149

Olson, J., & Hanchett, E. (1997). Nurse-expressed empathy, patient outcomes, and development of a middle-range theory. *Image: Journal of Nursing Scholarship, 29*(1), 71–76.

Parse, R. R. (2002). Mentoring moments. *Nursing Science Quarterly, 15*(2), 97.

Pavikoff, D., Tanner, A., & Pierce, S. T. (2005). Readiness of U.S. nurses for evidence-baed practice: Many don't understand or value research and have had little or no training to help them find evidence on which to base their practice. *American Journal of Nursing, 105*(9), 40–51.

Peterson, S. J., & Bredow, T. S. (2004). *Middle range theories: Application to nursing research*. Philadelphia: Lippincott Williams & Wilkins.

Phillips-Jones, L. (2001). *The new mentors and protégés: How to succeed with the new mentoring partnerships*. Grass Valley, CA: Coalition of Counseling Centers.

Prochaska, J. O., & DiClemente, C. C. (1983). Stages and processes of self-change of smoking: Toward an integrative model of change. *Journal of Consulting and Clinical Psychology, 51*(3), 390–395.

Puetz, B. E. (2007). Networking. *Public Health Nursing, 24*(6), 577–579.

Reynolds, K., & Magnan, M. A. (2005). Nurses' attitudes and beliefs toward human sexuality: Collaborative research promoting evidence-based practice. *Clinical Nurse Specialist, 19*(5), 255–260.

Rice, V. H. (2000). *Handbook of stress, coping, and health: Implications for nursing research, theory, and practice*. Thousand Oaks, CA: Sage.

Rojas-Guyler, L., Murnan, J., & Cottrell, R. R. (2007). Networking for career-long success: A powerful strategy for health education professionals. *Health Promotion Practice, 8*(3), 229–233. Retrieved from http://hpp.sagepub.com/cgi/content/abstract/8/3/229

Rosenstock, I. M. (1990). The health belief model: Explaining health behavior through expectancies. In K. Glanz, F. M. Lewis, & B. K. Rimer (Eds.), *Health behavior and health education: Theory research and practice* (pp. 39–62). San Francisco: Jossey-Bass.

Rosswurm, M., & Larrabee, J. (1999). A model for change to evidence-based practice. *Image: Journal of Nursing Scholarship, 31*(4), 317–322.

Roy, C., & Linendoll, N. M. (2006). Deriving international consensus on mentorship in doctoral education. *Journal of Research in Nursing, 11*(4), 345–353.

Sackett, D., Rosenberg, W., Gray, J., Haynes, R., & Richardson, W. (1996). Evidence based medicine: What it is and what it isn't. *British Medical Journal, 312*(7023), 71–72.

Spenceley, S. M., O'Leary, K. A., Chizawsky, L. L., Ross, A. J., & Estabrooks, C. A. (2008). Sources of information used by nurses to inform practice: An integrative review. *International Journal of Nursing Studies, 45*(6), 954–970.

Stetler, C. B., & DiMaggio, G. (1991). Research utilization among clinical nurse specialists. *Clinical Nurse Specialist, 5*(3), 151–155.

Titmus, C. (1999). Concepts and practices of education and adult education: Obstacles to lifelong learning. *International Journal of Lifelong Education, 18*(5), 343–354.

U.S. Department of Health and Human Services (DHHS). (1979). *The Belmont Report.* Retrieved from http://www.hhs.gov/ohrp/humansubjects/guidance/belmont.html

Walker, K. (2004). 'Double b(l)ind': Peer-review and the politics of scholarship. *Nursing Philosophy, 5*(2), 135–146.

Weaver, K., & Olson, J. K. (2006). Understanding paradigms used for nursing research. *Journal of Advanced Nursing, 53*(11), 459–469.

Whittemore, R. (2007). Top 10 tips for beginning a program of research. *Research in Nursing & Health, 30*(3), 235–237.

Yonge, O., Billay, D., Myrick, F., & Luhanga, F. (2007). Preceptorship and mentorship: Not merely a matter of semantics. *International Journal of Nursing Education Scholarship, 4*(1), Article 19. Retrieved from http://www.bepress.com/ijnes/vol4/iss1/art19

CHAPTER 5

DNP Involvement in Healthcare Policy and Advocacy

■ MARLENE H. MULLIN ■

"I am not discouraged, because every wrong attempt discarded is another step forward."

—Thomas Edison (1847–1931)

Our nation currently faces many challenges. In 2010, 48.6 million Americans of all ages (16%) were uninsured at the time of the National Health Interview Survey (NHIS) conducted by the Centers for Disease Control and Prevention's (CDC) National Center for Health Statistics (NCHS) (2011). According to the U.S. Department of Housing and Urban Development (HUD), an estimated 649,879 persons are homeless at any given night in the United States, with 109,920 being chronically homeless (U.S. Department of Housing and Urban Development, 2010). Disparities in health care, education, food distribution, and housing demand the attention of the DNP graduate.

Although the enormity of these problems may seem daunting and may cast doubts on how one can make a difference, DNP graduates possess the tools to make changes in our society. Knowledge and education are powerful instruments; DNP graduates possess both. DNP graduates also possess practical experience, leadership skills, and knowledge regarding research and evidence-based practice, which allows them to be powerful advocates for healthcare policies. Utilizing the gifts of knowledge, education, practice experience, leadership skills, and research to their full potential for the betterment of society is a challenge that all DNPs must undertake. Due to our nation's many challenges, it is imperative that DNP graduates become involved in shaping healthcare policy and promoting advocacy. DNP graduates are prepared to meet these challenges.

Nursing's Social Policy Statement (ANA, 1995) clearly states the nursing profession's commitment to society and the people who are served. Nursing's relationship with society is "based on an ethic of trust and the principle of justice" (Ballou, 2000, p. 178). Involvement in healthcare policy and advocacy that addresses issues of social justice and equity in health care are vital roles that all DNP graduates must assume to fulfill our responsibility to society (AACN, 2006).

It is also important for DNP graduates to remember that political decisions and social policy initiatives have an impact on the practice of nursing. DNP graduates need to attain a place at the table where policy decisions are made to have a say in the policies that govern nursing. DNP graduates are prepared to assume a leadership role in influencing and shaping policies that affect nursing practice.

This chapter provides a brief overview of the history of nursing's involvement in healthcare policy and advocacy. Specific strategies for becoming informed and involved in healthcare policy and advocacy are outlined. Two interviews with advanced practice registered nurses (APRNs) who have been active in healthcare policy and advocacy for many years are provided. The first interview is with Jeanette Wrona Klemczak, Michigan's Chief Nurse Executive. The second interview is with Nancy M. George, Assistant Director of the DNP Program and Assistant Professor of Nursing at Wayne State University College of Nursing. Dr. George is also President-Elect of the Michigan Council of Nurse Practitioners (MICNP) and Chairperson of the Michigan APRN Coalition. Finally, the chapter provides a specific case scenario that illustrates a DNP graduate's involvement in healthcare policy and advocacy.

■ Curriculum Standards

Essential V of the *Essentials of Doctoral Education for Advanced Nursing Practice* (AACN, 2006) provides specific curriculum standards for the DNP graduate related to healthcare policy and advocacy under the title Healthcare Policy for Advocacy in Health Care. Essential V states that DNP programs prepare graduates for the following activities related to healthcare policy and advocacy:

> DNP graduates are prepared to design, influence, and implement healthcare policies that frame health care financing, practice regulation, access, safety, quality and efficacy (IOM, 2001). Moreover, the DNP graduate is able to design, implement, and advocate for healthcare policy that addresses issues of social justice and equity in health care. The powerful practice experiences of the DNP graduate can become potent influencers in policy formation. Additionally, the DNP graduate integrates these practice experiences with two additional skill sets: the ability to analyze the policy process and the ability to engage in politically competent action. (O'Grady, 2004)

The DNP graduate has the capacity to engage proactively in the development and implementation of health policy at all levels, including institutional, local, state, regional, federal, and international levels. DNP graduates, as leaders in the practice arena, provide a critical interface between practice, research, and policy. Preparing graduates with the essential competencies to assume a leadership role in the development of health policy requires that students have opportunities to contrast the major contextual factors and policy triggers that influence health policy making at the various levels.

The DNP program prepares the graduate to:

1. Critically analyze health policy proposals, health policies, and related issues from the perspective of consumers, nursing, other health professions, and other stakeholders in policy and public forums.
2. Demonstrate leadership in the development and implementation of institutional, local, state, federal, and/or international health policy.
3. Influence policy makers through active participation on committees, boards, or task forces at the institutional, local, state, regional, national, and/or international levels to improve healthcare delivery and outcomes.
4. Educate others, including policy makers at all levels, regarding nursing, health policy, and patient care outcomes.
5. Advocate for the nursing profession within the policy and healthcare communities.
6. Develop, evaluate, and provide leadership for healthcare policy that shapes healthcare financing, regulation, and delivery.
7. Advocate for social justice, equity, and ethical policies within all healthcare arenas. (AACN, 2006, pp. 13–14)

▪ Historical Perspective

The modern nursing movement was started by Florence Nightingale in 1860 when she opened the first nurse training program at St. Thomas Hospital in England (Lewenson, 2007). "This landmark event signaled to the world that nurses required schooling for the work they did" (Lewenson, 2007, p. 23). Nightingale's concept that nurses should be trained, supervised, and managed by nurses themselves was a model adopted by many nurse training programs during this period. She believed that nursing and medicine should be separate disciplines. Most important, Nightingale believed nursing should organize and control itself. Nightingale's ambitious letter writing to influential people enabled her to obtain support for changes in health care and nursing education. She ultimately was able to garner support worldwide for her visionary ideas about sanitation, nursing education, and the separation of nursing from medicine.

In the United States, the modern nursing movement began with the opening of many Nightingale-influenced nurse training schools in 1873 (Lewenson, 2007). This also signaled the changing role of women in society. The nursing profession provided one of the first opportunities for women to work outside the home and financially support themselves. However, due to the fact that nursing's roots were in the church and military, patriarchal control existed (Lewenson, 2007). To overcome this issue, political action was necessary by nurses, as well as women in general, to obtain control over their education, work, and lives.

Between 1873 and 1893, many more nurse training schools opened, with the number rising to more than 1,129 by 1910 (Burgess, 1928). During this time, nursing was not regulated by any professional nursing group, which resulted in significant misuse of nurses. In fact, physicians and pharmacists controlled much of nursing practice, particularly in the private duty sector (Lewenson, 2007). Ultimately, this mistreatment and lack of control and regulation were the impetus for early nursing leaders to form professional nursing organizations (Lewenson, 2007).

The first professional nursing organizations were formed between 1893 and 1912. Although these organizations were originally formed to address the misuse and lack of representation for nurses, members ultimately became involved in social and political reforms that affected health issues in society. The first professional nursing organizations included what are now known as the National League for Nursing (NLN) and the American Nurses Association (ANA). The NLN originated in 1893, and its goal was to bring "uniformity in nursing curricula and standards of nursing practice" (Lewenson, 2007, p. 24). Nursing leaders of the NLN favored and encouraged collective action, which demonstrated the political and progressive nature of this group.

Nurse training programs nationally were encouraged to form alumnae associations to bring nurses together at the state level and ultimately at the national level (Lewenson, 2007). The ANA originally was an organization developed to unite the various alumnae groups that had been formed by nurse training programs across the country. All alumnae associations were encouraged to be involved in political action and social reform. Sophia Palmer, founding editor of the *American Journal of Nursing* (AJN), was one of the nursing leaders who spearheaded this effort. Palmer used the AJN, which was first published in 1900, to stimulate discussion among nurses about policy and political issues. The AJN also encouraged collective action on the part of nurses to influence legislation that affected the profession as well as the health of the public (Lewenson, 2007). The publication of the AJN was an important early political strategy undertaken by the ANA and the NLN to increase communication among nurses. Of interest, the AJN was originally funded by members of these two organizations (Lewenson, 2007).

One very important issue that was addressed by members of the ANA and discussed in the AJN was the registering of nurses. Significant political action and organization among nurses were taken to obtain recognition of nursing as a profession. The first state nurse registration act was passed in 1903, originally in the states of North Carolina, New York, New Jersey, and Virginia. This resulted in protecting the title "nurse" by law (Lewenson, 2007). Other states soon undertook registering nurses also.

During this time frame, the Spanish–American War erupted. Nurse leaders attempted to control which nurses were chosen to serve in the war. They were unsuccessful in their efforts against Anita Newcomb McGee, a physician and socialite from Washington. Much to the dismay of nursing leaders, McGee ultimately served as the leader and therefore chose which nurses served in the war. It was believed by many nursing leaders that this unfortunate outcome had occurred due to a lack of formal organization of nurses. Lessons were learned from this incident, and the need for political action to control and organize nursing was recognized more than ever (Lewenson, 2007).

Subsequently, two other nursing organizations were developed: the National Association of Colored Graduate Nurses (NACGN) and the National Organization for Public Health Nursing (NOPHN). NACGN arose out of the fact that African-American nurses were initially barred from membership in the ANA as a result of discrimination. NACGN was organized in 1908. Its focus included issues of discrimination, education, standards of practice, and nursing registration (Lewenson, 2007).

The nursing leaders of the ANA and the NLN formed the National Organization of Public Health Nursing (NOPHN) in 1912 to address substandard nursing practices in public health nursing. Public health nursing needs significantly increased in the beginning of the 20th century due to the overwhelming public health problems that occurred in the United States as a result of urbanization, industrialization, and immigration (Lewenson, 2007). NOPHN leaders recognized the importance of forming coalitions with other healthcare professionals as well as lay people to form a larger political base to advocate for changes to improve the health of the public (Lewenson, 2007).

The formation and organization of formal nursing organizations led to the involvement of nurses in other political issues, such as the campaign for suffrage. It was recognized that the ability to vote would enable nurses to have a voice in the laws that regulated practice, education, and health (Lewenson, 2007). Letters from the National American Woman Suffrage Association that requested support and articles about suffrage were published in the AJN. Initially, nurses were hesitant to participate in the suffrage movement due to fear that it would negatively influence efforts to obtain state nursing registration. In fact, at the 11th annual ANA convention in 1908, members opposed a resolution for the organization to support suffrage (Lewenson, 2007). Four years later, nursing leaders were successful in obtaining support from the nursing profession for women's suffrage. Political action to support women's suffrage was continued by the nursing profession until the 19th Amendment, which gave women the right to vote, was passed in the summer of 1920.

Finally, no history of nursing's involvement in political activities would be complete without mentioning two significant nurses who had an impact on public healthcare policy during this early period of the nursing profession. Lillian Wald and her colleague Mary Brewster opened the Henry Street Nurses' Settlement in 1893 in New York City. This was, in essence, the first nurse-run clinic in the United States (Fitzpatrick, 1975). Wald and her staff lived in this community and provided nursing care, health education, social services, and cultural experiences to clients who were seen in the clinic. The clinic gained world recognition for its success in addressing public health issues (Lewenson, 2007). Utilizing her knowledge and political savvy, Wald was able to influence and make many changes that affected the health of the residents and their community. She was influential in establishing the first park in New York City, which promoted children playing in a safe environment rather than the streets (Lewenson, 2007). Wald is also credited with advocating for the first school nurse after noting that many children missed school due to medical problems. Although the board of health initially hired a physician to examine the children, Wald ultimately was successful in convincing them to hire a public health nurse as well. Wald considered these nurses to be the first school nurses in the world. They were hired in 1902, and amazingly, their salary was $30,000 (Lewenson, 2007).

Another nurse, Margaret Sanger, revolutionized healthcare practice as a result of her political activism. Sanger led the struggle for legalizing birth control in the early 20th century. Sanger, a visiting nurse, was passionate that women should have control over their own bodies, specifically their reproductive functions. She was very politically savvy and sought support not only from nursing but from other organized groups of women, labor organizers, and philosophers (Lewenson, 2007). She met government resistance when she attempted to publish information about health issues such as syphilis. Sanger ultimately fled the United States in 1914 after being criminally convicted of writing an article that supported women separating procreation from the sexual act (Lewenson, 2007). She returned to the United States in 1915 following the death of her daughter. Ultimately, the government dropped the charges against Sanger due to public pressure. Sanger's efforts to provide birth control and health information to mothers continued when she opened a clinic in 1916 in New York City. Once again her efforts were met with resistance and she again faced arrest, prosecution, and imprisonment. Although Sanger was not successful, her efforts ultimately resulted in changes in the interpretation of the law, which influenced the founding of the Planned Parenthood organization (Lewenson, 2007).

Nursing's rich and fruitful political activism history in the 19th and early 20th century did not continue in the mid-20th century when the feminist movement began in the United States. Initially, nursing's involvement in this movement was basically nonexistent (Chinn & Wheeler, 1985). Although nursing was a female-dominated profession, nurses failed to become actively involved in the fight for equal rights for women until the 1970s. Two notable nursing leaders, Wilma Scott Heide and JoAnn Ashley, led the profession in recognizing the value of the feminist movement for the nursing profession. It became obvious to nurses that it was imperative to become involved in political activities that addressed the inequalities faced by women overall. It was also clear that nursing needed to assume a leadership role to promote changes in health care for the betterment of society. Nursing's support for the feminism movement was fully realized when the ANA supported the Equal Rights Amendment in the early 1970s (Lewenson, 2007). Two other pivotal events also occurred during this time. The National Organization for Women (NOW) was organized, and the Nurses Coalition for Action in Politics was established. The Nurses Coalition for Action in Politics was the first political action committee (PAC) for the nursing profession (Lewenson, 2007).

Although the political activities of nursing have continued from the late 20th century to the present, they have not been as vigorous as those of early nursing leaders. "Too often nurses are not included in policy decisions, not involved in policy making, or just not recognized at all" (Gordon, 1997 as cited in Lewenson, 2007, p. 31). It is obvious that much work is still needed by nursing to realize its full potential of influencing health care through health policy. Lewenson (2007) states that "nurses will learn that their extensive knowledge base and experience lend themselves to political activism" (p. 31). Early nursing leaders, such as Florence Nightingale, used the professional education of nurses to facilitate their political activism. Nursing has this opportunity once more with the advent of the Doctor of Nursing Practice (DNP) degree.

Involvement in political activities has always been an integral part of the role of nursing. Due to their expanded scopes of practice, it has been necessary for nurses to be involved in such issues as expanding nurse practice acts and obtaining third-party reimbursement and prescriptive authority. The shortage of physicians in primary care and medical residents in many areas has increased the demand and need for expanded roles in nursing. For this reason, more than ever, nurses need to be involved in political activities.

Of concern, the majority of political activities by nurses have focused on areas that expand and promote their practice (Oden, Price, Alteneder, Boardley, & Ubokudom, 2000). Given the dominance of medicine, this is not surprising; nevertheless, nursing involvement in health policy and advocacy to benefit the general population is imperative. DNP graduates are well prepared, as a result of their education and experience, for involvement in healthcare policy and advocacy. DNP graduates can serve as leaders in influencing and shaping healthcare policies and advocating for healthcare issues. In addition, DNP graduates can influence and shape policies that influence the practice of nursing.

The next section of this chapter discusses avenues for becoming informed and involved in political activities. Whether the DNP graduate chooses only to be knowledgeable about current political issues or chooses to run for a public office, some level of involvement is vital. DNP graduates are in the unique position to influence the future of health care through an array of positions and activities. It is also important to recognize that political activism may contribute to the long-term success and viability of DNP graduates in the healthcare arena.

■ Tips for Becoming Informed and Involved

Although the ideal method for learning to be politically savvy is through mentoring, role modeling, and practice, there are many catalysts for becoming informed and involved in politics. Due to our nation's current healthcare environment, there are a multitude of causes and issues that demand the attention of DNP graduates. It is the responsibility of all DNP graduates to become informed and involved to influence and shape healthcare policies as well as advocate for patients and the nursing profession.

A good way to get started is to first determine your areas of interest; find something you care about or find something new to care about. Next, determine the amount of time and energy you have to devote to political activism. Finally, be passionate and get started by being informed and involved!

Sources of Information

There exist many outstanding sources for obtaining information in our technologically advanced society. In addition to written materials, the Internet provides a wealth of information regarding healthcare policy and advocacy issues. Multimedia resources such as television and radio also are good sources for obtaining information. More in-depth information may be obtained through actual courses and continuing education offerings.

Professional Journals

Many professional nursing journals contain policy and political updates. Other sources for this information include medical journals and other healthcare professional journals. The names of nursing journals that frequently contain policy and political information may be found in **Table 5-1**.

Internet

The Internet provides endless access to information regarding public policies, health policies, government information, academic information, and government officials. In addition, many nursing associations provide specific information for nurses through the Internet. For example, the American Nurses Association website offers the *Online Journal of Issues in Nursing* (OJIN), and the National League for Nursing's website has a section titled Governmental Affairs.

Table 5-1 **Health Policy- and Advocacy-Related Journals**

- *American Journal of Nursing*, since 1900, has provided editorials, articles, and commentaries on political issues that affect nursing (monthly).
- *Journal of Professional Nursing*, the official journal of the AACN, provides information on public policy (bimonthly).
- *Nursing Economic$* provides a "Capitol Commentary," which examines current healthcare policy issues (bimonthly).
- *Journal of Nursing Scholarship*, the official publication of Sigma Theta Tau International Honor Society of Nursing, provides articles regarding health policy and systems (quarterly).
- *Policy, Politics & Nursing Practice* provides information regarding legislation that affects nursing practice, case studies in policy and political action, interviews with policy makers and policy experts, and articles on trends and issues (quarterly).
- Other journals with articles regarding health policy, health law, and ethics include *Yale Journal of Health Policy, Law, and Ethics*; *Journal of the American Medical Association*; *The New England Journal of Medicine*; *American Journal of Public Health*; *American Political Science Review*; *Health Affairs*; *Health Services Research*; *Journal of Health Politics, Policy and Law*; and *Journal of Public Health Policy*.

To start a search, there are several terms that are helpful for locating information on the Internet. These terms include administration, economics, law, management, policy, and statistics preceded by the terms health or medical. The utilization of these terms usually results in the successful location of health policy data. Tips for narrowing the search include enclosing the terms in quotation marks and utilizing conjunctions (i.e., and, or, and not). The use of a website's internal search engine is also highly recommended to refine the search. In addition, Google frequently provides an excellent beginning search and a vast array of information.

Table 5-2 lists several excellent websites for initiating a search. Take a moment to explore these websites for learning purposes as well as volunteer activities. Frequently, information regarding the advocacy and legislative programs for associations is available through their websites.

Textbooks

Several excellent textbooks are available for DNP graduates to increase their knowledge regarding politics and healthcare policy. The textbooks listed in **Table 5-3**

Table 5-2   Health Policy- and Advocacy-Related Websites

- Government-related websites:
  U.S. Department of Health and Human Services: http://aspe.hhs.gov/sp/nhii/faq.html
  World Health Organization: http://www.who.int/en
  GPO Access: http://www.access.gpo.gov
- Legislative websites:
  U.S. Legislation & Votes: http://clerk.house.gov/legislative/legvotes.aspx
  U.S. House of Representatives: http://www.house.gov
  U.S. Senate: http://www.senate.gov
- Academic websites:
  Duke Center for Health Policy, Law and Management (U.S. Health Policy Gateway):
      http://ushealthpolicygateway.wordpress.com
  National Health Policy Forum: http://www.nhpf.org
  Edmund S. Muskie School of Public Service, Cutler Institute for Health and Social Policy:
      http://muskie.usm.maine.edu/cutler
- Professional nursing association websites:
  American Nurses Association: http://nursingworld.org
  American Association of Colleges of Nursing: http://www.aacn.nche.edu
  National League for Nursing: http://www.nln.org
- Specialty association websites:
  American Association of Critical-Care Nurses: www.aacn.org
  American Academy of Nurse Practitioners: http://www.aanp.org
- Health professional association websites:
  National Multiple Sclerosis Society: http://www.nationalmssociety.org/government-affairs-
      and-advocacy/index.aspx
  American Heart Association: http://www.americanheart.org
  American Cancer Society: http://www.cancer.org

Table 5-3   Health Policy- and Advocacy-Related Textbooks

- Bodenheimer, T. S., & Grumbach, K. (2005). *Understanding health policy: A clinical approach* (4th ed.). New York: McGraw Hill.
  Provides a good overview of the basic principles of healthcare policy and how the healthcare system works.
- DeLaney, A. (2002). *Politics for dummies* (2nd ed.). New York: John Wiley & Sons.
  Good book for review of politics for both novices as well as those who are familiar with the political arena.
- Mason, D. J., Leavitt, J. K., & Chaffee, M. W. (2007). *Policy & politics in nursing and health care* (5th ed.). St. Louis, MO: Elsevier Saunders.
  Excellent textbook that provides a vast amount of information regarding nursing's history and progress in policy and politics.
- MoveOn. (2004). *MoveOn's 50 ways to love your country: How to find your political voice and become a catalyst for change.* Novato, CA: New World Library.
  Excellent resource for DNP graduates who want to make changes but don't know how.
- Weissert, C., & Weissert, W. (2006). *Governing health: The politics of health policy* (3rd ed.). Baltimore: The Johns Hopkins University Press.
  Provides an excellent review of the politics of healthcare policy making.

provide a start for the DNP graduate to become more informed and politically savvy, and **Table 5-4** provides a list of some multimedia resources.

Courses and Continuing Education

Many nursing associations offer courses specifically regarding healthcare policy and legislative issues. For example, the American College of Nurse Practitioners offers a "Policy Institute" every 2 years. For more information, go to their website at http ://www.acnpweb.org. Check national, state, and specialty nursing organization websites for information regarding healthcare policy meetings and conferences. For DNPs who are interested in a more in-depth program, the Robert Wood Johnson Foundation (RWJF) offers a Health Policy Fellowship Program. This yearlong fellowship

Table 5-4   Other Multimedia Resources

- Newspapers are a good source of information regarding international, national, state, and local politics as well as public policy issues. Two examples of newspapers that provide a significant amount of information on health policy issues include *The Wall Street Journal* (http://www.wsj.com) and *The New York Times* (http://www.nytimes.com).
- Network and cable television programs are a good source of information regarding political activities and public policy. C-SPAN and CNN are two networks that provide a vast amount of political information. C-SPAN broadcasts live government events. CNN has the talk show *Anderson Cooper 360°*, which provides political updates.
- National Public Radio (NPR) and C-SPAN radio are both excellent sources for public and political issues. DNP graduates can also listen to these radio stations through the Internet. NPR's website is at http://www.npr.org, and C-SPAN's website is at http://www.c-span.org. Many talk shows that address political issues are also available on radio.

brings health professionals to Washington, DC to experience an immersion in national health policy, primarily through working assignments in Congress (Michnich, 2007). For more information regarding the Robert Wood Johnson Health Policy Fellowship Program, go to their website at http://www.healthpolicyfellows.org.

Avenues for DNP Involvement in Healthcare Policy and Advocacy

Many outstanding opportunities exist for the DNP to be involved in shaping healthcare policy and advocating for patients. Membership and involvement in professional nursing organizations is an excellent source for initial involvement. The DNP graduate may also choose to use the workplace environment as well as educational and research-based endeavors to become involved in healthcare policy and advocacy. Some DNP graduates may choose to become more actively involved by seeking election for a public office.

Professional Nursing Organizations

Membership and participation in national, state, local, and specialty professional nursing organizations are critical for DNP graduates. Unity is vital for nurses if they wish to be successful in addressing problems in health care as well as in the nursing profession. Membership in these organizations provides nurses with a voice when healthcare issues are being discussed and changes are being proposed at all levels in healthcare policies. These associations also frequently provide legislative and public policy updates to members via newsletters or the Internet.

"Many professional nursing associations offer opportunities for volunteer services that lead to rich educational, mentoring and networking experiences" (Leavitt, Chaffee, & Vance, 2007, p. 42). DNP graduates who are members of the ANA may volunteer to participate in the Nurses Strategic Action Team (N-STAT) or the American Nurses Association Political Action Committee (ANA-PAC). N-STAT members act by being alerted by the ANA about critical healthcare issues and personally contacting their members of Congress as well as writing letters to them (Leavitt, et al., 2007). The ANA-PAC, which is the one of the top healthcare PACs in the United States, speaks for all 2.7 million registered nurses (Malone & Chaffee, 2007). The ANA-PAC is involved in direct and grassroots lobbying as well as "endorsing and supporting those candidates who have a record of supporting ANA policy interests or who have expressed positions that are consistent with ANA policy interests" (ANA, 2008). In addition, the ANA-PAC makes monetary contributions to candidates. PACs also exist in specialty, state, and local nursing professional associations. Their activities are similar to those of national associations. Many opportunities exist for involvement by DNP graduates in the political arms of these associations. "ANA-PAC is committed to increasing the number of RNs in public office at every level of government" (Malone & Chaffee, 2007, p. 772). The leadership skills and knowledge of DNP graduates make them excellent candidates for public offices. Visibility by involvement in these activities is vital for DNP graduates. Again, all it takes is interest, time, and energy!

Please see **Table 5-5** for ideas for how to become involved in professional nursing organizations and how to contact and communicate with legislators.

Table 5-5 Ideas for Involvement in Professional Nursing Organizations

- Support your national, state, specialty, and local nursing professional associations by joining them as a member.
- Be visible by attending association meetings.
- Volunteer to be on a PAC or other committees, task forces, or boards that are involved in healthcare policy, advocacy, or nursing practice issues.
- Volunteer to join a coalition.
- Volunteer to campaign for PAC-endorsed candidates.
- Offer to contact and write letters or e-mails to political officials regarding issues that influence healthcare policies and nursing practice and promote patient advocacy. Traditional letters and e-mails are highly effective tools to let public officials know what you think. To find the postal or e-mail address or phone number of your lawmaker, go to the websites for the Senate and the House of Representatives:
  - Senate: http://www.senate.yourstate.gov
  - House: http://www.house.yourstate.gov
- Speak with legislators and policy makers. As citizens of the United States, we have access to policy makers like no place else in the world. Tips for speaking effectively with politicians may be found on the websites of many of the professional nursing associations. In addition, when speaking to politicians, be sure to explain and promote the role of the DNP because many of them are not familiar with this new degree in nursing.
- Some general rules for writing, e-mailing, or speaking with your legislators include keeping your tone positive, being brief, staying focused on the subject, identifying the issue or specific bill being discussed, and, finally, presenting your position and giving sound rationale.

Workplace Involvement

The leadership skills of DNP graduates make them highly qualified for influencing and facilitating changes in the workplace environment. DNP graduates can serve as advocates to change and improve the policies and procedures that affect patients as well as nursing practice in their places of employment. DNP graduates can also serve as catalysts to implement new policies based on their vast knowledge and understanding of research and evidence-based practices. **Table 5-6** lists some examples of how DNPs can become involved in the workplace.

Involvement Through Education

The role of the DNP in education goes beyond the academic setting. One of the key methods to being a patient advocate is to develop and provide evidence-based, culturally relevant, and culturally sensitive patient education material. With our culturally

Table 5-6 Examples of Workplace Involvement

- Serve in leadership positions on policy and procedure committees.
- Serve in leadership positions on other committees or task forces that affect patient care and nursing practice.
- Serve in leadership positions when the workplace is undergoing reviews from accrediting agencies (e.g., The Joint Commission).
- Serve in leadership positions when the workplace is seeking Magnet status.
- Serve as a role model and mentor to staff members when changes are being implemented.

diversified nation, this is more important than ever. This is also one method to assist in correcting disparities in health care. Health promotion and advocacy through patient education continues to be a major focus for nursing as reflected in *Nursing's Social Policy Statement* (ANA, 1995). DNP graduates, as a result of their education and clinical expertise, are highly qualified to serve as leaders in developing and disseminating patient education material. There is also a multitude of ways for DNPs to be patient advocates through educational endeavors that involve public speaking and writing. Use your writing and speaking engagements for health promotion and advocacy for patients and families and to educate the public about DNP graduates and nursing. Please refer to **Table 5-7** for some examples of how to become involved through education.

Involvement Through Research

Diers and Price (2007) state that "research may be a tool to carve policy, if it is in the right hands and is carefully sharpened and skillfully applied" (p. 195). DNP graduates are knowledgeable regarding research and evidence-based practice. This knowledge can be applied to influence and initiate public, social, and health policies as well as advocate for patients. DNP graduates possess the knowledge to use research and evidence-based practices to influence the decision making of policy makers. In addition, DNP graduates may choose to be involved in research studies that influence organizational, health, and social policies. *Nursing's Social Policy Statement* (ANA, 1995) serves as a guide for nursing research efforts related to healthcare policy and advocacy. There is a wealth of opportunities for DNP graduates to use research to shape health and social policy and promote advocacy. Please refer to **Table 5-8** for examples of involvement through research.

Other Avenues for Involvement

Nursing is one of the most trusted professions in our nation (Feldman & Lewenson, 2000). DNP graduates can capitalize on this trust by becoming involved in many other

Table 5-7   Examples of Involvement Through Education

- Design education programs for staff members and other healthcare professionals.
- Serve as a leader in developing evidence-based, culturally relevant, and culturally sensitive patient education material.
- Serve as a leader in staff and patient education committees at the workplace.
- Facilitate evidence-based journal clubs that address cultural issues and health promotion, as well as other topics that promote quality patient care.
- Facilitate staff education programs regarding different methods of learning.
- Serve as a role model and mentor to staff regarding patient education.
- Facilitate patient support groups that are culturally relevant and culturally sensitive in your area of specialization.
- Seek opportunities to provide health education to the public via interviews on television and/ or radio shows. Share your expertise!
- Volunteer to write health articles for your local newspapers. Newspaper editors are always looking for experts to write articles regarding health topics!
- Volunteer to speak at support group meetings (e.g., cancer and MS support groups) regarding health topics. Support groups are always looking for speakers, particularly nurses, to provide health information to their participants.

Table 5-8   **Examples of Involvement Through Research**

- Present research to support policy and procedure changes in the workplace.
- Present research to initiate or support health or social policy initiatives at the local, state, or national level.
- Conduct research on topics that will advocate for patients and influence health and social policies. Publishing the research in a refereed journal is vital to increase the credibility of the study as well as disseminate the results to others.
- Facilitate evidence-based journal clubs for staff to promote evidence-based practice.
- Serve on institutional review boards (IRBs) to support nursing research and advocate for patients.

---

political activities to advocate for patients and shape health and social policies. As stated earlier, "ANA-PAC is committed to increasing the number of RNs in public offices at every level of government" (Malone & Chaffee, 2007, p. 772). The leadership skills and knowledge of DNP graduates make them excellent candidates for public offices, where they can gain visibility to educate politicians and the public regarding this new role and degree in nursing. To get started, first become familiar with the public policy and health policy issues that are currently under consideration at all levels of the government. Pay specific attention to the issues of interest at the desired level of involvement. Remember, all it takes to become involved is interest, time, and energy! **Table 5-9** provides some ideas for becoming involved through other avenues.

Table 5-9   **Examples of Other Avenues for Involvement**

- Vote! Exercise your right to vote on issues that promote advocacy and affect healthcare policies. Be aware of issues and vote in elections at all levels—local, state, and national.
- Volunteer to be on a local, state, or national committee, board, or task force. It is not necessary to be only on health-related committees. Consider other areas of interest for involvement.
- Familiarize yourself with the elected officials that represent you at all levels of government. Communicate with them. Educate them about DNP graduates. Share your expertise and perspectives regarding healthcare and nursing issues. Write letters that indicate your viewpoint and desired outcomes. See Table 5-5 (Items 6–8) for information about how to contact, write, and speak with your legislators.
- Volunteer to campaign for those elected officials who are supportive to health and nursing issues.
- Choose a political party affiliation. This is essential to obtain support for a political appointment.
- Seek opportunities for appointments. Most nurse and specialty associations offer appointment information. Another source for information is the League of Women Voters.
- Contact elected and appointed leaders, such as the governor and chief nurse executive, regarding involvement with task forces, boards, committees, and opportunities for appointments.
- Seek election for an office. To start, consider running for a local office, such as becoming a member of the school board or city council.
- Volunteer to be interviewed for newspapers, journals, and television and radio broadcasts regarding advocacy and health policy issues. Also, use these opportunities to promote and educate the public about DNP graduates and nursing.
- Respond to editorials and articles published in newspapers and journals regarding advocacy, healthcare policy, and nursing practice issues.

Interviews with Nurse Policy Makers and Advocates

Interview with Jeanette Wrona Klemczak

Jeanette Wrona Klemczak, RN, BSN, MSN is the first Chief Nurse Executive for the State of Michigan in Lansing. She was appointed to this position in 2002 by Governor Jennifer Granholm. She received her BSN from Madonna University and her MSN from Wayne State University. She has been active in politics, healthcare policy, and advocacy for many years. Ms. Klemczak played a key role in establishing funding for the first DNP program in Michigan at Oakland University in Rochester, Michigan. Ms. Klemczak was interviewed for this chapter to share her experience and expertise.

Ms. Klemczak, please describe your background and current position.

My background has been in psychiatric nursing as a clinical specialist in child and adolescent mental health. I have practiced as a staff nurse, nursing supervisor and administrator, public health administrator, founding director of a faculty clinical practice, and nursing professor. I am currently serving as Michigan's first Chief Nurse Executive, appointed in 2002 by Michigan's Governor, Jennifer Granholm. My charge from her is to serve as the focus for addressing Michigan's nursing shortage and to advise the governor on ways in which nurses can further impact the health of Michigan residents. The governor's vision for this position is to address nursing and healthcare issues through policy and legislation. We believe that institutionalizing change requires action and intervention in these arenas.

The key work of the Office of the Chief Nurse Executive is [to] engage the Michigan nursing community and healthcare stakeholders in the development of a strategic plan to address the needs of our nursing workforce. This plan was completed in collaboration with the Coalition of Michigan Organizations of Nursing (COMON) and serves as the blueprint for all of the healthcare community.

Ms. Klemczak, please describe specifically how you became involved in health and social policy activities.

I believe that advocacy is the core of our profession. My current role is part of a journey that began as a staff nurse at Detroit Receiving Hospital. As a staff nurse in pediatrics, I was struck at the lack of play activities and materials. We were able to work with the chief of pediatrics and hospital administration to institute a play therapy program. This was an impetus to pursue graduate work in child and adolescent mental health. I later returned to the hospital as a psychiatric clinical specialist in pediatrics.

This early experience working with Detroit's most vulnerable populations shaped the rest of my nursing career and commitment to social justice and advocacy.

It was my contact with Carol Franck, then executive director of the Michigan Nurses Association (MNA), that created the learning and experiences in more formal advocacy and policy work. Carol encouraged me to become an active member of the association. This included serving as a board member and then serving on the Political Action Committee (PAC) as a member and then chairperson. PAC work was informed by education about lobbying and allocation of the $100,000 for support of state legislative candidates. This education was provided by the lobbyists hired by MNA—Tom Hoisington and Becky Beckler of Public Affairs Associates. I was provided with opportunities to represent nursing and meet key state legislators at their fundraising events. We established interview surveys to determine candidates' positions on issues of importance to nurses and determined who received PAC funds and how much was offered. We were able to generously support nurses who were legislators or running for elected office. The MNA-PAC was the second largest health PAC in the state and had a seat at the table and a voice that was heard.

At Michigan State University College of Nursing, my dean, Dr. Marilyn Rothert, seized the opportunity to manage the Michigan Health Policy Forum at MSU. This forum invites key policy leaders to our state to discuss current healthcare issues and help educate and inform legislators, policy makers, and health professions educators. Dean Rothert appointed me as director of the forum. This provided collaboration with the two medical schools at MSU and partnership with Michigan healthcare organizations. In turn, I became a member of a group of states who also had policy forums under sponsorship with the Robert Wood Johnson Foundation. This was [an] opportunity to work at the national level on health policy issues with the National Health Policy Forum in Washington, DC.

Ms. Klemczak, please describe specific health and social policies you have initiated, influenced, etc.

In 2005 and 2006, I initiated work on legislation that facilitated the licensure of foreign-educated nurses wanting to practice in Michigan and legislation that created a new category of nursing licensure for nurses coming to Michigan from any state. These two pieces of legislation passed the legislative bodies and were signed by the governor in less than 1 year. This is record time for most legislation.

In 2007, at the governor's request, I created the Michigan Nursing Corps (MNC), a program to rapidly prepare nursing faculty at the master's and doctoral level. The white paper that shaped the MNC was entitled "The Bottleneck Proposal." The MNC was the centerpiece of the governor's 2007 State of the State message. She included funding for the MNC in her 2008 budget message to the legislature. I provided significant testimony for the House and Senate Appropriations Committees. In 2008, the MNC received $1.5 million. This was the year that the State of Michigan closed for 4 hours at the end of the budget year because there were not sufficient funds. It is a testimony to the bipartisan commitment of Michigan's legislators who still managed to find funding for this important nursing program.

In 2008, the legislature again stepped up, following my testimony, and appropriated $5 million for the MNC. I believe that educating our legislators is one of my most important priorities.

The House Health Policy Committee requested a briefing on the MI Strategic Plan for the Nursing Shortage. I provided that briefing and answered dozens of questions. They subsequently convened [a] special subcommittee to identify legislative actions to address the nursing shortage.

As chief nurse for Michigan's Children's Special Health Care Needs program, I was able to institute programs and policies to support home care of medically fragile children and respite services for parents and families.

At the Michigan Department of Public Health, I had the opportunity to work with legislative staff to develop the Michigan State Loan Repayment Program for health professions. My role was to assure that advanced practice registered nurses were included in the eligible professional groups for educational loan repayment. The first loan repayments were for nurse practitioners.

Ms. Klemczak, what do you view as the role of the nursing profession in advocacy and influencing and shaping health and social policies?

As I mentioned earlier, advocacy is the core of our profession. We are advocates beginning with the first patient we care for as a nursing student. One advocates for generic medications as a patient confides that she will not be able to afford to fill the fistful of prescriptions the physician has just left with the discharge orders. A nurse advocates for all the patients and the nurses on a unit that is dangerously understaffed. We are advocates when we work in a community to pass laws to prohibit smoking in restaurants. We are advocates when we work for child safety seats in our states. We are advocates when we vote for candidates that are committed to access to health care for all.

I believe one of the most effective vehicles for advocacy is the professional nursing organization. In Michigan, we have over 40 such organizations. I encourage every nurse and every nursing student to select one and become active in any way possible.

Ms. Klemczak, what do you view as the role of the DNP in advocacy and influencing and shaping health and social policies?

I believe the role of the DNP stems from unique knowledge and skills. The DNP is a new degree and is not yet known and understood by legislators and policy makers, as well as the nursing community at large. So, one of the first roles is to be able to articulate the DNP and what it brings to the dialogue. DNPs will need to develop an elevator message for their many advocacy audiences—that is, they must be able to describe what they can offer in the time it takes to ride an elevator five or six floors! DNPs can offer a framework for addressing healthcare issues using their knowledge of healthcare financing and economics along with their real-time experience with patients, families, and communities. A very effective strategy is to frame an issue using return on investment methods. For example, with the Michigan Nursing Corps, we were able to tell legislators that for every $1 they invested, the nurses educated and out in practice in their communities would return $1000 in economic benefit at the state and local levels.

Ms. Klemczak, what activities do you recommend for DNPs to become involved in to influence and shape health and social policies?

Again, one is most effective in the collective. DNPs can advocate for access to health care through several state professional organizations. There are also statewide coalitions for insurance initiatives, such as Michigan Health Insurance Access Advisory Council (MHIAC). DNPs can provide testimony at hearings for specific legislation by offering data, evidence/research, and anecdotal experiences.

DNPs can approach legislators and policy makers (such as the director of the Michigan Department of Community Health) to introduce needed policies and programs. Michigan is very involved in redesigning primary care. There are advisory groups and committees where DNPs can provide expertise. It is critical to stay informed and in the know so that when task forces and other advisory groups (such as the Patient Safety Commission) are formed, DNPs will have a place at the table.

Ms. Klemczak, how do you foresee DNPs having an impact on the future of health care through their role in advocacy and health and social policy activities?

DNPs will be uniquely positioned at a unique time and circumstance in our nation's healthcare environment. We have a new administration in Washington led by President Barack Obama. Both political parties know that there must be change in our healthcare policies and delivery systems. However, most change will take place at the state and local level. Michigan will rapidly approach the federal government for a Medicaid waiver to enable over 500,000 currently uninsured individuals to have healthcare coverage. At the same time, we are facing severe shortages of primary care physicians. DNPs, along with other nursing colleagues, are prepared to offer solutions that are initiated at the health policy tables.

It is important to have nurses, especially DNPs, in elected office. Nurses and physicians are almost automatically assigned to health policy committees in the Michigan House and Senate. These are incredible opportunities for shaping health and social policy. The road to such an elected office may begin as a local school board member, county commissioner, or even the library board. The state political party leadership is very interested in recruiting and grooming potential candidates. DNPs should consider the political party of their choice and become involved in the county party group as a beginning step.

Interview with Dr. Nancy M. George

Nancy M. George, PhD, FNP-BC is Assistant Director of the DNP Program and Assistant Professor of Nursing at Wayne State University College of Nursing. Dr. George is also President-Elect of the Michigan Council of Nurse Practitioners and Chairperson of the Michigan APRN Coalition. She received her BS from Michigan Technological University in Biological Sciences, Diploma in Nursing from Bronson School of Nursing, and MSN and PhD from the University of Michigan. Her interest in policy was nurtured in her nurse practitioner and doctoral studies.

Dr. George, please describe specifically how you became involved in health and social policy activities.

My interest in policy and politics began in a bipartisan household with political discussions over the dinner table. My mother ran for township clerk as a Democrat in a Republican-dominated township. My mother demonstrated that it is always important to be involved in the policy process and stay true to your beliefs. She instilled in me the importance of voting and staying informed about the decisions that are being made for me at the local, state, and national level. When I was in the Peace Corps in Kenya, I learned firsthand the importance of a free and elected government and the impact it can have on the people. I believe that these activities influenced my thinking when it comes to nursing and nurse practitioner practice environments. I had several influential nurse practitioner mentors when I was new in my career who got me involved with our state nursing organization. That was the start of being involved and staying involved in the health and social policy issues that impact nursing.

Dr. George, please describe specific health and social policies you have initiated, influenced, etc.

I have been involved in the past two attempts to get nurse practitioners (NPs) prescriptive authority in Michigan. I helped draft language, attended hearings, and met with legislators. In our last attempt, I testified regarding the educational preparation of NPs regarding pharmacological education. In our current attempt to gain autonomous plenary authority, I have been on the APRN Coalition as we started to draft not only prescriptive authority language but also to bring the statutes in Michigan in line with APRN Consensus Model language supported by the National Council of State Boards of Nursing (NCSBN) and many other professional organizations. I currently am the Chairperson of the APRN Coalition as we continue to move forward the agenda of the two bills (HB 4774 and SB 481) that were introduced to the Michigan House of Representatives and Senate this summer. I work tirelessly to bring the APRN groups (NPs, CNSs, CNMs) together as we move forward. Our main charges have been to have a consistent message, show a united front, and work hard to bring Michigan regulatory environment into the 21st century. These duties include producing brochures and pamphlets with my APRN colleagues and meeting with legislators, regulators, and other influential health groups in Michigan. While these activities have, I believe, had the most direct impact on policy, my role as a nurse educator has had a significant impact on future and current NPs. I believe if I can influence five students who were not previously active in the policies that impact their profession then I have succeeded in assisting my chosen profession.

Dr. George, what do you view as the role of the nursing profession in advocacy and influencing and shaping health and social policies?

I think that nursing gets a reputation of not being politically active but I think our history tells a different story. Nurses have always been politically active . . . we only have to look at the work of Florence Nightingale, Lavinia Dock, Margaret Sanger, Dorothea Dix, and many others to see the influence that nursing has had on health and health policy. I believe that there are many of us that continue to work on the health issues that impact our patients/clients on a daily basis. Some of us are more visible in our activities. If you believe that part of nursing's role is to advocate for patients/clients then how can we not view being active in health policy as a piece of the advocacy. Good health policy allows for good patient care. So nurses need to be involved, even if that means that only activity is voting in every election. We need a strong nursing voice in health policy for the patients and we can't have that if we don't have nurses interested and involved in health policy.

Dr. George, what activities do you recommend for DNPs to become involved in to influence and shape health and social policies?

The first activity is to be informed. Use your talents of understanding and disseminating complex information to inform and shape health policy. Use your passion for nursing and the people that we care for to direct you to the health and social policies that you could influence. Policy is the penultimate way to roll all the skills you have learned or are learning as a DNP into an action plan. Taking the advocacy for patients to the next level and making a difference on a broader scale is vital. So the real question is where do I start . . . join your professional organizations. Find out what needs these organization have; there is usually more work than can be completed by a few individuals. Work on policy or political campaigns. Many NPs/CNSs/CNMs are working on the passage of HB 4774/SB 481, including meeting with legislators, some of them for the first time, so don't be afraid to step into an area in which you are unfamiliar. Think about running for office. There are too few nurses in the legislature and individuals with little health and nursing knowledge are making decisions that impact your lives. Think about becoming influential providers in the systems you work in . . . ever thought of being Chief Nursing Officer or Chief Executive Officer? As the health arena changes, DNPs can be at the forefront of new systems. . . . nurse owned and run hospitals? Be involved, because if you aren't driving the bus someone else will and you will just be along for the ride.

Dr. George, what do you view as the role of the DNP in advocacy and influencing and shaping health and social policies?

DNPs have the ultimate skills in being the movers and shakers of health and social policy. DNPs have the educational background that prepares them for making a difference. Skills in communication, research, clinical practice, and leadership are geared to prepare the leaders for the future of nursing and advanced practice nursing. As DNPs you will have the skills necessary to make some of the changes that need to be made. The advent of the IOM report on the *Future of Nursing* and many other reports have put APRNs in the forefront of health care. DNPs should have read these documents and could use them to support the need for change in our healthcare system that will improve the outcomes for all.

Dr. George, how do you foresee DNPs impacting the future of health care through their role in advocacy and health and social policy activities?

I believe that as more DNPs are in the clinical arena using research to make the needed evidence-based clinical changes, they will become leaders of the emerging new healthcare system. As the DNP numbers increase, there will be more individuals with the credentials, communication skills, and knowledge to be leaders in advocating for changes to the health and social systems that impact so many Americans. Further, legislators, policy makers, and regulators will have nursing professionals who can provide accurate evidence-based information regarding the quality outcomes of health care that are so needed to improve our health system. Perhaps most important is that with increased policy activity many of these DNPs will actually decide to run for office. The horizons are bright for the DNP who becomes active in the policy arena.

■ Case Scenario: DNP Involvement in Healthcare Policy and Advocacy

Dr. K. is a 2007 DNP graduate who is employed as an adult nurse practitioner specializing in the care of cardiac surgery patients at a large teaching hospital. Additionally, Dr. K. has a special interest in homelessness. For the past several years, Dr. K. has volunteered at a local shelter once per week each month. The shelter where she volunteers is a nonprofit program that focuses on providing shelter, education, and counseling to rehabilitate homeless individuals. Participation in the program is on a voluntary basis. Candidates for the program undergo intense intake interviews before being accepted. Individuals who are accepted into the program must be drug free and willing to undergo random drug testing. The program is very structured and rigorous; therefore, only those individuals who truly want to change are accepted. A major focus of the program is to provide participants with assistance in acquiring employment and permanent housing. Thirty individuals are accepted into the program every 60 days.

Participants receive meals, shelter, education, and counseling for a maximum of 60 days. Funding for the program is provided by government agencies (60%) and private contributions (40%).

Dr. K. provides health education to participants; therefore, she generally becomes well acquainted with each of them. During the years that Dr. K. has been volunteering at the shelter, she has noticed that many individuals repeat the program. Several of the returnees have told Dr. K. that they believe they would have been successful the first time they were enrolled if they had been given more time. Dr. K. shares these discussions and her concerns with Ms. T., the program director. Ms. T. indicates that the program has a recidivism rate of approximately 20% yearly. Dr. K. suggests that perhaps the length of the program should be individualized because some participants need more time and others need less. Ms. T. indicates that to her knowledge no clear guidelines exist regarding the optimal length of programs to rehabilitate homeless individuals. She states that the 60-day stay is based on networking with programs that have similar goals and objectives. Dr. K. is concerned that there are no clear guidelines regarding the length of a program. Dr. K. offers to perform a search to find out if there is any new information regarding rehabilitating homeless individuals. Ms. T. is skeptical but agrees to have Dr. K. investigate the matter.

Dr. K. starts the search to determine if there is any evidence-based information regarding the rehabilitation of homeless people. First, Dr. K. does an extensive review of the literature at the hospital library where she is employed. Next, she does an Internet search using the terms "homelessness and rehabilitation." Dr. K. then decides to go to the websites of various government agencies, such as the U.S. Department of Health and Human Services, to investigate rehabilitation of homeless people. Although there is not a great deal of information regarding the subject, she is successful in locating several research articles regarding homelessness rehabilitation. One of the articles is a research study performed by one of the professors at the local university. Dr. K. contacts the professor, Dr. S., who provides her with additional research articles regarding rehabilitating homeless individuals. Ultimately, Dr. K.'s search uncovers several articles that provide evidence-based practice information about rehabilitating homeless people. Three specific articles discuss individualizing the length of the program to decrease rates of recidivism.

Dr. K. shares her findings with Ms. T. She also provides Ms. T. with the names and phone numbers of the programs that are discussed in the research articles. Ms. T. agrees to review the information and contact the other programs. Several weeks later, Ms. T. approaches Dr. K. and asks for her assistance in developing a plan to individualize the length of the program for participants. A formal plan is developed, including specific intake criteria and methods for evaluating the ongoing progress of participants. Ms. T. seeks Dr. K.'s assistance in presenting this information to the shelter's board of directors. The board of directors is very impressed with Dr. K.'s and Ms. T.'s presentation, which includes information regarding research and evidence-based practice. As stakeholders in the program, they are very interested in decreasing the rate of recidivism to rehabilitate new homeless individuals rather than work with repeat participants. From the stakeholder's perspective, this will make the program more efficacious and cost effective. Additionally, if participants do not require the entire 60-day stay, cost savings may be realized. The board of directors overwhelmingly approves the plan to individualize the length of stay for shelter participants starting with a trial of 1 year. The policy and procedures for the program are temporarily revised.

The new program is implemented with careful monitoring over the next year. Dr. K. continues volunteering at the shelter and hears many positive remarks from participants regarding the individualization of the program. Some remarks include, "I feel like I have more control," and "I think I am ready to go out on my own." Dr. K. notices that there are fewer repeat participants, and this is verified when Ms. T. tells her the rate of recidivism is down to 10%. The board of directors is very pleased with the results and approves continuation of the individualized program. The policy and procedures for the program are permanently revised.

Dr. K. decides to conduct a research study with Dr. S. (PhD) regarding homeless individuals who participate in the program. The focus of the study is on factors that contribute to the participant's success or failure with the program. Funding for the study is obtained from the U.S. Department of Health and Human Services. This information will be used by the shelter to assist and support future participants.

This case study demonstrates the role of the DNP as an advocate and influencer of policy. It demonstrates the DNP's utilization of research and evidence-based practice to affect access to care and quality of care, shape policy, implement change, and influence healthcare financing. Finally, it demonstrates collaboration between a DNP and PhD in conducting clinical research.

SUMMARY

- *Nursing's Social Policy Statement* clearly states the nursing profession's commitment to society and the people who are served (ANA, 1995).
- Involvement in advocacy and healthcare policy is a natural extension of nursing's responsibilities and activities.
- Essential V of the *Essentials of Doctoral Education for Advanced Nursing Practice* provides specific curriculum standards for DNP programs related to healthcare policy and advocacy.
- DNP graduates possess the knowledge and education as well as leadership skills and practice experience to be powerful advocates for patients and to shape healthcare policy.
- Nursing has a rich and fruitful history of political activism beginning with Florence Nightingale in 1860 and continuing through the present. However,

it is evident that nursing still has much work to do to realize its full potential of influencing health care through health policy.

■ Tips for DNP graduates who are getting started in advocacy and healthcare policy include determining areas of interest, determining the amount of time and energy available to devote to political activism, and becoming informed and involved.

■ There are multiple sources for DNP graduates to become informed regarding advocacy and healthcare policy, including professional journals, Internet searches, textbooks, policy courses, newspapers, and television and radio programs.

■ Avenues for involvement by DNP graduates in advocacy and shaping healthcare policy include membership in professional nursing organizations, workplace involvement, educational endeavors, and research endeavors.

■ Nursing is one of the most trusted professions in our nation (Feldman & Lewenson, 2000). DNP graduates can capitalize on this trust by becoming involved in political activities that advocate for patients and shape healthcare policies. DNP graduates are excellent candidates for public offices based on their knowledge and leadership skills.

REFLECTION QUESTIONS

1. Do you believe it is important for DNP graduates to be involved in advocacy and shaping healthcare policy? Why or why not?
2. What do you see as the role of DNP graduates in advocacy and shaping healthcare policy?
3. Do you see yourself assuming a leadership role in advocacy and healthcare policy? If yes, how? If not, why?
4. What are your areas of interest regarding advocacy and healthcare policy?
5. What are some specific ways you have advocated for patients? Recall specific instances where you made a difference for a patient and/or family through advocacy.
6. What are some specific policies you have designed, influenced, or implemented? Be sure to include institutional policies, community policies, etc.
7. Do you think it is important to be a member of professional nursing organizations? If yes, to what organizations do you belong? If no, what organizations could enhance your interests and allow you to become more politically involved?
8. What do you believe is the role of education and research in advocacy and healthcare policy?
9. Are you active in workplace committees, such as education and research committees? If not, in what ways do you think you can become involved in education and research in your workplace?
10. Would you be comfortable seeking election for a public office? Why or why not?

EDITOR'S NOTE

The author of this chapter is an excellent example of a DNP graduate in a health policy role. Dr. Marlene Mullin has been on the Board of Directors for Hope Warming Center in Michigan since March 2010 and also serves as the Treasurer for the Board of Directors. Dr. Mullin has also volunteered to provide health care, meals, clothes, etc. to the homeless since 2005. Dr. Mullin is also currently President-Elect of the Metro Detroit Chapter of MICNP (Michigan Council for Nurse Practitioners), the largest chapter in the State of Michigan with over 460 proud members. She assumes the presidency in January 2012. As President of the Metro Chapter, she will oversee all activities of the chapter in collaboration with the other board members, which include a President-Elect, Secretary, Treasurer, and Education Coordinator. The Detroit Metro chapter also provides monthly educational sessions and participates in fundraisers for various healthcare organizations. Dr. Mullin has also been a member of the APRN Coalition since 2009, which has been actively lobbying to make legislative changes for APRNs in the State of Michigan. The proposed legislative changes include adding a definition of APRNs to the public health code, granting the Board of Nursing the authority to issue an APRN license, creating an APRN task force as a subcommittee of the Board of Nursing, adding APRNs to the list of licensed healthcare providers who are able to prescribe medications independently including Schedule 2–5 controlled drugs, and the ability to prescribe physical and speech therapy. Dr. Mullin has also personally met with her area senator and representative to garner support for the bill. Dr. Mullin is indeed a DNP graduate affecting practice through active involvement in health policy and advocacy, and I am proud to call her my colleague.

REFERENCES

American Association of Colleges of Nursing (AACN). (2006). *Essentials of doctoral education for advanced nursing practice.* Retrieved from http://www.aacn.nche.edu/publications/position/DNPEssentials.pdf

American Nurses Association (ANA). (1995). *Nursing's social policy statement.* Washington, DC: Author.

American Nurses Association (ANA). (2008). *ANA-PAC 2008 Election Action.* Retrieved from http://www.nursingworld.org/HomepageCategory/NursingInsider/Archive_1/2008NI/Oct08NI/ANAPAC2008Action.aspx

Ballou, K. A. (2000). A historical-philosophical analysis of the professional nurse obligation to participate in sociopolitical activities. *Policy, Politics, & Nursing Practice, 1*(3), 172–184.

Burgess, M. A. (1928). *Nurses, patients, and pocketbooks.* New York: Committee on the Grading of Nursing Schools.

Centers for Disease Control and Prevention (CDC), National Center for Health Statistics (NCHS). (2011). *Health insurance coverage: Early release of estimates from the national health interview survey, 2010.* Hyattsville, MD: Author.

Chinn, P. L., & Wheeler, C. E. (1985). Feminism and nursing: Can nursing afford to remain aloof from the women's movement. *Nursing Outlook, 33*(2), 74–76.

Diers, D., & Price, L. (2007). Research as a political and policy tool. In D. J. Mason, J. K. Leavitt, & M. W. Chaffee (Eds.), *Policy & politics in nursing and health care* (5th ed., pp. 195–207). St. Louis, MO: Elsevier Saunders.

Feldman, H. R., & Lewenson, S. B. (2000). *Nurses in the political arena: The public face of nursing.* New York: Springer.

Fitzpatrick, L. (1975). *The National Organization for Public Health Nursing, 1912–1952: Development of a practice field.* New York: NLN Press.

Institute of Medicine (IOM). (2001). *Crossing the quality chasm: A new health system for the 21st century.* Washington, DC: National Academies Press.

Leavitt, J. K., Chaffee, M. W., & Vance, C. (2007). Learning the ropes of policy, politics, and advocacy. In D. J. Mason, J. K. Leavitt, & M. W. Chaffee (Eds.), *Policy & politics in nursing and health care* (5th ed., pp. 34–52). St. Louis, MO: Elsevier Saunders.

Lewenson, S. B. (2007). A historical perspective on policy, politics, and nursing. In D. J. Mason, J. K. Leavitt, & M. W. Chaffee (Eds.), *Policy & politics in nursing and health care* (5th ed., pp. 21–33). St. Louis, MO: Elsevier Saunders.

Malone, P. S., & Chaffee, M. W. (2007). Interest groups: Powerful political catalysts in health care. In D. J. Mason, J. K. Leavitt, & M. W. Chaffee (Eds.), *Policy & politics in nursing and health care* (5th ed., pp. 766–777). St. Louis, MO: Elsevier Saunders.

Michnich, M. (2007). The Robert Wood Johnson health policy fellowship. In D. J. Mason, J. K. Leavitt, & M. W. Chaffee (Eds.), *Policy & politics in nursing and health care* (5th ed., pp. 52–57). St. Louis, MO: Elsevier Saunders.

Oden, L. S., Price, J. H., Alteneder, R., Boardley, D., & Ubokudom, S. E. (2000). Public policy involvement by nurse practitioners. *Journal of Community Health, 25*(2), 139–155.

O'Grady, E. (2004). Advanced practice nursing and health policy. In J. Stanley (Ed.), *Advanced practice nursing emphasizing common roles* (2nd ed., pp. 374–394). Philadelphia: Davis.

U.S. Department of Housing and Urban Development. (2010). *Annual homeless assessment report to Congress* (HUD No. 07-0685). Washington, DC: U.S. Government Printing Office.

CHAPTER 6

The DNP Graduate as Educator

▪ Karen McBroom Butler ▪

"Do not go where the path may lead; go instead where there is no path and leave a trail."

—Ralph Waldo Emerson (1803–1882)

A clinical doctorate provides graduates with enhanced knowledge to improve nursing practice and patient outcomes; advanced competencies for extremely complex clinical, faculty, and leadership roles; enhanced leadership skills; and parity with other professions (American Association of Colleges of Nursing [AACN], 2004a). All these functions are essential for educators. However, despite the practice doctorate (Doctor of Nursing Practice [DNP]) preparation, the role of nurse educators is not emphasized or recognized as fully as other roles for the degree.

The *AACN Position Statement on the Practice Doctorate in Nursing* (AACN, 2004a) states that the practice doctorate should be the graduate degree for advanced nursing practice, including but not limited to the four current advanced practice roles: clinical nurse specialist, nurse anesthetist, nurse–midwife, and nurse practitioner. An additional recommendation was that practice doctorate programs, as in research-focused doctoral programs, offer additional course work and practicums that would prepare graduates to fill the role of nurse educator (AACN, 2004a).

The traditional view is that nurses who are prepared with a research doctorate (PhD, DNS, DSN, or DNSc) should be nurse educators and function in faculty roles, particularly in research-intensive institutions. Certainly their role is extremely valuable to both nursing education and to the generation of new knowledge. However, there is a history of valuing individuals with professional doctorates in nursing education as well. Many schools of nursing employ faculty with a professional education doctorate (EdD), which is different from the PhD in education. These individuals have and continue to play an important role in collegiate nursing education (Hathaway, Jacob, Stegbauer, Thompson, & Graff, 2006).

The DNP prepares nurses with advanced skills and specialized knowledge in an identified area of nursing practice, including translation of science into practice. This preparation is important for the educator role. In addition, the discipline of education, which encompasses a completely separate body of knowledge and competence, is important. Graduates of research-focused and practice-focused doctoral programs may need additional preparation in teaching methodologies, curriculum design and development, and program evaluation methodologies if those areas of preparation have not been addressed in the students' original programs of study (AACN, 2006b). With preparation in teaching methodologies and curriculum, graduates of both practice- and research-focused programs can function effectively as nursing faculty members. More important, together they contribute alternate, complementary approaches and expertise to the educator role. The pairing of professional and academic degrees within a discipline is common practice in academics, both inside and outside of health sciences (Hathaway, et al., 2006).

This chapter provides a case for the DNP graduate in a nurse educator role and explains how nursing can be influenced and strengthened as a result. Specific case scenarios about DNP graduates in educator roles are included to illustrate how they can effectively contribute to the traditional education, research, practice, and service roles in nursing education.

■ Curriculum Standards

The *Essentials of Doctoral Education for Advanced Nursing Practice* (AACN, 2006b, Table 1) discusses curriculum standards but does not speak directly to the role of nurse educator (please refer to **Table 6-1**). However, there is content inherent to nursing education as well as advanced nursing practice, which is broadly defined by the AACN (2004a) as "Any form of nursing intervention that influences health care outcomes for individuals or populations, including the direct care of individual

Table 6-1   **Curriculum Standards: Essentials of Doctoral Education for Advanced Nursing Practice**

1. Scientific underpinnings for practice
2. Organizational and systems leadership for quality improvement and systems thinking
3. Clinical scholarship and analytical methods for evidence-based practice
4. Information systems/technology and patient care technology for the improvement and transformation of health care
5. Healthcare policy for advocacy in health care
6. Clinical scholarship and analytical methods for evidence-based practice
7. Clinical prevention and population health for improving the nation's health
8. Advanced nursing practice

Source: Adapted from AACN, 2006b.

patients, management of care for individuals or populations, administration of nursing and health care organizations, and the development and implementation of health policy" (p. 2).

DNP Essentials and National Initiatives

Certainly, nurse educators who are experts in advanced nursing practice are needed and timely, given the initiatives by the Institute of Medicine (IOM; Greiner & Knebel, 2003; IOM, 2011) and the National Research Council (2005). These reports call for nursing education that prepares individuals for interdisciplinary practice, information systems, quality improvement, and patient safety expertise. Not only are these essential skills for DNP graduates, they are important skills for nurse educators to possess, teach, and role model for students.

In the introduction to the *Essentials of Doctoral Education for Advanced Nursing Practice* (AACN, 2006b), additional IOM recommendations are referenced that include promotion of health care that is safe, effective, client centered, timely, efficient, and equitable; it also recommends education of healthcare professionals that includes delivery of patient-centered care while working on interdisciplinary teams and an emphasis on evidence-based practice, quality improvement, and informatics. The best prepared senior nurses should be in key leadership positions and should participate in executive level positions. DNP-prepared educators serve as key leaders in nursing and as such are positioned to make a powerful impact on health care that addresses the IOM recommendations. Such an impact could be made through education of students, professional role modeling, and clinical practice opportunities.

DNP Essentials and the Educator Role

Although the *Essentials of Doctoral Education for Advanced Nursing Practice* (AACN, 2006b) do not speak directly to the educator role, there are competencies in every Essential that are important and relevant to nurse educators. The introduction to the Essentials document contains a section titled "DNP Graduates and Academic Roles," which states that DNP graduates "will seek to fill roles as educators and will use their considerable practice expertise to educate the next generation of nurses" (AACN, 2006b, p. 7). The major focus of DNP educational programs, as in other practice disciplines, will be centered on practice specialization. Those who desire an educator role should have additional preparation in pedagogy to enhance their ability to teach the science of the profession they practice and teach. Some of this formal course work may occur within the context of the DNP program (AACN, 2006b).

■ The Nursing Faculty Shortage

When considering the role a DNP graduate may assume as a nursing faculty member, it is important to examine the context in which the conversation takes place. This is particularly pertinent now when we are facing a national shortage of registered nurses.

Exacerbating the overall nursing shortage is the increasing deficit of full-time master's and doctorally prepared nursing faculty members.

The Shortage of Nurses and Nursing Faculty

A national conversation about the DNP graduate as nurse educator is both essential and timely. Literature in professional journals and publications, as well as the popular press, is full of stories about the dwindling supply and resulting increased demand for registered nurses (RNs). Buerhaus, Potter, Staiger, and Auerbach (2009) suggest that the shortage of registered nurses in the United States could be as high as 50,000 by 2025, with demand for RNs expected to grow by 2% to 3% annually. The current and future shortage of registered nurses has been reported extensively (AACN, 2011; Aiken, Clark, Sloane, Sochalski, & Silber, 2002; Berliner & Ginzberg, 2002; Buerhaus, Staiger, & Auerbach, 2000; Buerhaus, Potter, Staiger, & Auerbach, 2009; Goodin, 2003; Greiner & Knebel, 2003). Recently, more attention has been given to a critical factor in resolving the problem: the availability of adequate numbers of appropriately educated, highly qualified nursing faculty to teach students. Indeed, this very shortage of faculty in nursing programs may negatively affect the number of qualified applicants accepted to both basic and advanced practice nursing education programs. Difficulty in filling nursing faculty positions may be the most crucial factor affecting the future supply of nurses (Brendtro & Hegge, 2000).

History of the Nursing Faculty Shortage

Nursing educational institutions have always had a shortage of doctorally prepared faculty, partly due to this academic norm occurring later in nursing than other professions. A substantial decrease in nursing school enrollments in the 1980s led to a decrease in faculty positions (Brendtro & Hegge, 2000). As early as the 1980s, concerns were being expressed about nursing faculty shortages (Fitzpatrick & Heller, 1980). One study (Zebelman & Olswang, 1989) found that students in doctoral programs became more focused on research than on faculty roles and preparation as they progressed through their programs; these authors voiced concern that this approach might have a negative impact on the supply of doctorally prepared nursing faculty. Likewise, Princeton (1992) looked at the development and status of graduate nursing education for teachers and argued that the numbers of graduate programs should be increased to deal with the faculty shortage. De Tornyay (1989) wrote that the environment of graduate programs discouraged students from seeking teaching positions. The 1980s predictions of a faculty shortage became a reality as opportunities for those with PhDs in nursing extended beyond educational institutions (Mullinix, 1990). The National Sample Survey of Registered Nurses databases estimated that in 1992, 1996, and 2000 the proportion of nurses with nursing doctorates who were employed in schools of nursing with baccalaureate and higher degrees showed steady declines, going from 68% in 1992 to 49% in 2000 (Division of Nursing, 2001).

Faculty Shortage Impacts on Student Enrollment

The AACN reports that 67,563 qualified nursing school applicants were turned away from baccalaureate and graduate programs in 2010 because of the insufficient number of faculty, clinical sites, classroom space, and clinical preceptors, as well as budget concerns and restraints. Nearly two-thirds of the nursing schools that responded to this survey identified the faculty shortage as a primary reason for not accepting all qualified applicants into entry-level nursing programs (AACN, 2010b). The AACN estimates that the national nurse faculty vacancy rate is 6.9% in baccalaureate and/or graduate programs, with almost 93% of the vacancies being faculty positions requiring or preferring a doctoral degree (AACN, 2010a). The problem is not limited to university nursing programs. A National League for Nursing (NLN, 2006) report found that the total average faculty vacancy rate was 5.6% at associate degree in nursing program colleges and 7.9% in bachelor's degree in nursing and higher degree programs.

In a Southern Regional Education Board (SREB) survey of 491 institutions in 16 states, researchers found more than 425 unfilled faculty positions, and 86 institutions reported that they did not have enough faculty to cover the undergraduate and graduate programs offered. The data also revealed that 144 faculty members retired in that academic year, and more than 550 resignations had been received in the current academic year or were expected in the coming 2 years. In terms of educational preparation, most of the 6,322 nurse educators had master's degrees in nursing (SREB, 2003).

Related Factors

There are additional factors that contribute to the nursing faculty shortage. For example, the average age of faculty members is increasing, thus reducing the number of productive years nurse educators can teach (AACN, 2011). The average age of doctoral-prepared faculty holding the ranks of professor, associate professor, and assistant professor were 60.5, 57.1 and 51.4 years, respectively. A complicating issue is that nurses enter academia later in their careers (AACN, 2005).

Data suggest there is an oncoming wave of faculty member retirements over the next decade. Some researchers project that for individuals who were faculty members in 2001, between 200 and 300 will be eligible for retirement annually from 2003–2012. The average age of nursing faculty at retirement is 62.5 years (Berlin & Sechrist, 2002).

Higher compensation in the clinical arena is becoming more available and increasingly attractive to current and potential faculty members. Average salaries for clinical nursing positions have risen more than those for nursing faculty positions, probably because most universities are constrained in their ability to increase faculty salaries (AACN, 2005; Brentro & Hegge, 2000). In fall of 2004, the median-calendar year salaries for teaching faculty with doctoral degrees in the rank of associate and assistant professors were $77,605 and $73,333, respectively; those with master's degrees had median salaries of $62,778 and $58,567, respectively (Berlin, Wilsey, & Bednash, 2005). In comparison, the 2004–2005 median salaries for a nurse anesthetist, head of nursing (executive and management) and nursing director were $121,698, $157,754, and $104,191, respectively (Berlin, et al, 2005). The American Academy of Nurse Practitioners reports that the average salary of nurse practitioners, across all settings and specialty areas, is $89,579 (Rollet, 2010), contrasted with master's-prepared faculty serving as associate professors, earning an annual average salary of $78,155 (AACN, 2011)

Although the number of doctoral programs has increased from 54 in 1992 to 93 in 2004 (Berlin, Bednash, & Alsheimer, 1993; Berlin, Wilsey, & Bednash, 2005), this has not resulted in an increase in graduates. In 2010, the AACN found that 10,223 qualified applications were turned away from master's programs and over 1,200 qualified applicants were turned away from doctoral programs. The primary reason given for these numbers was a shortage of faculty (AACN, 2010a). The ultimate consequence is further reductions in doctorally prepared nurse educators available for faculty positions.

An adverse effect of the faculty shortage is an increase in faculty workload, with added likelihood of stress, burnout, and attrition. Researchers report faculty members' ages are increasing steadily, shortening the length of time to likely retirement and a loss of younger faculty (AACN, 2005; Berlin & Sechrist, 2002). The use of part-time or less-qualified faculty members or assigning faculty members to teach outside their areas of specialization may result in lower quality programs. Schools may hire more master's-prepared clinical experts with little or no preparation for teaching (Brendtro & Hegge, 2000). Princeton (1992) described this type of "on-the-job training" as a costly "hit-and-miss situation" (p. 35). Other issues related to the nursing faculty shortage include a decline in the percentage of younger faculty (Berlin & Sechrist, 2002), tuition and loan burden for graduate study (Peterson's Colleges of Nursing Database, 2002), workload and role expectations (Brendtro & Hegge, 2000), and alternate career choices (AACN, 2011).

The nursing faculty shortage cannot be viewed separately from the overall nursing shortage, but the implications of decreasing numbers of faculty members are twofold; both are of equal importance. First, it is essential to have faculty members with the knowledge and skills needed for good teaching; there is a pressing need for scholars and researchers in education (Tanner, 1999). Second, institutions must have nursing faculty members with the requisite education and skills to be researchers to continue to generate and advance the scientific knowledge base for nursing (Hinshaw, 2001). This author contends that DNP graduates can have a significant impact on these concerns.

■ DNP Graduates Can Fill the Nursing Faculty Gap

The AACN (2006b) states that DNP graduates will seek to fill roles as educators and use their wealth of practice expertise to educate the next generation of nurses. With additional work in pedagogy, DNP graduates are uniquely qualified to help fill the nursing faculty gap.

Nursing Leadership and the Shortage

Many strategies have been proposed to address the overall nursing and nursing faculty shortage. Among these are federal and state funding initiatives; strategic partnerships with private corporations; national media campaigns (AACN, 2011); career progression initiatives to reach out to students early; moving nursing graduates through graduate studies more rapidly; identification of a range of options beyond entry-level roles of faculty, researcher, and administrator; and fostering competitive salaries and improved work environments (AACN, 2001). Berlin and Sechrist (2002) state that nurse educators must rapidly arrive at both short- and long-term solutions that may require examination of some of the sacrosanct traditions of nursing education as well as an unbiased scrutiny of faculty work environments. They suggest a streamlined educational process and consideration of adoption of a broader-based view of the educational preparation for faculty status.

National and state nurse leaders and deans of schools of nursing, along with nursing faculty members and others, have a great opportunity to work in collaborative leadership to affect the nursing faculty shortage. Heifetz (1994) writes of working together as partners in shared leadership to face current issues, create a new paradigm, and stimulate action to create a desired future. If ever there was a time for nursing leaders in education to work together to create a preferred future, this is certainly the era.

Strategic Leadership with DNP-Prepared Educators

The DNP degree offers education that prepares graduates for leadership roles at the highest level, with clinical expertise and the knowledge and skills necessary to translate research findings into practice. These are all areas that can be used to build a successful career in nursing education. Depending on a specific curriculum, graduates may need additional preparation in pedagogy. This is not different than graduates of many PhD programs. According to the NLN (2002), all nurse educators need core knowledge and skills that entail the ability to enhance learning, advance the total development and professional socialization of students, design appropriate learning experiences, and evaluate learning outcomes.

One strategy that has been cited to reverse the nursing faculty shortage includes career progression initiatives that move nurses through graduate school more quickly. The AACN (1999) recommended that education be compressed to become more attractive. The AACN's *Essentials of Doctoral Education for Advanced Nursing Practice* (2006b) recommends that DNP programs be 3 calendar years (36 months of full-time study, including summers) or 4 academic years. This recommendation is for those programs that offer a BSN–DNP option, and it is much more streamlined than the time and expense necessary to obtain the two previously required degrees (master's and doctorate). It also gives the student a doctoral education with an appropriate number of academic credits. For those who already have a master's degree, the time to completion of a DNP program would be even shorter with less expense incurred.

A second proposed strategy to reduce the nursing faculty shortage is to encourage students to return to graduate school at an earlier age. This is a paradigm change; no longer is it feasible to recommend that students work for years in clinical settings between degrees. Undergraduate students should be encouraged to return to master's programs early after graduation; master's students should be encouraged to obtain doctorates earlier in their careers as well (Anderson, 2000). Because the DNP degree will, in many cases, replace master's degree programs that prepare nurses for advanced nursing practice, it follows that students will be entering DNP programs at an earlier age than students in prior doctoral programs, with the additional benefit of students being doctorally prepared in 3 years. Not only could these efforts increase the number of younger nurses with advanced degrees, but doctorally prepared faculty members would enter the workforce at earlier ages, thus increasing the amount of time they have available for productive academic careers.

A third proposed strategy to reduce the nursing faculty shortage is the development of more flexible degree programs. Distributed learning and online courses would increase the availability of graduate education to those who may not live near a school that offers doctoral programs. Accelerated career pathways, such as BSN to DNP, may entice those who have a limited number of years and/or money to invest in graduate education. Current clinically focused, master's-prepared faculty members should be encouraged to pursue a DNP degree. Such new programs make graduate opportunities available to those who do not wish to be researchers but are interested in clinical leadership and expertise, often in educational settings (Marion, et al., 2003).

Another way to stretch available resources is to adequately prepare faculty members to use technology (Boyden, 2000). DNP graduates will begin preparation for this role as addressed in the AACN's *Essentials of Doctoral Education for Advanced Nursing Practice* (2006b). The use of information technology will be incorporated into DNP curricula and will set the stage for additional work with teaching technology.

A New Paradigm

With decreasing numbers of nursing faculty have come more responsibility for those left behind. Traditionally, faculty roles have been threefold: education, research, and service. Perhaps it is time to reexamine those roles and, at least in some cases, separate them to create more realistic work expectations (Brendtro & Hegge, 2000). For example, a faculty member who is an expert in teaching may be allowed to teach most of the time without doing research; a researcher may be given the majority of his or her time to concentrate on generating new knowledge; and a DNP graduate may be given the opportunity to teach, function in clinical practice leadership roles, and/or work as a member of a research team in partnership with research-focused colleagues to translate findings into practice. This is being done by some schools of nursing already, yet for others—particularly parent institutions in which schools of nursing reside—the paradigm shift is pending.

To promote such a paradigm shift, it is important to think outside of the box about those who may be able to fulfill faculty roles and obligations. The creative use of diversely prepared faculty members is a good option; the strengths of the individual and his or her educational preparation should be capitalized upon. It may take a real paradigm change for nursing educators to accept that there are those without PhDs in nursing who can successfully teach student nurses. Nurse leaders need to work together to establish a place and a role for these professionals and to incorporate them effectively into nursing education.

Undergraduate Education

DNP graduates are prepared to teach at the undergraduate level. Fitzpatrick (2002) states that "expert clinicians are needed to teach clinicians" (p. 57). Further, she proposes that nursing faculty members who teach at the basic (as well as advanced practice) level principally need expert clinical skills paired with skills in teaching; therefore, the best preparation for teaching these clinicians is the clinical doctorate (Fitzpatrick, 2002).

Baccalaureate nursing students love clinical practice; it is the foremost reason they come to nursing school, and it is their primary framework for nursing. DNP-prepared educators can make a real difference in the education of these young nurses, both in the classroom and clinical settings. Because DNP graduates are expert clinicians, they can clearly explain and demonstrate clinical phenomena. In addition, they can write realistic case studies and have the expertise and experience to answer difficult, complex clinical questions.

DNP graduates are excellent nursing role models for undergraduate students, both in advanced nursing practice utilizing expert clinical skills and as doctorally prepared educators who are dedicated to nursing practice. National scholars recognized this potential when writing *Advancing the Nation's Health Needs: NIH Research Training Programs* (Committee, 2005). The authors state that "the need for doctorally prepared practitioners and clinical faculty would be met if nursing could develop a new nonresearch clinical doctorate, similar to the MD and PharmD in medicine and dentistry" (p. 74).

Graduate Education

DNP graduates are prepared to teach at the graduate level. Particularly for faculty members who teach in clinically focused graduate programs, clinical teaching necessitates advanced clinical knowledge and enhanced practice skills. DNP graduates are master teachers in clinical practice and are role models for advanced nursing practice. The AACN's *Essentials of Doctoral Education for Advanced Nursing Practice* (2006b) states that faculty members who teach in DNP programs should have diverse backgrounds and scholarly perspectives in the specialty areas for which they are preparing graduates. Broad faculty expertise is needed, which includes doctorally prepared, research-focused faculty as well as doctorally prepared, practice-focused faculty with expertise to support the educational program.

In addition, there is a need for a group of faculty members who are actively engaged in practice as part of their faculty roles, because active practice provides the same type of applied clinical learning environments for DNP students that active research programs provide for PhD students (AACN, 2006b). Faculty members should have current experience by participating in clinical practice and/or monitoring current nursing practice to prepare students to enter the complex world of health care (Sperhac & Goodwin, 2003). Through faculty practice, there is a learning environment that models rapid translation of new knowledge into practice and evaluation of practice-based models of care (AACN, 2006b). Additionally, the development and implementation of programs of scholarship that represent knowledge development from original research for some faculty members and application of research in practice for others is recommended (AACN, 2006b).

Diverse Opportunities

There are many opportunities for DNP graduates to pursue and fulfill academic roles. These are not restricted to research-intensive institutions. There are regional universities, community colleges, and other institutions that offer nursing education programs. All of these venues are in need of doctorally prepared nursing faculty. The possibilities are there for those who choose to pursue them, and nursing will be better for the inclusion of educational diversity among its faculty ranks. **Table 6-2** lists tips for DNP graduates who are interested in pursuing a career in academia. Case scenario 3 (later in this chapter) illustrates the successful career of a DNP-prepared faculty member who teaches at both the undergraduate and graduate levels at a regional state university.

■ Promotion and Tenure

Conversations about DNP graduates in faculty roles generally involve discussion about promotion and tenure. Although criteria for promotion and tenure are determined mostly by individual institutions, there are some commonalities. Strategies used by someone with a clinically focused doctorate to achieve promotion and tenure may be somewhat different than those used by someone with a research-focused doctorate, but it is possible to attain both promotion and tenure, even at many research-intensive institutions. (See case scenarios 1 and 2 for illustrative examples.)

Practice Doctorates: A Case for Tenure

Promotion and tenure are primarily institutional decisions, for both eligibility and standards. The AACN (2004b) voices confidence that a DNP-prepared faculty member will compete favorably with faculty members who hold other practice doctorates in tenure and promotion decisions. This is the case in law, education, physical therapy, pharmacy, public policy and administration, public health, and other disciplines (AACN, 2004b). It is common for institutions to have policies that enable those with professional doctorates to attain tenure (Hathaway, et al., 2006).

There are institutions of higher learning that offer different types of tenure, such as a regular title series (the traditional, research-based format) and alternate options,

Table 6-2 **Tips for DNP Graduates Who Are Interested in Pursuing a Career in Academia**

■ Do your homework! The requirements for faculty roles are different at every institution. What is expected of the faculty? What are the options and specifications for attaining promotion and tenure? What is the emphasis: Is it a community college with the primary goal of educating students or a research-intensive university that values grant funding and scholarly productivity? Is it a mix of these things? If so, where would you fit into the mix?

■ Know what your interests and talents are (teaching, implementation of evidence-based clinical practices, faculty practice, partnering with researchers, etc.). Match your interests with the priorities and strengths of the institution.

■ If you are primarily interested in education, are there other nurse educators at the institution who will support you in this role? Is there support for continuing work in curriculum development, teaching strategies, and student outcomes evaluation?

■ If you are interested in teaching undergraduates, what is the school's NCLEX pass rate for the past 5 years? If you are interested in teaching at the graduate level, what programs are available, and how many of the students are successful in attaining certification in their specialties?

■ If you are interested in faculty clinical practice, are clinical sites that fit your expertise associated with the institution? Are the sites willing to consider a joint appointment?

■ If you are interested in partnering with researchers, is there a researcher or a research team with interests similar to yours? Are they willing to discuss partnering opportunities and support you in your role, including assistance with meeting the criteria for promotion and tenure? Remember, academic scholarship should include the application of knowledge, and you are an expert in this area.

■ Market what you can do! DNP preparation and roles are relatively new, and many parent institutions do not understand the competencies that a DNP-prepared faculty member brings to the role. Be specific about what you can offer, and provide this information in writing when you apply for a faculty position.

■ Don't give up! There are many opportunities for DNP-prepared faculty members to serve and flourish. Finding the right fit is essential and will create a path for a successful, satisfying career in academia.

such as clinical or special title series, in which requirements for tenure may be based more on clinical practice or teaching excellence. It is important for DNP graduates to be fully cognizant of the opportunities and requirements at a particular institution before accepting employment.

The AACN's *Essentials of Doctoral Education for Advanced Nursing Practice* (AACN, 2006b) lists indicators of productive programs of nursing practice scholarship, many of which may be used toward promotion and tenure in various settings. These include:

extramural grants in support of practice innovations; peer reviewed publications and presentations; practice-oriented grant review activities; editorial review activities; state, regional, national, and international professional activities related to one's practice area; policy involvement; and development and dissemination of practice improvement products such as reports, guidelines, protocols and toolkits. (p. 21)

The DNP graduate is educationally prepared with the relevant knowledge and skills to accomplish these indicators and thereby should be considered for tenure-track positions at academic institutions that host schools of nursing. Inclusion of these skills in written communications when applying for academic positions may be helpful both to the applicant and the employer.

Hathaway et al. (2006) argue that having the ability to earn a practice doctorate will enhance many nursing faculty members' scholarly productivity and have a positive impact on their ability to earn tenure. Many schools employ master's-prepared nursing faculty members who are important to the educational mission and devoted to clinical practice. These faculty members may not wish to pursue research doctorates, or, if they do, they may not use their research preparation, thereby limiting their scholarly productivity and the ability to earn tenure. This is supported by data showing that only 11% of doctorally prepared nurses are working in research-intensive institutions (AACN, 2006a; Health Resources and Services Administration, 2004). Earning a practice doctorate, such as a DNP degree, will provide knowledge and skills to faculty members who are clinically focused and contribute to their ability to earn tenure (Hathaway, et al., 2006).

The Scholarship of Application

Scholarship application has been described by Boyer (1990). Although the generation of new scientific knowledge and scholarly publication are appropriate performance criteria for research faculty, Boyer (1990) argues that application of knowledge through professional practice should also be valued. This definition of scholarship legitimizes nonresearch endeavors by emphasizing that application of knowledge engages scholars who must determine how knowledge can be applied to problems, how it can be helpful to stakeholders outside of the institution, and how social or clinical problems can create an agenda for future research. New understanding can come from application of knowledge. When this occurs, theory and practice interact, and each renews the other. According to Boyer (1990), the logical conclusion is that if the institution values clinical practice, the scholarship of application must be considered in tenure decisions.

A Valuable Partnership: Research and Clinical Practice

One creative approach involves having DNP graduates partner with researchers, either individually or as part of a research team. Researchers are skilled in the generation of new knowledge, and DNP graduates are prepared to translate this new knowledge into practice as well as evaluate outcomes (thereby generating new research questions). This is a perfect marriage of interest, education, and talents, and it also puts the theory–research–practice loop that has been advocated for many years into active practice (Fawcett, 2005; Fawcett, Watson, Neuman, Walker, & Fitzpatrick, 2001; Hathaway, et al., 2006; Neuman & Fawcett, 2001).

Hinshaw (2001) states that there must be nursing faculty with the requisite education and skills to be researchers to continue the generation and advancement of the scientific knowledge base for nursing. This author contends that there must also be nursing faculty with the requisite education and skills to be expert clinicians to apply new knowledge and evaluate outcomes. Through the development of such teams of faculty, the scientific knowledge base for nursing can be generated, applied, refined, and advanced. Examples of such partnering opportunities are illustrated in the first two case scenarios at the end of this chapter.

■ Conclusion

Education is a part of every nurse's role, whether we are educating our patients, their families, our colleagues, or students. This chapter has made a case for why DNP graduates are uniquely prepared to function as nursing faculty in diverse settings and how this fits into the current context of nursing education and the nursing faculty shortage. The creative use of diversely prepared faculty is essential and will capitalize on the strengths of individuals and their educational preparation while bringing alternate, complementary approaches and expertise to the role.

It may take a real paradigm change for those in nursing education to accept that there are those without research-focused doctorates in nursing who can successfully teach nursing students at all levels and fulfill the roles necessary to attain promotion and tenure. Nurse leaders must work together to establish a place and a role for these DNP-prepared professionals and to incorporate them effectively into nursing education.

■ Case Scenarios: The DNP Graduate as Nurse Educator

It is useful for DNP students and graduates who are interested in pursuing nursing faculty roles to see illustrative examples of those who have been successful in this quest. The following three case scenarios are examples of how three DNP graduates are working to successfully fulfill nursing faculty roles, both in research-intensive and regional state universities.

Case Scenario 1: A DNP Graduate in a Faculty Role in a Research-Intensive State University

Dr. B. is a 2006 DNP graduate who is employed as a nursing faculty member at a large, public, research-intensive land grant university in the southeastern United States. Prior to graduation from her DNP program, she was an undergraduate course coordinator, lecturer, and clinical instructor (nontenure track) in the College of Nursing for 5 years. Upon graduation, her rank was changed to assistant professor, special title series (tenure track). Her additional new responsibilities include teaching leadership in the school's DNP program and serving as a faculty associate in the university's Tobacco Policy Research Program (TPRP).

Dr. B. is well suited for these new responsibilities. In practice prior to teaching, she held several high-level nursing administrative positions in the medical center. Therefore, not only is she well versed in the leadership literature from her DNP curriculum, she has actual practice experience in leadership roles, which enhances her ability to teach the content and illustrate its use. Dr. B. has taken advantage of continuing education opportunities and has used peer review to hone her teaching skills.

In addition, she functions as a leader in the College of Nursing as chairperson for several committees and as undergraduate course coordinator, and she leads in the broader university setting by serving on committees and partnering with faculty from other departments for specific projects. Dr. B. also advises DNP students and chairs their doctoral committees. She serves as a leader in the community by donating her time and expertise to various health-related interest groups. She is a reviewer for several professional journals and has served on statewide professional committees. Leadership in the form of serving the College of Nursing, university, profession, and community satisfies a commonly held tenure requirement of service.

Dr. B.'s baccalaureate students are intensely interested in her practice doctorate; clinical nursing is their primary framework for nursing. They love that when they ask clinically oriented questions she has the expertise to answer them and can illustrate the answer with real-life clinical experiences. They are fascinated that she has a doctorate focused on clinical nursing practice and strive to learn more about this option. Through her, they are able to see a role model who loves clinical nursing as they do and who also has the professional accomplishment of obtaining a doctoral degree. Dr. B. received an Outstanding Undergraduate Faculty Award in 2006 and a Teacher Who Made a Difference Award in 2011.

Dr. B. has a great interest in health promotion for college students based on almost 20 years of working with them. Her DNP capstone project involved the creation and publication of an evidence-based toolkit to prevent meningococcal meningitis in college students. Upon completion of her DNP program, she joined the Tobacco Policy Research Program, knowing that both tobacco use and exposure to secondhand smoke are significant threats to health. The mission of the TPRP is to reduce tobacco use and exposure to secondhand smoke through research, education, and policy development.

The TPRP is made up of professionals with diverse backgrounds: research, biostatistics, health administration, public health, social work and counseling, and clinical expertise, among others. Dr. B. has been mentored by and partners with the other members and participates in program planning, implementation, and evaluation, and writing of grants, abstracts, and manuscripts, as well as presentation of work at professional meetings. She has a particular interest in tobacco use prevention and tobacco dependence treatment, and she works on programming in this area. One example of these efforts includes designing cessation programming for hospital employees, patients, and visitors prior to the medical campus becoming entirely smoke free.

An additional area of interest lies in educating nursing students to assist their patients with tobacco use prevention and tobacco dependence treatment. She designed, implemented, and evaluated a tailored, evidence-based curriculum to educate nursing students to assist patients through the use of national guidelines. The findings of this research project were published in a national refereed journal.

Since her 2006 graduation, Dr. B. has many other scholarly accomplishments. She has most recently worked with community partners to reduce the health and economic burden of tobacco use in rural populations. Dr. B. was the principal investigator (PI) on a research study using community engagement strategies with local health department personnel, cooperative extension agents, and other community members to develop evidence-based interventions to motivate rural smokers to consider quitting. She was nominated by her colleagues for a national Community Engagement Award in 2011. She is also the Co-PI on a grant funded by the Centers for Disease Control and Prevention through the Kentucky Department of Public Health to address tobacco prevention and cessation issues. Her scholarly work has been peer reviewed and presented in local, state, national, and international venues, as well as published in a variety of refereed professional journals including the *Journal of Nursing Education, Nursing Leadership Forum, Worldviews on Evidence-based Nursing, Family and Community Health, Public Health Nursing, Preventive Medicine,* and *Policy, Politics and Nursing Practice.*

Since completing the DNP program she has had 13 manuscripts published or in press (8 are first-authored with 2 more under review) as well as 2 textbook chapters. Dr. B. has also had 34 abstracts peer reviewed and accepted for publication and/or presentation at regional, national, and international professional meetings, 25 of which are first authored.

On a 7-year tenure trajectory, Dr. B. has successfully completed her 2- and 4-year tenure reviews. Feedback has been overwhelmingly positive and she looks forward to preparing final tenure materials for submission next year.

Recognition of excellence in teaching, scholarly achievements, nomination for a national Community Engagement Award, and evidence of university and public service will be the basis of Dr. B.'s achievement of promotion and tenure. Her clinical experiences and DNP education laid the foundation for all of these accomplishments.

Case Scenario 2: A DNP Graduate in a Faculty Role That Includes Clinical Practice in a Research-Intensive State University

Dr. H.P. is a 2006 DNP graduate who is employed as a nursing faculty member at a large, public, research-intensive land grant university in the southeastern United States. Prior to graduation from her DNP program, she was an assistant professor, clinical title series (nontenure track), and served as an undergraduate course coordinator and clinical instructor, as well as an instructor in the master's program in the College of Nursing. Upon graduation, her rank was changed to assistant professor, special title series (tenure track). She is in the fourth year of the tenure process, due to achieve tenure status at year 7.

Dr. H.P. now serves as the coordinator of the DNP Program Acute Care Nurse Practitioner Track, which is an administrative position for curriculum development and implementation. She also is the lead faculty for other core DNP and master's-level courses. Dr. H.P. assumes full faculty membership on multiple university academic and governance committees while maintaining an active practice as an acute care nurse practitioner intensivist in a private hospital setting. Through her practice she manages the care of critically ill adult and geriatric patients within an interdisciplinary practice environment.

Dr. H.P. is the primary investigator for an outcomes evaluation study of the advanced practice registered nurse (APRN) intensivist role. She is also the principal investigator for a funded translational research project designed to explore the relationship between inflammation, cardiac function, and weaning from mechanical ventilation in order to gather pilot data in preparation for a larger grant submission in the future. This project is aimed at developing an intervention to implement in practice. She is a co-investigator for another study to evaluate characteristics of mechanically ventilated patients via retrospective chart audits. She is an associate with the Rich Heart Research Group and is being mentored by a PhD-prepared faculty member in this effort.

Dr. H.P. is well prepared for these new responsibilities. For many years she has worked as a leader in tertiary care clinical settings as an acute care APRN, planning and implementing clinical research projects. Now she is also well versed in the leadership literature from her DNP curriculum and can add outcomes evaluation to her toolkit of skills. This enhances her ability to make meaningful changes in clinical practice and also to teach the content and illustrate its use. Dr. H.P. functions as a leader in the College of Nursing and the broader university by serving on program and governance committees. Dr. H.P. assumes regional and national leadership roles by serving as a grant reviewer for organizations such as Health Resources and Services Administration (HRSA), Sigma Theta Tau, and the American Association of Critical-Care Nurses. She is a textbook author and editor and reviews manuscripts for numerous professional nursing journals. Leadership in the form of serving a clinical site, the College of Nursing, the university, and the profession satisfies the tenure requirement of service.

Dr. H.P. is a role model for undergraduate and graduate students who are very interested in her role as an acute care nurse practitioner. Students respect her expertise and her willingness to enthusiastically share her experiences with them. They are interested in how she decided to obtain a practice doctorate and how she uses it in her everyday experiences. She is a role model who loves clinical nursing as they do and who also has the professional accomplishment of obtaining a doctoral degree. Dr. H.P. has an undergraduate research intern working with her, spending 4 hours a week participating in data collection. She is excited to be able to mentor undergraduate students in this role, and they are fortunate to benefit from her expertise. Dr. H.P. also chairs multiple doctoral committees for DNP students and is a member of one PhD committee. These doctoral students desire to work with Dr. H.P. because of her practice and research expertise. She hosts visiting scholars who are interested in conducting research in critically ill patients at her clinical practice site.

Dr. H.P. has a great interest in the care of critically ill adult patients, particularly those who are mechanically ventilated. She has planned, implemented, and evaluated clinical studies to look at the association between specific variables and ventilator-associated pneumonia. Her DNP capstone project involved the implementation and evaluation of a ventilator care protocol that included an evidence-based oral care guideline she developed during her DNP course work. Following graduation, she began to collaborate with her PhD-prepared mentor on research initiatives that involve mechanically ventilated patients. Besides her funded project, Dr. H.P., along with her mentor, involves graduate students in a retrospective study where students review the medical records of mechanically ventilated adults to build a large data set from which to launch future investigations. Dr. H.P. has presented scholarly presentations at professional meetings as a result of her work.

Dr. H.P. has created a collaborative model between herself as a DNP-prepared nurse and her mentor, who is PhD prepared. Her DNP preparation has enabled her to provide the leadership needed to build a collaborative program in the acute care hospital setting. Her work will have a significant impact on clinical practice, focusing on mechanically ventilated patients.

Dr. H.P. is often called upon to consult on the research and development of medical equipment and to serve as an expert witness in litigation cases. These examples are evidence of broadening recognition of her practice expertise and influence.

Since her 2006 graduation, Dr. H.P. has accomplished many scholarly endeavors. She serves as editor and author for a popular critical care nursing textbook. She also has a first-authored manuscript in press, two under revision, and several others in preparation. Dr. H.P. has had numerous peer-reviewed abstracts accepted for publication and presentation in regional, national, and international venues. These scholarly achievements, along with recognition of excellence in teaching, as evidenced by student evaluations and an outstanding clinical practice in acute care, will help Dr. H.P. to achieve promotion and tenure. Her clinical experiences and DNP education laid the foundation for her success.

Case Scenario 3: A DNP Graduate in a Faculty Role at a Regional State University

Dr. P. is employed as a nursing faculty member at a regional state university in the southeastern United States, which has both baccalaureate and graduate nursing programs. Prior to achieving the DNP degree, Dr. P. served as assistant faculty in a nontenure-track position, teaching mental health nursing at the baccalaureate level. After graduation with her DNP degree in 2006, Dr. P. was promoted to a tenure-track position, and her responsibilities were expanded to include a position as graduate faculty. She now teaches nursing research at the master's level and will be teaching evidence-based practice in the university's newly developed DNP program.

Dr. P.'s prior nursing experience included clinical work in medical–surgical areas, home health, and hospice care. After achieving a master's degree in psychiatric/mental health nursing and earning accreditation through the American Nurses' Credentialing Center (ANCC) as a clinical nurse specialist, she worked at a large state hospital, where her duties included staff supervision and support, clinical case management, and staff education. Although she has a full-time teaching position, she continues to work at the hospital several hours each week, developing curricula for and leading clients in psychoeducational groups.

The combination of her extensive nursing experience and the education she received in the DNP program has provided Dr. P. with a solid basis for teaching both undergraduate and graduate students. She believes the DNP emphasis on evidence-based practice has been especially helpful in her teaching as well as in clinical practice; she also has an increased ability to evaluate and discuss current healthcare issues with students. Because they have heard different views of the practice doctorate, Dr. P.'s students are interested in discussing the program with her. In addition, she has been able to demonstrate the value of the DNP degree to other faculty and to emphasize to them the benefits of having faculty members with both clinically based and research-based doctoral degrees. It is significant that the university recently began a Doctor of Nursing Practice Program (in which Dr. P. will also be teaching).

Since her graduation, Dr. P.'s article describing her capstone project has been published by a peer-reviewed psychiatric nursing journal. Her other recent scholarly activity includes development and presentation of a continuing education module about evidence-based practice and a presentation about implementation of the recovery model in mental health care at a regional psychiatric nursing conference. She recently developed a 3-hour continuing education offering on domestic violence for the continuing education department. She also serves as a reviewer of articles for a major peer-reviewed nursing journal. She keeps current in her knowledge about mental health nursing, as well as nursing education, by reading and evaluating current nursing research and literature and attending relevant nursing workshops and conferences, and she also maintains her accreditation as an advanced practice registered nurse. The DNP degree emphasis on leadership has also enabled Dr. P. to serve successfully in significant positions in the local American Nurses Association as well as in the local Sigma Theta Tau chapter. Notably, Dr. P. attained tenure at her institution, a significant accomplishment that would not have been possible without her DNP education.

SUMMARY

- Education is a part of every nurse's role. A DNP degree provides graduates with enhanced knowledge to improve nursing practice and patient outcomes; advanced competencies for extremely complex clinical, faculty, and leadership roles; enhanced leadership skills; and parity with other professions, but nurse educator is still a less-recognized role of the DNP graduate.
- Graduates of research-focused and practice-focused doctoral programs may need additional preparation in pedagogy, but both can function effectively as nursing faculty members and bring alternate, complementary approaches and expertise to the role.
- Although the *Essentials of Doctoral Education for Advanced Nursing Practice* (AACN, 2006b) does not speak directly to the educator role, there are

competencies in every Essential that are important and relevant to nurse educators.

■ The shortage of registered nurses in the United States could be as high as 50,000 by 2025. Difficulty in filling nursing faculty positions may be the most crucial factor affecting the future supply of nurses.

■ There are multiple factors associated with the nursing faculty shortage: aging of current faculty members, entering academia later in life, discouragement of students from careers in academia, compensation, workload, and work environment.

■ Innovative strategies and the ability to think outside of the box about those who may be able to fulfill faculty roles are needed. Creatively using diversely prepared faculty members and capitalizing on the strengths of individuals' educational preparation are good options. DNP graduates are uniquely positioned to fill the nursing faculty gap.

■ Clinical teaching at both undergraduate and graduate levels necessitates advanced clinical knowledge and enhanced practice skills. The DNP graduate is a master teacher and a role model in the area of advanced clinical nursing practice.

■ Promotion and tenure are primarily institutional decisions, but a DNP faculty member should be able to compete favorably with faculty members who hold other practice doctorates. A possible strategy is the partnering of DNP graduates with research-focused faculty to marry the generation of new knowledge with the translation of new knowledge into clinical practice.

REFLECTION QUESTIONS

1. What education preparation and experience do you think is important for a nurse educator to have to teach at the undergraduate level and the graduate level?
2. What education preparation and experience do you think is important for a nurse educator to have to pursue scholarly interests?
3. What kinds of scholarly contributions do you think a DNP-prepared faculty member could make?
4. How important do you think it is for nurse educators to have current clinical expertise, either through practice or research?
5. What are some creative ways that DNP-prepared nursing faculty members can partner with research-prepared nursing faculty members to improve nursing practice and patient health outcomes?
6. What contributions can DNP-prepared nursing faculty members make in schools of nursing that are not research intensive, for example, those that offer associate, BSN, or MSN degrees in regional universities?
7. Despite the factors that contribute to the nursing faculty shortage, serving as a nurse educator offers opportunities to impact many lives, not only the lives of every student but also those whose lives and care are ultimately entrusted to

the students throughout their nursing careers. Can you see nursing education in your future? If so, how can you make a unique contribution in an educator role, utilizing the knowledge and skills gained from your DNP education?

AUTHOR'S NOTE

The author would like to thank Drs. Melanie Hardin-Pierce and Leandra Price for their friendship as well as assistance in the writing of this chapter.

This work is dedicated to my husband, John Allen Butler, my parents, Charles Samuel McBroom and Eugenia Hunt, and my brothers, Kraig and Kelly McBroom, who give me unconditional love and support in all I do. Any positive influence I have on my students and ultimately the many lives they will touch in the future is in honor of my family.

REFERENCES

Aiken, L., Clark, S., Sloane, D., Sochalski, J., & Silber, J. (2002). Hospital nurse staffing and patient mortality, nurse burnout, and job dissatisfaction. *Journal of the American Medical Association, 288,* 1987–1993.

American Association of Colleges of Nursing (AACN). (1999). *Faculty shortages intensify nation's nursing deficit* (Issue Bulletin). Washington, DC: Author. Retrieved from http://www.aacn.nche.edu /Publications/Issues/IB499WB.htm

American Association of Colleges of Nursing (AACN). (2001). *Strategies to reverse the new nursing shortage.* Retrieved from http://www.aacn.nche.edu/publications/position/tri-council-shortage

American Association of Colleges of Nursing (AACN). (2004a). *AACN position statement on the practice doctorate in nursing.* Washington, DC: Author. Retrieved from http://www.aacn.nche.edu/dnp /position-statement

American Association of Colleges of Nursing (AACN). (2004b). *Doctor of nursing practice programs: Frequently asked questions.* Retrieved from http://www.aacn.nche.edu/dnp/faqs

American Association of Colleges of Nursing (AACN). (2005). *Faculty shortages in baccalaureate and graduate nursing programs: Scope of the problem and strategies for expanding the supply.* Washington, DC: Author.

American Association of Colleges of Nursing (AACN). (2006a). *Custom data report: Nursing faculty.* Washington, DC: Author.

American Association of Colleges of Nursing (AACN). (2006b). *Essentials of doctoral education for advanced nursing practice.* Retrieved from http://www.aacn.nche.edu/publications/position /DNPEssentials.pdf

American Association of Colleges of Nursing (AACN). (2010a). *Special survey of AACN membership on vacant faculty positions.* Washington, DC: Author.

American Association of Colleges of Nursing (AACN). (2010b). *2010–2011 enrollment and graduations in baccalaureate and graduate programs in nursing.* Washington, DC: Author.

American Association of Colleges of Nursing (AACN). (2011). *Nursing shortage fact sheet.* Retrieved from http://www.aacn.nche.edu/media-relations/fact-sheets/nursing-shortage

Anderson, C. A. (2000). Current strengths and limitations of doctoral education in nursing: Are we prepared for the future? *Journal of Professional Nursing, 16*(4), 191–200.

Berlin, L., Bednash, G., & Alsheimer, O. (1993). *1992–1993 enrollment and graduations in baccalaureate and graduate programs in nursing.* Washington, DC: American Association of Colleges of Nursing.

Berlin, L. E., & Sechrist, K. R. (2002). The shortage of doctorally prepared nursing faculty: A dire situation. *Nursing Outlook, 50*(2), 50–56.

Berlin, L., Wilsey, S., & Bednash, G. (2005). *2004–2005 salaries of instructional and administrative nursing faculty in baccalaureate and graduate programs in nursing.* Washington, DC: American Association of Colleges of Nursing.

Berliner, H. S. M., & Ginzberg, E. (2002). Why this hospital nursing shortage is different. *Journal of the American Medical Association, 288,* 2742–2744.

Boyden, K. M. (2000). Development of new faculty in higher education. *Journal of Professional Nursing, 16*(2), 104–111.

Boyer, E. L. (1990). *Scholarship reconsidered: Priorities of the professoriate.* San Francisco: Jossey-Bass.

Brendtro, M., & Hegge, M. (2000). Nursing faculty: One generation away from extinction? *Journal of Professional Nursing, 16*(2), 97–103.

Buerhaus, P., Potter, V., Staiger, D., & Auerbach, D. (2009). *The future of the nursing workforce in the United States: Data, trends, and implications.* Sudbury, MA: Jones and Bartlett.

Buerhaus, P., Staiger, D., & Auerbach, D. (2000). Implications of an aging registered nurse workforce. *Journal of the American Medical Association, 283,* 2948–2954.

Committee for Monitoring the Nation's Changing Needs for Biomedical, Behavioral, and Clinical Personnel, Board on Higher Education and Workforce, National Research Council. (2005). *Advancing the nation's health needs: NIH research training programs.* Washington, DC: National Academies Press.

de Tornyay, R. (1989). Who will teach the future nurses? *Journal of Nursing Education, 28*(2), 52.

Division of Nursing, Bureau of Health Professions, HRSA. (2001). *The registered nurse population: National sample survey of registered nurses* (unpublished special reports generated for the American Association of Colleges of Nursing).

Fawcett, J. (2005). *Contemporary nursing knowledge: Analysis and evaluation of nursing models and theories* (2nd ed.). Philadelphia: Davis.

Fawcett, J., Watson, J., Neuman, B., Walker, P. H., & Fitzpatrick, J. J. (2001). On nursing theories and evidence. *Journal of Nursing Scholarship, 33,* 115–119.

Fitzpatrick, J. (2002). The balance in nursing: Clinical and scientific ways of knowing and being. *Nursing Education Perspectives, 23*(2), 57.

Fitzpatrick, M. L., & Heller, B. R. (1980). Teaching the teachers to teach. *Nursing Outlook, 28*(6), 372–373.

Goodin, H. J. (2003). The nursing shortage in the United States of America: An integrative review of the literature. *Journal of Advanced Nursing, 43,* 335–343.

Greiner, A. C., & Knebel, E. (Eds.). (2003). *Health professions education: A bridge to quality.* Washington, DC: National Academies Press.

Hathaway, D., Jacob, S., Stegbauer, C., Thompson, C., & Graff, C. (2006). The practice doctorate: Perspectives of early adopters. *Journal of Nursing Education, 45,* 487–496.

Health Resources and Services Administration. (2004). *The registered nurse population: National sample survey of registered nurses March 2004. Preliminary findings.* Retrieved from http://bhpr.hrsa.gov /healthworkforce/rnsurveys/rnsurvey2004.pdf

Heifetz, R. A. (1994). *Leadership without easy answers.* Cambridge, MA: Harvard University Press.

Hinshaw, A. (2001). A continuing challenge: The shortage of educationally prepared nursing faculty. *Online Journal of Issues in Nursing, 6*(1). Retrieved from http://www.nursingworld.org /MainMenuCategories/ANAMarketplace/ANAPeriodicals/OJIN/TableofContents/Volume62001 /No1Jan01/ShortageofEducationalFaculty.aspx

Institute of Medicine (IOM). (2011). *The future of nursing: Leading change, advancing health.* Washington, DC: National Academies Press.

Marion, L., Viens, D., O'Sullivan, A., Crabtree, K., Fontana, S., & Price, M. (2003). The practice doctorate in nursing: Future or fringe? *Topics in Advanced Nursing e-Journal, 3*(2). Retrieved from http://www .medscape.com/viewarticle/453247_1

Mullinix, C. F. (1990). The next shortage—the nurse educator. *Journal of Professional Nursing, 6*(3), 133.

National League for Nursing (NLN). (2002, May 18). *Position statement: The preparation of nurse educators.* Retrieved from http://www.nln.org/aboutnln/PositionStatements/prepofnursed02.htm

National League for Nursing (NLN). (2006). *Nurse educators 2006: A report on the faculty census survey of RN and graduate programs.* New York: National League for Nursing Press.

National Research Council. (2005). *Advancing the nation's health needs: NIH research training programs.* Washington, DC: National Academies Press.

Neuman, B., & Fawcett, J. (Eds.). (2001). *The Neuman systems model* (4th ed.). Upper Saddle River, NJ: Prentice Hall.

Peterson's Colleges of Nursing Database. (2002). (Special database created for AACN internal research purposes). Lawrenceville, NJ: Peterson's, a part of The Thomson Corporation.

Princeton, J. C. (1992). The teacher crisis in nursing education—revisited. *Nurse Educator, 17*(5), 34–37.

Rollet, J. (2010). *2009 National Salary and Workplace Survey.* Retrieved from http://nurse-practitioners-and-physician-assistants.advanceweb.com/Features/Top-Story/2009-National-Salary-and-Workplace-Survey-Results.aspx

Southern Regional Education Board (SREB). (2003). *SREB study indicates serious shortage of nursing faculty.* Atlanta, GA: Author. Retrieved from http://publications.sreb.org/2003/02N03-Nursing_Faculty.pdf

Sperhac, A., & Goodwin, L. (2003). Using multiple data sources for curriculum revision. *Journal of Pediatric Health Care, 17,* 169–175.

Tanner, C. A. (1999). Developing the new professorate. *Journal of Nursing Education, 38*(2), 51–52.

Zebelman, E., & Olswang, S. (1989). Student career goal changes during doctoral education in nursing. *Journal of Nursing Education, 28*(2), 53–73.

CHAPTER 7

The DNP Graduate as Ethical Consultant

■ Lisa Astalos Chism ■

"Act in such a way that you treat humanity, whether in your own person or in the person of any other, always at the same time as an end and never merely as a means to an end."

—*Immanuel Kant (1724–1804)*

The DNP graduate may integrate several roles such as leader, researcher, clinician, policy advocate, and educator. Within each of these roles, the DNP graduate will likely encounter various ethical scenarios. Many DNP curricula are currently including ethics coursework to prepare the DNP graduate with the skills necessary to evaluate ethical issues. Peirce and Smith (2008) believe that "there is a need for an expanded view of required ethics content in the curriculum of Doctor of Nursing Practice programs nationwide" (p. 270).

Ethics is defined as the principles of conduct governing an individual or group (Merriam-Webster, 2011b). An ethicist is one who specializes in or is very concerned with ethics (Merriam-Webster, 2011a). Although it may be presumptuous to describe a DNP graduate as an ethicist, a DNP graduate will likely be regarded as an ethical consultant in his or her setting. The DNP graduate may be consulted regarding research, clinical, leadership, and professional ethical scenarios (Peirce & Smith, 2008). Therefore, it is necessary for DNP graduates to develop an understanding of ethical content, including terms, inquiry, and theories. A review of ethical content will enable DNP graduates to evaluate ethical scenarios they may encounter within their setting and specific roles.

This chapter is not inclusive of the ethical content necessary for every potential ethical scenario a DNP graduate may evaluate. Instead, this chapter is intended to introduce or review certain ethical terms, inquiry, and theories that will give DNP graduates the tools to recognize ethical scenarios and obtain the information necessary for evaluation of these scenarios.

Highlighted concepts in bioethics are also reviewed. Nursing ethics is described, including a toolkit DNP graduates should be familiar with to evaluate ethical scenarios in their setting. Important content regarding ethical leadership is reviewed as well. Ethical standards regarding Internet and telehealth, also a concern of DNP graduates, are discussed. Finally, specific scenarios are reviewed to assist DNP graduates with ethical discussions.

■ First a Story . . .

Ethical dilemmas have been debated for centuries among philosophers and scientists. Over the last century, certain events have triggered bioethical concerns. One such event in 1951 involved a young African-American woman named Henrietta Lacks who was a tobacco farmer from Southern Virginia.

The granddaughter of slaves, Henrietta was raised by her grandfather on a tobacco farm. When she was 30 years old and had given birth to her fifth child, Henrietta began experiencing abdominal pain and knew something was wrong. Finally, she asked her husband to drive her to Johns Hopkins Hospital. At the time, Johns Hopkins was the only hospital in the area that would see African-American patients for free.

Henrietta was evaluated and a biopsy confirmed cancer of her cervix. She began radiation treatment, which required her to stay overnight in the hospital twice a month. During her stay, doctors removed several pieces of tissue from her cervix and began growing and studying the tissue. This was done without Henrietta's or her family's consent.

Attempts to grow cancerous tissue outside the body had been made several times without success. The hope was that these cells would help determine what caused cancer and contribute to the development of a cure. Henrietta's cells astonished doctors and scientists by surviving outside her body and continuing to divide. These cells were later named HeLa cells after Henrietta Lacks.

Unfortunately, the doctors could not save Henrietta and she succumbed to cervical cancer 6 months after she was diagnosed. Her cells, however, continued to thrive and reproduce and were found to be the first "immortal" cells discovered. Her family was not informed of this discovery until several years later.

HeLa cells led to several landmark developments in science and medicine. HeLa cells were later used to test a polio vaccine that led to the development of a treatment that saved and protected millions of people. Some of the HeLa cells were found to behave differently than others. Scientists learned how to isolate specific HeLa cells, multiply them, and create a new cell line. This discovery led to developments that became the basic techniques for in vitro fertilization and cloning. HeLa cells also were used to discover that humans have 46 chromosomes in 23 pairs, not 48. Because of this discovery, the basis of genetic testing and diagnosis was developed. Finally, anticancer drugs are currently in clinical trials due to the discovery that HeLa cells used an enzyme to repair their DNA.

It was 25 years after the cells were discovered that a scientist contacted Henrietta's family to obtain cell samples from them for further testing. Henrietta's husband had a third-grade education and did not understand what was being explained to him. This event led to a controversial, confusing journey for the family, who never knew Henrietta's cells had been taken. Her cells were in fact the first cells to be bought and sold for research and eventually led to a multibillion dollar industry.

This story may stir many emotions and raise multiple ethical questions. The people who took the cells had the best intentions in mind and many wonderful, life-changing discoveries were made as a result of Henrietta's cells. However, cells come from people who may have certain feelings and thoughts about their tissue being used.

Was the means justified by the end? Were Henrietta or her family harmed by the doctors taking the cells? What about all the people who have benefited from HeLa cells and the discoveries that were developed? This true story may help DNP graduates examine their own positions through self-reflection and review of ethical content.

To learn more about Henrietta Lacks's story, please refer to *The Immortal Life of Henrietta Lacks* by Rebecca Skloot (2010).

■ Back to the Basics

Developing an understanding of ethics will lead to "anticipating and recognizing health care dilemmas and making good judgments and decisions based on universal values that work in unison with the laws of the land, and our constitution" (Pozgar, 2010, p. 3). Further, ethics guides caregivers to "make right judgments as guided by using wisdom to do good" (Pozgar, 2010, p. 3). This section of the chapter provides DNP graduates with a review of basic ethical content including selected ethical terms, inquiry, and theories.

Ethical Terms

Ethics has been broadly defined as the principles of conduct governing an individual or group. More specifically, Butts and Rich (2008) define ethics as "the study of ideal human behavior and ideal ways of being" (p. 4). Butts and Rich (2008) also describe ethics as a process, or "doing ethics," whereby one's beliefs are supported by sound reasoning justified by "logical, theoretically based arguments" (p. 5). Ethics emphasizes "the rightness and wrongness of actions, as well as the goodness and badness of motives and ends" (Pozgar, 2010, p. 2). Ethics is also considered a moral philosophy, or discipline, concerned with what is morally right or wrong (Pozgar, 2010, p. 2).

Morals, on the other hand, are "specific beliefs, behaviors, and ways of being derived from doing ethics" (Butts & Rich, 2008, p. 5). The opposite of morality is immorality, which describes "behavior in opposition to accepted societal, religious, cultural or professional ethical standards and principles" (Butts & Rich, 2008, p. 5). Morals may be rooted in culture or religion. The evaluation of morality requires the DNP graduate to reach a decision of what is right or wrong within an ethical scenario.

A code of ethics describes standards of conduct and states certain principles regarding responsibilities and duties of those professionals to whom they apply (Pozgar, 2010). Professionals frequently subscribe to specific values or moral standards written into formal documents referred to as codes of ethics. The American Nurses Association (ANA) *Code of Ethics for Nurses* and the International Council of Nurses' (ICN) *Code of Ethics for Nurses* are examples of nursing codes of ethics and should be used as a resource for DNP graduates when evaluating ethical scenarios. These codes of ethics are discussed more fully later in the chapter.

Values have been defined as "ideals, beliefs, customs, modes of conduct, qualities, or goals that are highly prized or preferred by individuals, groups, or societies" (Burkhardt & Nathaniel, 2008, p. 83). Values may influence judgments one may make and reflect what one believes is good or bad. Values may also influence how one behaves or thinks; they may be learned and incorporated at an early age and continue to develop throughout one's life. This may occur through formal teaching by parents, teachers, or professional leaders. More informal values may be developed through socialization and role modeling (Burkhardt & Nathaniel, 2008).

Reasoning describes the "use of abstract thought processes to think creatively, to answer questions, solve problems, and to formulate strategies for one's actions and desired ways of being" (Butts & Rich, 2008, p. 9). Moral reasoning relates to reasoning that focuses on moral or ethical issues. Socrates believed that moral reasoning was "inherent to rational beings, waiting to be drawn forth" (Forman, & Ladd, 1991, p. 1). Conversely, Forman and Ladd believed "one learns to recognize good reasons by engaging in discussion and debate, considering opposite views, and questioning oneself and others" (p. 1).

Ethical Inquiry

The study of ethics includes various types of ethical inquiry. Normative ethics involves prescribing values, behaviors, and ways of being that are considered right or wrong when deciding what to do in a specific situation (Butts & Rich, 2008). This type of ethical inquiry involves evaluating what is right, what is good, and what is genuine (Pozgar, 2010). When applying normative ethics, one is applying accepted moral standards and codes. One form of accepted moral standard is common morality. "Common morality consists of normative beliefs and behaviors that the members of society generally agree about and are familiar to most human beings" (Butts & Rich, 2008, p. 6).

Applied ethics may attempt to explain moral problems common in health care such as assisted suicide and euthanasia. Meta-ethics involves applying the understanding of the language of morality through the meaning of related concepts such as virtuous and good (Butts & Rich, 2008). Contrary to normative ethics, meta-ethics does not apply what ought to be done "because it is right" but instead is concerned with the meaning of what a "good" outcome would be. Descriptive ethics is more concrete and describes what one thinks about morality or moral behavior (Butts & Rich, 2008). Descriptive ethics is also referred to as comparative ethics and describes what one believes is right or wrong (Pozgar, 2010). Descriptive ethics also pertains to professional moral values and behaviors that can be examined through research.

Ethical Theories

Ethical theories serve as guidelines when individuals question what they should do or how they ought to be. Ethical theories also provide justification for why one chooses to do something a certain way, especially when faced with a moral dilemma. The following theories discussed are highlighted ethical theories from Butts and Rich's (2008) nursing ethics textbook titled *Nursing Ethics: Across the Curriculum and Into Practice*. These theories were chosen due to their relevance when discussing nursing ethics and the DNP graduate.

Virtue Ethics

Virtue ethics emphasizes the "excellence of one's character and considerations of sort of person one wants to be" (Butts & Rich, 2008, p. 18). Virtue ethics focuses on the inherent character of a person rather than on specific actions (Pozgar, 2010). This particular theory is closely linked to the beliefs of Aristotle, who thought a person of virtue was one who was an excellent friend, critical thinker, and citizen. Plato and Hume also described similar approaches to value ethics. Plato described the four virtues of prudence, fortitude, temperance, and justice (Butts & Rich, 2008). Hume related that virtues stemmed from "the natural human tendency to be sympathetic and benevolent toward other people" (Butts & Rich, 2008, p. 19).

Beauchamp and Childress (2009) describe five focal virtues of the healthcare professional: compassion, discernment, trustworthiness, integrity, and conscientiousness. Compassion as a virtue is focused on others and involves concern regarding others' pain, suffering, disability, and misery. Discernment involves the recognition and insight one exhibits when deciding the appropriate action to take in a given situation (Burkhardt & Nathaniel, 2008). Trustworthiness entails the belief that another will act with the right motives consistent with moral norms (Beauchamp & Childress, 2009). Integrity includes soundness, reliability, wholeness, and integration of moral character (Beauchamp & Childress). Conscientiousness describes one being motivated to do the right thing because it is right and extends the appropriate effort to do so (Beauchamp & Childress).

Natural Law Theory

Natural law theory stems from the philosophy of St. Thomas Aquinas. This theory emphasizes that the "law of reason is implanted in the order of nature (usually thought to be implanted by God)" and provides the rules of human nature (Butts & Rich, 2008, p. 21). Natural law theory is frequently associated with Judeo-Christian ethics.

Deontology

Deontology, or the study of duty, is an ethical theory that focuses on duties and rules. Deontology also describes the view that the "rightness or wrongness of an act depends upon the nature of the act, rather than its consequences" (Burkhardt & Nathaniel, 2008, p. 39). The term "deontology" is Greek for "duty." Deontology is sometimes referred to as Kantianism after Immanuel Kant. Immanuel Kant (1724–1804) was a German philosopher who prescribed that individuals' moral worth is determined by their dutiful actions. Moreover, if acting from Kant's philosophy, one is bound to duty over love. Many professional codes of ethics are based on Kant's principles such as the ethical codes used in nursing. These principles within the ANA *Code of Ethics for Nurses* and the ICN *Code of Ethics for Nurses* are so inherent to nursing, they are often unnoticed (Butts & Rich, 2008). Deontology is a useful ethical theory in that it provides clear guidelines for evaluating the wrongness or rightness of an action.

Principlism

Principlism uses principles that serve as rules for conduct dictated by duty. Common principles include beneficence and autonomy. Principlism is reflected in the basis of bioethics as well as positions related to patients' rights.

Utilitarianism

Simply broken down, utilitarianism describes actions that are judged by their utility. When employing the theory of utilitarianism, emphasis is placed on promoting the greatest good and inflicting the least amount of harm possible (Butts & Rich, 2008). Utilitarianism is also described as a "moral theory that holds that an action is judged as good or bad in relation to the consequence, outcome, or end result that is derived from it" (Burkhardt & Nathaniel, 2008, p. 33). Further, the greatest good of groups, rather than individuals, is emphasized.

Casuistry

Casuistry describes considering specific situations individually when making ethical decisions. Additionally, outcomes or similar cases in the past are considered when making ethical decisions. Casuists emphasize the importance of past cases, history, precedents, and past circumstances (Beauchamp & Childress, 2009). Social consensus is formed around past cases and this consensus becomes authoritative for new cases (Beauchamp & Childress). Current healthcare ethics committees utilize this theory when considering individual ethical issues related to patients (Butts & Rich, 2008).

Narrative Ethics

Similar to casuistry, narrative ethics is a story-based approach to making ethical decisions. Narrative ethics focuses on personal life narratives interacting with others' personal life narratives (Butts & Rich, 2008). When evaluating an ethical scenario using this theory, an individual's personal narrative stories are considered when making ethical decisions.

Critical Theory

Critical theory broadly describes "theories and worldviews that address the domination perpetrated by specific powerful groups of people and resulting in the oppression of other specific groups of people" (Butts & Rich, 2008, p. 27). For example, feminist ethics is utilized to examine how ethical situations affect women. An ethic of care, frequently utilized by nurses, is based on the ethical experiences of women and feminist ethics. Specifically, an ethic of care emphasizes traits considered feminine such as love, compassion, sympathy, and concern for the well-being of other people (Butts & Rich, 2008). Beauchamp and Childress (2009) also describe an ethic of care as traits valued in intimate, interpersonal relationships such as fidelity and love. Caring is further defined as "to care for, emotional commitment to and deep willingness to act on behalf of persons with whom one has a significant relationship" (Beauchamp & Childress, 2009, p. 36). This theory is familiar ground for many in the nursing profession and therefore relevant for DNP graduates as a basis of ethical decision making.

■ Bioethics: Expanding the Basics

Throughout the 20th century, numerous scientific advances, scarcity of medical resources, and unethical research studies led to the development of a branch of ethics termed bioethics. Bioethics is defined as "the philosophical study of ethical controversies brought about by advances in biology, research, and medicine" (Pozgar, 2010, p. 403). The following section of this chapter reviews bioethical principles relevant for DNP graduates.

The Birth of Bioethics

Among the many events that led to the birth of bioethics, the Tuskegee Syphilis Experiment led to the establishment of the Office for Human Research Protections (OHRP) and the federal regulation requiring institutional review boards for the protection of human subjects enrolled in research studies (OHRP, 2005). The Tuskegee Syphilis Experiment was a clinical study conducted between 1923 and 1972 in Tuskegee, Alabama developed by the U.S. Public Health Service to study the progression of untreated syphilis. The study subjects included 399 impoverished African-American sharecroppers from Mason County, Alabama who were infected with syphilis. The men were not informed of the purpose of the study, nor that they had syphilis. Instead, they were told they had "bad blood," a local term describing several medical illnesses (NPR, 2002). For their participation in the study, the men were given free medical care, free meals, and free burial services. In the 1940s, penicillin was found to be effective in the treatment of syphilis but many still did not receive this treatment in order to prolong the study and observe full, long-term progression of the disease. In fact, to ensure that men would continue with the painful spinal taps used in the study, a misleading letter was sent out titled "Last Chance for Special Free Treatment." Their burial expenses were not paid for until an autopsy was done for further investigation (CDC, 2011).

In 1972, the Tuskegee Syphilis Study was made public by a whistleblower who leaked information to the press and the study ended. At that time, 74 of the men were still alive, 28 had died of syphilis, 100 had died from complications related to syphilis,

40 of their wives had become infected with syphilis, and 19 of their children were born with congenital syphilis (CDC, 2011). The public knowledge of this study led to a series of developments related to bioethics.

In 1974, Congress passed the National Research Act to regulate studies involving human participants. In 1997, President Clinton apologized on behalf of the nation for the tragic consequences of the Tuskegee Syphilis Study. In 2001, the President's Council on Bioethics was formed. The Centers for Disease Control and Prevention provided $10 million in 2004 for the Tuskegee University National Center for Bioethics in Research and Health Center, and in 2006, the Bioethics Center at Tuskegee University was formally opened (CDC, 2011).

As a result of the National Research Act, a commission was created to define the principles supported for research involving human subjects and a 4-day conference was held at the Belmont Conference Center at the Smithsonian. In 1976, the commission released its report titled "The Belmont Report." This report outlined three principles for all human subject research: respect for persons, beneficence, and justice (National Commission, 1978). The principle of nonmaleficence, or to do no harm, was described in the Belmont Report under the principle beneficence.

Soon after the Belmont Report was released, in 1979 Beauchamp and Childress published their book *Principles in Biomedical Ethics*, which is currently in its sixth edition. Beauchamp and Childress (2009) outline four biomedical principles described as autonomy, beneficence, nonmaleficence, and justice. These principles are used today when ethical principlism is invoked to analyze and resolve many health care–related ethical scenarios.

Autonomy

Beauchamp and Childress (2009) refer to the ethical principle autonomy as respect for autonomy. Personal autonomy has been defined as "self-rule that is free from controlling interference by others and from certain limitations such as inadequate understanding that prevents meaningful choice" (Beauchamp & Childress, 2009, p. 103). Respect for autonomy involves more than simply noninterference from others. It includes "building up or maintaining others' capacities for autonomous choice and other conditions that destroy or disrupt autonomous action" (Beauchamp & Childress, 2009, p. 103). According to Beauchamp and Childress (2009), specific moral rules are supported by respect for autonomy. These moral truths include: "1) Tell the truth, 2) Respect the privacy of others, 3) Protect confidential information, 4) Obtain consent for interventions with patients, 5) When asked, help others make important decisions" (Beauchamp & Childress, 2009, p. 104).

Informed consent describes the "process by which patients are informed of possible outcomes, alternatives, and risks of treatment, and are required to give their consent freely" (Burkhardt & Nathaniel, 2008, p. 58). Informed consent involves respecting the person's autonomy to make their decisions based on the appropriate information given to them regarding a specific circumstance or potential outcome. Respect for autonomy clearly emphasizes the importance of informed consent.

From a cultural perspective, Dayer-Berenson (2011) relates that "how much or how little autonomy a patient wishes to express is culturally mediated" (p. 113). In an effort to be culturally sensitive to a patient's autonomy, the process of informed consent should involve meaningful discussion regarding healing methods and expected or desired outcomes as opposed to a one-sided explanation of specific risks and benefits of a treatment or procedure (Dayer-Berenson, 2011). This process includes the cultural perspectives of others and allows for informed decision making by patients and their families.

Beneficence

The principle of beneficence refers to "the moral obligation to act for the benefit of others" (Beauchamp & Childress, 2009, p. 197). Beneficence describes the acts that are generally doing good, helping others, and showing compassion (Pozgar, 2010). Beyond simply doing good for others, beneficence requires that one knows the beliefs, cultures, and values of others in order to act in their best interest.

Paternalism is a form of beneficence that involves individuals or institutions believing they know what is best for the patient/person and thus making decisions for them (Pozgar, 2010). Beauchamp and Childress (2009) define paternalism as "the intentional overriding of the person's preferences or actions by another person, where the person who overrides justifies this action by appeal to the goal of benefiting or of preventing or mitigating harm to the person whose preferences are overridden" (p. 208). Paternalistic acts may include deception, manipulation of information, lying, nondisclosure of information, or use of force or coercion (Beauchamp & Childress, 2009).

Nonmaleficence

The principle of nonmaleficence describes the obligation to "do no harm." Nonmaleficence is concerned with avoiding the infliction of harm on others. Beauchamp and Childress (2009) make a specific distinction between beneficence and nonmaleficence where beneficence is a more active principle that requires one to take an active role to help others by preventing harm, removing harm, or promoting good. Nonmaleficence simply requires intentionally refraining from doing harm.

Justice

The principle of justice refers to "fairness, treating people equally and without prejudice, and with the equitable distribution of benefits and burdens" (Butts & Rich, 2008, p. 48). Justice involves treating all persons in similar circumstances similarly. Social justice describes how all people should have the same rights, benefits, and opportunities (Butts & Rich, 2008).

■ Nursing Ethics

Nursing ethics has been defined as an extension of bioethics where ethical issues are viewed from a nursing perspective (Butts & Rich, 2008). Nursing ethics draws from traditional bioethics and extends the meaning of these principles to scenarios nurses are often faced with in their profession. Further, the focus of nursing ethics is relationship based and involves issues that are related to relationships between nurses and their patients or nurse and their colleagues (Butts & Rich, 2008).

ANA Code of Ethics for Nurses

The American Nurses Association (ANA) *Code of Ethics for Nurses with Interpretive Statements* is considered the standard for nurses to refer to as their code for ethical behavior. The ANA *Code of Ethics* "makes explicit the primary goals, values, and obligations of the profession" (ANA, 2001, p. 9). The ANA *Code of Ethics* serves the following purposes:

1. "It is a succinct statement of the ethical obligations and duties of every individual who enters the nursing profession;
2. It is the profession's nonnegotiable nursing standard;
3. It is an expression of nursing's own understanding of its commitment to society." (ANA, 2001, p. 9)

The code reflects several approaches to evaluating ethical scenarios such as using ethical theories, ethical principles, and cultivating virtues.

The ANA *Code of Ethics for Nurses* includes nine provisions accompanied by interpretive statements that give more specific interpretations for practice. This code provides a framework for nurses to use in ethical evaluation and decision making. The ANA *Code of Ethics* is essential for all DNP graduates to use when evaluating ethical scenarios. The entire ANA *Code of Ethics for Nurses with Interpretive Statements* may be viewed at http://www.nursingworld.org/MainMenuCategories/EthicsStandards/CodeofEthicsforNurses.aspx. Certain provisions of the code are highlighted for DNP graduates as they are considered to have focal importance to the ethical scenarios DNP graduates may encounter. However, DNP graduates should become familiar with every provision of the ANA *Code of Ethics for Nurses*, along with interpretive statements.

Provision 1

"The nurse, in all professional relationships, practices with compassion and respect for the inherent dignity, worth, uniqueness of every individual, unrestricted by considerations of social or economic status, personal attributes, or nature of health problems" (ANA, 2001, p. 11).

Interpretive statements within this provision include respect for human dignity, relationship to patients, nature of health problems, right to self-determination, and relationships with colleagues and others (ANA, 2001). DNP graduates will likely reflect on this provision when evaluating patients' individual needs, rights, and values. This provision may also be used as a guide when DNP graduates are evaluating clinical ethical scenarios within their clinician roles. This provision will be essential to informed consent in the clinical setting. Finally, this provision provides guidance when evaluating scenarios related to interprofessional collaboration among colleagues.

Provision 2

"The nurse's primary commitment is to the patient, whether an individual, family, group, or community" (ANA, 2001, p. 14).

The interpretive statements within this provision include primacy of patients' interests, conflict of interest for nurses, collaboration, and professional boundaries (ANA, 2001). DNP graduates in leadership roles should reflect on this provision when evaluating ethical scenarios related to community programs or resources. Also, DNP graduates in leadership, clinician, education, or research roles will be concerned with conflicts of interest when allocating resources or spending within an organization. Clinicians will also be concerned with this provision when billing directly for services. Collaboration will also be a concern of DNP graduates when evaluating ethical scenarios related to interprofessional collaboration such as participation in multidisciplinary team meetings or ethics committees.

Provision 3

"The nurse promotes, advocates for, and strives to protect the health, safety, and rights of the patient" (ANA, 2001, p. 16).

Interpretive statements within this provision include privacy, confidentiality, protection of participants in research, standards and review mechanisms, acting on questionable practice, and addressing impaired practice (ANA, 2001). DNP graduates in all roles will be concerned with this provision. Potential ethical scenarios for which DNP graduates may use this provision as a guide include any violation to patients' privacy, confidentiality, and informed consent to participate in research. Additionally, DNP graduates in clinical and leadership roles may encounter ethical scenarios related to addressing impaired or questionable practice and use this provision to guide ethical evaluation.

Provision 5

"The nurse owes the same duties to self as to others, including the responsibility to preserve integrity and safety, to maintain competence, and to continue personal growth and professional growth" (ANA, 2001, p. 23).

The interpretive statements within this provision include moral self-respect, professional growth and maintenance of competence, wholeness of character, and preservation of integrity (ANA, 2001). DNP graduates may use this provision as a guide when evaluating ethical scenarios related to the maintenance of specialty certification for advanced practice registered nurses. Personally, DNP graduates may reflect on this provision when evaluating their own contributions to the nursing profession. DNP graduates may also use this provision as a guide when threats to personal integrity are evident such as verbal abuse from patients or coworkers.

Provision 7

"The nurse participates in the advancement of the profession through contributions to practice, education, administrative, and knowledge development" (ANA, 2001, p. 27).

Interpretive statements within this provision include advancing the profession through active involvement in nursing and healthcare policy; advancing the profession by developing, maintaining, and implementing professional standards in clinical, administrative, and educational practice; and advancing the profession through knowledge development, dissemination, and application to practice (ANA, 2001). DNP graduates may use this provision as a guide when evaluating ethical scenarios related to the DNP degree itself. DNP graduates in administrative roles may use this provision when evaluating ethical scenarios related to professional standards when employing nurses. Finally, DNP graduates may use this provision as a guide when evaluating scenarios related to scientific inquiry in nursing and related issues.

Provision 9

"The profession of nursing, as represented by associations and their members, is responsible for articulating nursing values, for maintaining the integrity of the profession and its practice, and shaping social policy" (ANA, 2001, p. 29).

The interpretive statements within this provision include assertion of values, profession carries out its collective responsibility through professional associations, intra-professional integrity, and social reform (ANA, 2001). The DNP graduate is charged with upholding nursing organizations' values and ethical standards. Further, DNP graduates have a role in shaping policy and social reform. Therefore, DNP graduates may use this provision as a guide when evaluating ethical scenarios related to socio-cultural issues such as homelessness, hunger, violence, and the stigma of illness.

ICN Code of Ethics for Nurses

The International Council of Nurses *Code of Ethics for Nurses* was initially adopted by the ICN in 1953. The code has been revised several times, most recently in 2005. This ICN code should also be used as a guide for DNP graduates when evaluating ethical scenarios. The ICN code is based on the four responsibilities of nurses: "to promote health, to prevent illness, to restore health, and alleviate suffering" (ICN, 2006, p. 1). The ICN *Code of Ethics for Nurses* has four principal elements that outline the standard of ethical conduct:

Elements of the Code

1. Nurses and People
   - The nurses' primary professional responsibility is to people requiring nursing care. In providing care, the nurse promotes an environment in which the human rights, values, customs, and spiritual beliefs of the individual, family, and community are respected.
   - The nurse ensures that the individual receives sufficient information on which to base consent for care and the related treatment.
   - The nurse holds in confidence personal information and uses judgment in sharing this information.

- The nurse shares with society the responsibility for initiating and supporting action to meet the health and social needs of the public, in particular those of vulnerable populations.
- The nurse also shares responsibility to sustain and protect the natural environment from depletion, pollution, degradation, and destruction.

2. Nurses and Practice

- The nurse carries personal responsibility and accountability for nursing practice, and for maintaining competence by continual learning.
- The nurse maintains a standard of personal health such that the ability to provide care is not compromised.
- The nurse uses judgment regarding individual competence when accepting and delegating responsibility.
- The nurse at all times maintains standards of personal conduct that reflect well on the profession and enhance public confidence.
- The nurse, in providing care, ensures that use of technology and scientific advances are compatible with the safety, dignity, and rights of people.

3. Nurses and the Profession

- The nurse assumes the major role in determining and implementing acceptable standards of clinical nursing practice, management, research, and education.
- The nurse is active in developing a core of research-based professional knowledge.
- The nurse, acting through the professional organization, participates in creating and maintaining safe, equitable social and economic working conditions in nursing.

4. Nurses and Coworkers

- The nurse sustains a cooperative relationship with coworkers in nursing and other fields.
- The nurse takes appropriate action to safeguard individuals, families, and communities when their health is endangered by a coworker or any other person.[1]

Nursing's Social Policy Statement

Nursing's Social Policy Statement is a document that nurses can use as a framework for understanding nursing's relationship with society and nursing's obligation to those who receive nursing care (ANA, 2010b). Silva and Ludwick (2006) questioned whether or not the DNP degree itself was ethical in relation to *Nursing's Social Policy Statement*. In their discussion, they questioned why *Nursing's Social Policy Statement* was not used when the DNP degree's foundational framework was developed. *Nursing's Social Policy Statement* is indeed another tool DNP graduates should use as a guide when

---

[1]Reprinted with permission of the ICN.

evaluating ethical scenarios, especially when faced with social issues. The values of the nursing profession and social responsibility are described within *Nursing's Social Policy Statement*. Additionally, nursing's scope of practice and regulation of nursing practice are described within this statement, which may be needed when DNP graduates in clinical or leadership roles evaluate ethical scenarios related to practice and regulation of practice.

Nursing Ethics Summary

The ANA *Code of Ethics for Nurses*, the ICN *Code of Ethics for Nurses*, and *Nursing's Social Policy Statement* are all necessary elements of the DNP graduate's nursing ethics toolkit. Although every ethical scenario will be unique, DNP graduates should use these tools as guides to ensure that the ethical standards of the nursing profession are upheld. Ways to access the ANA *Code of Ethics for Nursing*, the ICN *Code of Ethics for Nurses*, and *Nursing's Social Policy Statement* are detailed in **Table 7-1**.

▪ Ethical Leadership Tools for the Ethical Leader

DNP graduates will likely be in leadership roles within their clinical setting or academic environment or in more formal leadership roles within healthcare organizations. Gallagher and Tschudin (2009) describe three levels of leadership in which nurses may engage that will require a grasp of ethical leadership. These three levels are noted to be consistent with the envisioned leadership roles that DNP graduates will likely be engaged in. Gallagher and Tschudin (2009) described these levels as:

> "The micro-level, where nurses provide leadership as role models in their work with individuals and teams; the meso-level, where nurses contribute to organizational discussions and policy development; and the macro-level, where nurses engage politically, lobbying politicians and ensuring their voice is heard in national and international forums." (p. 225)

Table 7-1   **Resources for the DNP Ethical Consultant**

- International Council of Nurses *Code of Ethics for Nurses*, http://www.icn.ch/about-icn /code-of-ethics-for-nurses
- American Nurses Association *Code of Ethics for Nurses*, http://www.nursingworld.org /MainMenuCategories/EthicsStandards/CodeofEthicsforNurses.aspx
- *Guide to the Code of Ethics for Nurses* (2010), American Nurses Association, http://www .nursesbooks.org/Main-Menu/Ethics/Guide-to-the-Code-of-Ethics-for-Nurses.aspx
- *Nursing's Social Policy Statement, Third Edition* (2010), American Nurses Association, http://www .nursesbooks.org/Main-Menu/Foundation/Nursings-Social-Policy-Statement.aspx
- *Principles of Biomedical Ethics* (2009), Beauchamp and Childress, Oxford University Press
- *Nursing Ethics: Across the Curriculum and Into Practice* (2008), Butts and Rich, Jones & Bartlett Learning
- *eHealth Code of Ethics*, eHealth Ethics Initiative, http://www.ihealthcoalition.org /ehealth-code

DNP graduates within leadership roles must have a firm understanding of ethics content (reviewed earlier in the chapter), traits of ethical leaders, ethical decision-making models, and methods to prevent ethical conflicts. Piper (2007) relates that healthcare leaders need specific knowledge of ethics. This knowledge should include a "definition of ethics, ethical conflict and ethical dilemmas, along with a methodology to examine ethics within an organization" (Piper, 2007, p. 249).

Traits of Ethical Leaders

Paul B. Hofmann, DrPH, FACHE, president of the Hofmann Healthcare Group, presented at an ethics program titled "Rising to the Ethical Challenges of Healthcare Leadership" in the fall of 2008. He described what specific behavioral traits are essential for an ethics leader. These six traits were described as:

1. "Ethically conscious, having an appreciation for the ethical dimensions and implications of one's daily actions and decisions;
2. Ethically committed, being completely committed to doing the right thing;
3. Ethically competent, having the knowledge and understanding necessary to make ethically sound decisions;
4. Ethically courageous, acting upon these competencies even when the action may not be accepted with enthusiasm or endorsement;
5. Ethically consistent, establishing and maintaining a high ethical standard without making or rationalizing inconvenient exceptions. Also, be able to rebuff the pressures to equivocate, to accommodate and to justify an action or decision that is ethically flawed;
6. Ethically candid, being open and forthright about the complexity of reconciling conflicting values, be willing to ask uncomfortable questions and be an active, not a passive, advocate of ethical analysis and ethical conduct." (Hofmann, 2008, as cited in Buell, 2009, p. 54)

These six traits are admirable and noteworthy traits that DNP graduates should strive to embody when encountering ethical scenarios in leadership positions. DNP graduates in leadership roles should reflect regularly on these traits in an effort to ensure they are practicing ethical leadership.

Ethical Decision-Making Model

A model for ethical decision making that may be applicable to various scenarios DNP graduates may encounter is reviewed later in the chapter. However, ethical decision making for leaders is somewhat more unique and requires an approach that considers "stakeholders" and "organizational" effects of the ethical decision. When discussing the ethical leader, Sanford (2006) reviews specific "Steps to Ethical Management Decisions." This model takes into account the effect on organizational politics that leaders making ethical decisions will have to consider. This model also notes that many "stakeholders" are involved in the decisions made. Sanford describes this model in seven steps:

1. "Identify the issue/question;
2. Identify the stakeholders who will be affected by the solution/answer. These may include customers/patients, staff/employees, the organization, the community, medical staff, and others;
3. List possible solutions/answers;
4. Evaluate each stakeholder's viewpoint, consider which decision will do the most harm or good today and in the future;
5. Identify the organization's decision-making rules;
6. Make the decision including evaluating if you can explain why you made this decision and would you be proud of this decision if it was on the front page of your local newspaper;
7. Act and reflect on the action including evaluating the results of the action and learning from the evaluation to improve ethical decision making in the future." (2006, p. 9)

Sanford also offers this insightful advice DNP graduates should note regarding ethical leadership: "Ethical leaders realize that a short term 'win' at the expense of the future is not a 'win' at all but smoke and mirrors used to make the manager look good today" (2006, p. 7).

Ethical Conflict

In addition to evaluating ethical scenarios, DNP graduates in leadership roles will also have a responsibility to prevent ethical conflict within an organization. Although many ethical conflicts are unavoidable, Piper (2007) proposed recommendations to prevent ethical conflicts. These recommendations ensure that an ethical culture exists within the organization thereby preventing potential ethical conflicts.

First, Piper (2007) suggests that "great people" with "ethics as a key principle of their values" are necessary to ensure that ethical conduct is practiced by everyone in the organization (p. 253). Second, "great leadership" is necessary to set the example of ethical conduct (Piper, p. 253). The leader must hold everyone in the organization accountable for ethical behavior and create an organizational culture of ethics. Third, a "great governing board" is necessary to hold the standards of ethical conduct and support the leadership in creating a culture of ethics (Piper, p. 253). Fourth, an "ethics policy" should be developed that "addresses ethical behavior and how to address ethical conflicts" (Piper, p. 253). The policy should outline a definition of ethics and the principles and guidelines used to handle ethical conflicts. Fifth, an "ethics consultant" with expertise in this area should perform an ethics evaluation (Piper, p. 253). This evaluation of the leadership, policies, and procedures would examine the justice and fairness in various departments within the organization such as human resources, finance, and healthcare delivery (Piper).

Summary of Ethical Leadership

The DNP graduate may engage in leadership roles ranging from role modeling in a practice environment to chief nursing officer of a large organization. Therefore, tools for ethical leadership are imperative for the DNP graduate to successfully evaluate ethical scenarios in leadership roles. These tools include traits necessary for ethical leadership, an ethical leadership decision-making tool, and recommendations for avoiding ethical conflicts. These tools are not inclusive of those necessary for DNP graduates to evaluate ethical leadership scenarios but rather provide exemplars for the DNP graduate to begin the process of ethical leadership.

■ Telehealth Ethics: Ethical Concerns in the 21st Century

The 21st century presents unique ethical scenarios for the DNP graduate with the development of telehealth. Telehealth, sometimes referred to as telemedicine, encompasses all healthcare delivery that involves information technology. Telehealth spans the use of information technology from electronic medical records to patients seeking information on the Internet. Telenursing is more specifically "the provision of nursing care utilizing any form of electronic media" (Burkhardt & Nathaniel, 2008, p. 172). With the advent of telehealth comes unique ethical scenarios DNP graduates will likely encounter.

Electronic Medical Records

An electronic medical record (EMR) is defined as a computer application that electronically stores individually identifiable health data (Layman, 2008). The development of EMRs has raised certain ethical scenarios, most dealing with privacy. It is therefore prudent to make the distinction between "ethics" and "regulation." Ethics has been defined as the principles of conduct governing an individual or group (Merriam-Webster, 2011b). "Codes of ethics are not legally binding but rather voluntary standards a profession or industry adopts" (Simpson, 2005, p. 179). Regulations "include laws and the official policies the healthcare organizations employ" (Simpson, 2005, p. 179).

However, there are scenarios where ethics and regulations are intertwined and violating an ethical principle may result in legal consequences. The Health Insurance Portability and Accountability Act of 1996 (HIPAA) is an example of a law born from an ethical principle. HIPAA has also been referred to as the Privacy Rule. "A major goal of the Privacy Rule is to assure that individuals' health information is properly protected while allowing the flow of health information needed to provide and promote high quality health care and to protect the public's health and well being" (U.S. Department of Health and Human Services, 2011). The Privacy Rule attempts to protect patients' medical information, both paper and online.

The development of EMRs has prompted ethical discussions related to certain ethical principles. EMRs have been noted by most to be beneficent and purported to do good for others (Layman, 2008). However, EMRs have raised concerns regarding the principle of autonomy. Autonomy "requires that the clinician do all he or she reasonably can to respect the patient's right to make an informed decision pertaining to actions the clinician may or may not take on their behalf and to have personal information protected" (Fleming, Edison, & Hon Pak, 2009, p. 798).

Protecting patients' health information is much more challenging with the development of EMRs. EMR data can be "accessed by almost anyone, simultaneously, at anytime, from anywhere" (Phillips & Fleming, 2009, p. 329). EMR may contain highly sensitive information such as social and family history, lifestyle, medications, medical conditions, and genetic information. HIPAA requirements include restrictions regarding user IDs and passwords to access this information, but unfortunately, these regulations are sometimes violated and so is patient privacy.

EMRs may also be used to promote or hinder the ethical principle of justice. EMRs may be viewed as a source of health information that can increase patients' compliance and self-management (Layman, 2008). However, where inequity exists, such as families and patients who cannot afford a computer, this information may not be accessible. In this instance, lack of access to EMRs may be viewed as injustice (Layman, 2008).

Internet Information Seeking

Patients frequently seek information from the Internet to manage their own health. Patients can access everything from healthcare plans to healthcare providers, insurers, and healthcare facilities (Butts & Rich, 2008). Unfortunately, many cannot adequately evaluate health information on the Internet and healthcare professionals are faced with helping patients safely navigate the Internet and the vast amount of health information available. The Internet Healthcare Coalition published an *eHealth Code of Ethics* in an effort "to ensure that people worldwide can confidently and with full understanding of known risks realize the potential of the Internet in managing their own health and the health of those in their care" (Healthcare Coalition, 2010). This code of conduct is used by "marketers, health professionals, and creators of Web sites in an attempt to enhance a trustworthy environment for consumers of health information, products, and services" (Butts & Rich, 2008, p. 109). The *eHealth Code of Ethics* consists of eight principles based on autonomy, or respect for persons. These principles are as follows:

Candor: Disclose only information that is beneficial to the consumer. Sites should clearly indicate who owns or has an interest in the site or service and the purpose of the site or service.

Honesty: Be truthful and not deceptive. Clearly distinguish content intended to promote or sell a product, service, or organization from educational or scientific content.

Quality: Provide health information that is accurate, easy to understand, and up to date that allows users to make their own judgments about the health information, products, or services provided by the site.

Informed Consent: Respect users' right to when and how their personal data may be collected, used, or shared.

Privacy: Respect and protect the privacy of others.

Professionalism in Online Health Care: Respect ethical obligations to patients and inform and educate patients about the limitations of healthcare information on the Internet.

Responsible Partnering: Evaluate the trustworthiness of the organizations and websites.

Accountability: Provide the opportunity for users to give feedback, evaluate the website, and monitor the compliance of the *eHealth Code of Ethics*.

The *eHealth Code of Ethics* can be accessed at http://www.ihealthcoalition.org /ehealth-code. DNP graduates should become familiar with and use this code when evaluating ethical scenarios related to consumer information on the Internet.

Tweeting, Facebooking, and Chatting: Ethical Perils of Social Networks

The advent of social networks presents a whole new threat to patient privacy. DNP graduates will likely encounter ethical scenarios related to social networking. Unfortunately, violators of patient privacy may involve patients, consumers, and healthcare providers.

Facebook offers subscribers the ability to connect electronically to friends and colleagues all over the world. Facebook has approximately 800 million users worldwide (Facebook Press Release, 2011). Healthcare professionals using social networks must be mindful of professional boundaries and patients' rights to privacy. The Privacy Rule, or HIPAA, "applies to any healthcare provider who electronically transfers information in connection with certain transactions including both institutional and individual providers" (Hader & Brown, 2010, p. 271). The Privacy Rule protects any health-related information in paper, electronic, or oral form. Posting patient information, even when seemingly not identifiable, is still a violation of HIPAA and of a patient's autonomy.

The ANA *Code of Ethics for Nurses*, the ICN *Code of Ethics for Nurses*, and the basic principles of bioethics clearly support the need to protect patients' privacy. Blogging, posting, tweeting, or chatting about patients or patients' personal health information is a clear violation of ethics and the law. Due to the novelty of social networks, it is imperative that DNP graduates remain mindful of this new exchange of information and ensure responsible social networking among themselves and their colleagues.

Telehealth and Ethics Summary

The 21st century has brought wonderful advances to information technology and health care. With these advances come new challenges and responsibilities for DNP graduates. Specifically, DNP graduates have a responsibility to be aware of new ethical scenarios and develop the skills to evaluate these scenarios. DNP graduates need not only a grasp of ethical content but also an understanding of information technologies and new developments within telehealth. Fleming, Edison, and Hon Pak (2009) stated "Technology is neither ethical nor unethical . . . rather it is the intent and means by which the technology is implemented that impacts the question of appropriate utilization" (p. 797).

■ Ethical Decision-Making Model

As previously stated, due to their positions in leadership, research, clinical practice, and academia, DNP graduates will likely be asked to evaluate various ethical scenarios within their roles. Once a basic understanding of ethical, bioethical, and nursing ethics content is developed, DNP graduates are equipped to begin the process of critically evaluating ethical scenarios. However, evaluation of ethical scenarios is a *process* that DNP graduates will need to develop throughout their careers. With experience, understanding of ethical content, and a diligent commitment to upholding the ethical standards of the nursing profession, DNP graduates will become more proficient at this process.

Burkhardt and Nathaniel (2008) developed an ethical decision-making model that may be useful for DNP graduates when an ethical scenario is presented. This model is based on the premise that ethical decision making is "a process that overlays other dynamic biological, psychological, and social processes—layer upon layer" (Burkhardt & Nathaniel, 2008, p. 128). Further, the process of ethical decision making requires ongoing evaluation and assimilation of information, making way for an evolving perspective that may change over time. This model allows for evolving perspectives as one moves toward a resolution or decision.

Step One: Articulate the Problem

Burkhardt and Nathaniel's (2008) first step of their model involves clearly describing the ethical problem that has been identified. This is followed by identifying desired goals. Identifying goals will allow movement toward step three of the model, developing strategies. Burkhardt and Nathaniel (2008) relate that because strategies are often dramatic, identifying goals at this time will reduce conflict later in this process. Further, by clearly identifying the problem, the problem will be defined as an ethical or practical dilemma.

Step Two: Gather Data and Identify Conflicting Moral Claims

Once the ethical problem is clearly identified, one should gather the necessary information or facts to provide clarification of the issues involved. Burkhardt and Nathaniel (2008) relate that throughout this process, attention should be paid to the societal, religious, and cultural values and beliefs of those involved. In addition, one should identify the participants' ethical perspectives. This is when an understanding of basic ethical content, theories, principles, and perspectives is imperative.

Step Three: Explore Strategies

Identifying the problem and gathering data is followed by identifying possible strategies. Burkhardt and Nathaniel (2008) state that "various options begin to emerge throughout the assessment process" (p. 130). In an effort to eliminate unacceptable alternatives, the proposed alternatives should be evaluated as to how they best fit the identified goals, beliefs, lifestyles, and values (Burkhardt & Nathaniel, 2008). This step of the ethical decision-making process may take time to develop acceptable strategies as well as eliminate unacceptable strategies. Further, once a strategy is adopted, one must be ready and willing to act upon it (Burkhardt & Nathaniel, 2008).

Step Four: Implement the Strategy

Once a strategy is adopted, it is implemented. However, Burkhardt and Nathaniel (2008) relate that this may be the most difficult step of the model. Those involved in this process must feel empowered to make a difficult decision. The emotions that are surely stirred by implementing the strategy should be acknowledged by those involved and accepted as part of this difficult process (Burkhardt & Nathaniel, 2008).

Step Five: Evaluate Outcomes

Burkhardt and Nathaniel (2008) state that upon acting on the decision, "reflective evaluation sheds light on the effectiveness and validity of the process" (p. 132). The effects of the strategy on those involved in the process should be evaluated. This step of the model may involve ongoing evaluation of additional ethical problems that may arise as the situation changes and new data are gathered (Burkhardt & Nathaniel).

▪ Putting It All Together: Ethical Scenarios with Discussion

As stated earlier in the chapter, DNP graduates are not *ethicists* but rather experts in nursing practice who will encounter ethical scenarios within their settings. It is the DNP graduate's responsibility to become familiar with ethical content as well as nursing's ethical standards for practice. The following are possible ethical scenarios DNP graduates may encounter within their various roles.

Scenario 1

Dr. A. is a DNP-prepared nurse practitioner within a multidisciplinary breast center. As part of her role, Dr. A. cares for patients with breast health issues, including breast cancer. When a new patient in the breast center is evaluated, Dr. A. orders and discusses diagnostics tests with the patient, and, if need be, orders a breast biopsy. The breast center's philosophy of care is designed to be seamless and potentially takes the patient from assessment and evaluation to diagnostics and biopsy—all in the same day. One would think this is an ideal scenario.

On one particular day, Dr. A. sees her first new patient of the day. She assesses the 39-year-old mother of two who is under a great deal of stress due to lack of child care at home. The patient, Ms. B., relates that she found a lump in her breast about 6 months ago but due to her schedule and lack of child care, has been unable to come in to the breast center. She has never had a mammogram and has no family history of breast cancer.

As per standard of care, Dr. A. examines Ms. B., orders a mammogram and ultrasound, and awaits the results. In the meantime, Ms. B. receives a call that her babysitter is late for an appointment and needs to leave soon. Stressed and worried, Ms. B. undergoes the ordered diagnostic testing. While in the ultrasound room, she is informed by the radiologist that there is a mass in her breast that is worrisome and requires a biopsy. In an effort to provide seamless care, the room is prepped. Ms. B., confused and in a hurry, consents to the procedure. While she waits for the radiologist to perform the biopsy, her mind is racing. She wishes her husband had come, she wishes she had made different child care arrangements, she might have gotten a second opinion regarding the biopsy. But, she thinks, the doctors and nurses know best. They told me I needed the biopsy today so I should have it. Tears stream down her face and she wishes she wasn't there alone. At the end of a 4-hour appointment, seamless care has been provided and precious time is saved by having the biopsy performed so quickly. Ms. B. is diagnosed a week later with Stage One breast cancer and she begins receiving treatment within 1 week of presenting to the clinic.

Discussion

Upon reviewing this scenario, one may note that from a deontological theory, Dr. A. performed her duty to the patient and did what was right by diagnosing cancer and initiating the necessary treatment as soon as possible. However, with regard to beneficence, or doing what benefits the patient, the answers are not so clear. The patient benefitted from an early diagnosis, but at what cost? One should note that the actions of the multidisciplinary team were paternalistic in that the decision was made for Ms. B. that it would be best if she had her biopsy on the same day as her first visit to the breast center. One may consider that Ms. B. was actually emotionally harmed by the paternalistic actions and nonmaleficence was not supported.

How could this scenario have been handled differently by Dr. A.? Do you think Dr. A. is aware that her actions could be viewed as paternalistic, or do you think she is acting purely out of duty? What would you do if you encountered this scenario?

Scenario 2

Dr. B. is a DNP-prepared clinical nurse specialist working in an urban healthcare center serving a multicultural population. Dr. B.'s role includes counseling patients and their families regarding end-of-life care. One of his patients, Ms. C. on the renal transplant floor, is suffering from end-stage renal disease and has been denied a second transplant. Dr. B. knows from previous admissions that Ms. C. does not wish to be resuscitated and has previously signed advance directive paperwork. However, during this new admission, the advance directive must be signed again. Ms. C. is from a Middle Eastern country and speaks little English. Her family has been present and translating for her.

Dr. B. is consulted by the nursing staff to renew the advance directive due to the fact that the family is currently refusing to sign the paperwork. Dr. B. arrives on the unit, is met by the English-speaking son of Ms. C. (Ms. C.'s power of attorney) who states, "She is confused; she doesn't know what she wants." Dr. B. tries to counsel Ms. C.'s son and reassure him that this is what Ms. C. had wanted.

Unfortunately, the next day, Ms. C.'s condition worsens and she is placed on a ventilator. Ms. C.'s son continues to refuse to sign the advance directive. Dr. B. consults with the medical team who continues aggressive medical care. Ms. C.'s health declines and she becomes comatose. Ms. C. remains unresponsive and on a ventilator for several more days. She is eventually determined to have minimal brain activity and is finally removed from the ventilator.

Discussion

This particular scenario involves many ethical concerns ranging from the provision of culturally sensitive care to respect for the patient's autonomy. First and foremost, whenever there is a language barrier, respect for autonomy and informed consent require a translator be present for all medical decision-making discussions. This ensures that all information is appropriately shared with the patient.

At times, healthcare professionals may feel they need to override a patient's autonomous choice in order to practice nonmaleficence (or do no harm). This involves the art of ethics and requires careful deliberation and ethical reflection. The healthcare providers made decisions based on a deontological perspective—they felt it was their "duty" to save Ms. C.'s life. In this situation, however, the patient had made her wishes clear in a previous advance directive. "Nurses have multiple ethical obligations, sometimes competing, sometimes conflicting, including those to the patient, the organization or institution in which they work, or other healthcare professionals, and the nursing profession" (Davis, 2010, p. 15). Importantly, the ANA *Code of Ethics for Nurses* makes clear that the nurse's primary obligation is to the patient. Nurses may need courage to act when dealing with the consequences of an ethical decision (Davis, 2010).

What should Dr. B. have done when the family members refused to sign the advance directive for Ms. C.? Would an ethics committee have a role in this scenario? What would you do in this scenario? What ethical principles would you feel took precedence in this scenario?

Scenario 3

Dr. C. is a vice president of nursing at a large tertiary care hospital. She has been having trouble recruiting and keeping nursing staff and as a result is short staffed for some of the units in the hospital. She is faced with making a choice regarding allocation of resources. She may spread the nurses around the hospital with few nurses

202 ■ CHAPTER 7 The DNP Graduate as Ethical Consultant

on each unit or close certain units and staff the open units adequately. If she closes units, the patients already admitted would be cared for but this decision would limit how many patients could be admitted in the future (Davis, 2010).

Discussion

Evaluating this ethical scenario requires reflection on the principles of justice, non-maleficence, and beneficence. The principle of justice must be considered when resources are limited or managed (Davis, 2010). Distributive justice refers to "the sharing of burdens and benefits in the allocation of resources, sometimes, but not always, under conditions of scarcity or rationing" (Davis, 2010, p. 17). Dr. C. should consider what solution would promote the most good while inflicting the least harm. Under the conditions she is faced with scarcity of resources, and Dr. C. must evaluate what option promotes the care of the patients in her institution.

Would you close some units and provide better staffing for the patients currently admitted? What would you do regarding the lack of open beds for new admissions? What ethical principles would you rely on to evaluate this scenario?

Scenario 4

Dr. D. is an associate professor in a large university-based school of nursing. Dr. D. teaches students who are second-degree students, or those with a bachelor's degree in another field, and returning to school for a degree in nursing. The majority of Dr. D.'s students are in midlife and have experienced layoffs related to a declining economy within their area.

Many of Dr. D.'s students are doing well in the program and expressing a love for the nursing profession. However, Dr. D. occasionally has a student who clearly is looking for job security rather than expressing a commitment to the profession. These particular students do mediocre work academically and meet the minimal requirements in their clinical rotations but lack any passion for caring for patients.

Dr. D. struggles regularly regarding these students and seeks assistance from the administration. She and her colleagues counsel these students regarding their career choice but many stay in the program, graduate, and enter the nursing profession. Despite her best efforts in her academic setting, Dr. D. is disillusioned regarding teaching and wonders if she should stay in this setting and what she can do about this ethical scenario.

Discussion

Although there may be nothing Dr. D. can do regarding students who entered the profession for job security, she may reflect on the ANA *Code of Ethics* Provision 5: "The nurse owes the same duties to self as to others, including the responsibility to preserve integrity and safety, to maintain competence, and to continue personal and professional growth" (ANA, 2001, p. 23). This provision will remind her that her responsibility to the profession is to ensure competence in the profession. Her students must meet the academic requirements but she cannot ensure that they love their chosen profession.

Dr. D. is responsible to vigorously counsel students who don't seem to "fit" with nursing and offer alternate career choices that may better suit these students. She may also decline to give letters of recommendation after graduation (Fowler, 2010). It is Dr. D.'s responsibility to ensure competence, but not her responsibility to ensure that these students stay within the profession.

How would you counsel these students? What would you do if your students expressed a lack of passion or actual disdain for the nursing profession?

Scenario 5

Mr. E. is a busy certified registered nurse anesthetist practicing in a labor and delivery unit within an academic hospital. He has been considering returning to school for a DNP degree and has been researching DNP degree programs. As part of his decision making, he met with his director to discuss reducing his hours in order to allow time for returning to graduate school. He was met with resistance and questioned why he needed "yet another degree." Mr. E. explained the DNP degree to his director as well as the reasons why he wanted to expand his knowledge base and improve his overall practice.

After this meeting, Mr. E. was somewhat discouraged, and despite the fact that he was committed to advancing his profession and his own professional development, he is now struggling with his decision.

Discussion

Reflecting on the ANA *Code of Ethics for Nurses* may help Mr. E. with his decision to pursue a DNP degree. Provision 7 states: "The nurse participates in the advancement of the profession through contributions to practice, education, administration, and knowledge development" (ANA, 2001, p. 27). Commitment to this provision does not necessarily mean everyone must return to graduate school; however, this provision supports nursing contributing to the profession through ongoing educational efforts and development of nursing's body of knowledge.

The ANA *Code of Ethics for Nurses* states that "administrators must create an environment that is supportive of the ongoing educational needs of nurses and conducive to rapid implementation and innovation" (Drought & Epstein, 2010, pp. 90–91). The nursing profession can advance only through the commitment of nurses who are willing to learn and incorporate new knowledge (Drought & Epstein, 2010). Provision 7 of the ANA Code for Nurses and Mr. E.'s commitment to his profession should help him evaluate his decision to return to school for a DNP degree.

How would you respond to your director if you encountered resistance regarding returning to graduate school? What ethical perspectives would drive your decision to return to school despite meeting resistance?

Interviews with Nurse Ethicists: Wisdom from the Field

Drs. Janie Butts and Karen Rich are nurse ethicists and nursing professors at the University of Southern Mississippi School of Nursing. Their interviews provide valuable insights regarding ethics in nursing and implications for DNP graduates.

Dr. Butts/Dr. Rich: Could you describe your background including education and nursing/academic experience, as well as your current position?

Dr. Butts: My career as a registered nurse involves a 32-year era of my life thus far, occurring in advancing stages. In the first stage of my nursing career, I was an associate degree-prepared, then a baccalaureate-prepared, clinical practice nurse with a focus in adult health nursing, in labor and delivery, and finally in emergency nursing. In my current and second stage, I have been a nursing educator since 1990—for 21 of my 32 years of nursing—from 1993 to present at The University of Southern Mississippi School of Nursing and my earlier teaching years from 1990 to 1993 at William Carey University. My love for knowledge and being a nursing educator with a master's of science degree in nursing led me down a path of lifelong learning. A doctor of science degree in nursing (DSN) was earned in 1998 from the University of Alabama at Birmingham School of Nursing with a focus in nursing education and curriculum, clinical intervention research with elders, and behavioral intervention research with at-risk adolescents. In 2002 as I began teaching in the PhD program of nursing, my focus turned sharply to ethics, bioethics, and theory. In response to these areas of interest, I attended several summer seminars and earned certificates in ethics and bioethics at the Kennedy Institute of Ethics at Georgetown and at the University of Washington at Seattle, Departments of Law, Medicine, and Allied Health Care. Then in 2002 I earned a certification in ethics from Rush University in Chicago. A significant amount of my learning came from a self-taught approach of reading, daily reflection and journaling, and studying philosophy, ethics, bioethics, and theory development. The most recent research is a qualitative content analysis on adults who have lost their adult siblings. I have numerous articles in journals and many book chapters in others' books. Dr. Rich and I are coauthors of two books, one nonedited nursing ethics book in its second edition with a third edition forthcoming and one new edited book with a variety of book chapters by distinguished nursing and nonnursing authors. In my current position at the university, I teach ethics courses and theory development and analysis courses in the baccalaureate, master's, DNP, and PhD programs at differing levels of complexity.

Dr. Rich: I have been a nurse for 31 years. I began my career as an associate degree nurse and quickly realized that I wanted to pursue higher education in nursing. I have earned a master's in public health nursing, a post-master's as a psychiatric-mental health nurse practitioner, and a doctorate in nursing with an emphasis in ethics. Although my plan was to practice as a psychiatric nurse practitioner while I pursued that degree, I became captivated with philosophy and ethics during my doctoral education and my career took a different direction. Actually, Dr. Butts was one of my teachers and played a big role in my academic development during my doctoral program. We began collaborating on scholarly writing projects, and I became a teacher at The University of Southern Mississippi. Now, I teach public health, ethics, professional development, research, and graduate classes in quality improvement. I absolutely love being a teacher.

Dr. Butts/Dr. Rich: Could you describe how you define "nurse ethicist," including how you became a nurse ethicist?

Dr. Butts: The nurse ethicist role can be described in different ways according to the working environment and context. The nurse ethicist is an advanced practice registered nurse with a degree or advanced certification in ethics education and with ethics expertise. The nurse ethicist in clinical settings manages the ethical issues of professional nursing practice. For instance, one large healthcare system—Clarian Health in collaboration with the Fairbanks Center for Medical Ethics and the Indiana University School of Nursing—created the nurse ethicist role for "creating and sustaining programs in clinical ethics and nursing ethics education with the goal of empowering the ethical lives of nurses in the context of the interdisciplinary environments in which they work" (Wocial, Bledsoe, Helft, & Everett, 2010, p. 287).

In academia, we are realizing the need for curricula with more concentrated content in ethics, bioethics, and ethical decision making for the express function of improving and maintaining ethical clinical practice. We are seeing a significant emphasis on students' capacity to show evidence of ethical expertise in their nursing practice integrated throughout the AACN baccalaureate essentials (2008), the master's level essentials (2011), and the doctoral essentials for advanced nursing practice (2006) documents and the current NCLEX plan (2010). The IOM (2010) published recommendations for the future of nursing, emphasizing a higher level of education and expertise in collaboration, which includes ethical collaboration with other healthcare disciplines. I have discovered that students and many faculty are intensely interested in the topics of moral integrity in their personal lives and ethical decision making in nursing practice, one reason being that they are experiencing and observing increased moral distress, indicating ethical conflicts in practice.

I have already described my personal progression of ethics education in the first interview question. My curiosity in and pursuance of ethics and bioethics grew from my interest in ethical issues with at-risk adolescents, such as confidentiality issues and the right to choose or refuse treatment. Studying, teaching, and writing about ethical analysis and decision making have helped me to develop the skills of "making an argument," that is, providing justification for my stance, both theoretically and pragmatically.

Dr. Rich: I define a nurse ethicist as a nurse with a master's or doctoral degree who has had advanced educational preparation in bioethics and nursing ethics in the form of a specific degree or certificate. A nurse ethicist should have a clear research, scholarship, and practice track focused on nursing ethics. Before I became a nurse educator, one of my favorite practice roles was being a discharge planner at a teaching hospital in the heart of New Orleans. I worked as a team member within the hospital's social services department and took on the role of interacting with, teaching, counseling, and advocating for patients and families during a wide range of physical, social, and psychological stages and conditions related to health and illness. Many of the patients and families with whom I worked were coping with end-of-life care and decisions, which were very ethical in nature. Other ethics-related issues in my work involved accessing care and resources, addressing issues of social justice, being an intermediary between patients and families and the nursing and medical staff at the hospital, and trying to appropriately confront problems related to autonomy and paternalism. When I began working in home care, I found that many of the same basic ethical issues existed, only in a different type setting. When I entered my PhD in nursing program with an emphasis in ethics, the content felt natural to me. I was thrilled to be able to link theories and concepts to the issues that I had experienced in my practice. One of the things that I always have pondered in my career is why some nurses "go the extra mile" to help patients and families while other nurses want to do the bare minimum. Why do some nurses seem to "tune out" rather than to "tune in" on being caring, present, and compassionate? Studying ethics helped me find a scholarly way to consider my unanswered questions.

Dr. Butts/Dr. Rich: Do you believe that ethics education is important in nursing education for nurses and advanced practice registered nurses, and if so why?

Dr. Butts: Yes, I believe that ethics is not *just* important but is also mandatory and should be deliberately placed content at all levels of nursing education, whether as a separate course or integrated into all courses across each and all levels. The American Nurses Association's *Code of Ethics with Interpretive Statements* (2001) and *Nursing: Scope and Standards of Nursing Practice* (2010a) denote that nurses are morally obligated and committed to manifest evidence of a solid ethical practice with far-sighted decision making rooted from knowledge and contemplated judgments. To accomplish this level of ethical practice entails that nurses remain well informed, competent, and engaged in clinical skills, professional ethics, bioethics issues, and research.

Dr. Rich: I absolutely believe that ethics education is important for all levels of nursing. Nursing, to me, is an inherently moral endeavor. Consequently, to practice nursing well, nurses need to work on positively developing their character and moral intellect as well as nursing praxis.

Dr. Butts/Dr. Rich: Do you think that nursing curricula prepare nurses and advanced practice registered nurses in education sufficiently for professional ethical practice? Specifically, is there any fundamental ethical content missing from ethics education in nursing?

Dr. Butts: I believe that nurses and advanced practice registered nurses are not educationally adept in ethics for professional ethical practice for two reasons. One rationale is that the implementation of ethics education has been sluggish because of not being recognized as a prominent foundation for nursing education. Nursing faculty traditionally prefer to stick with what has been a blueprint for student and faculty success, which has translated to a slow implementation of ethics education. Ethics typically has been considered as only a small portion of the essential content within the typical specialties of graduate nursing education and the subspecialties of undergraduate nursing education (that is, adult health, childbearing mothers, newborns, child family health, psychiatric-mental health, and public health care). I believe this approach is quickly changing as new and different nursing, medical, and organizational demands and societal expectations for ethical practice are brought to the forefront of health care.

The second rationale has to do with the complexity and density of ethical practice. Novice nurses do not yet have the capacity for the full range of complex considerations required for ethical practice, analysis, and decision making—either because of the very nature of graduates being a novice nurse without depth in clinical experience, or because in nursing school they often receive only limited ethics education from which to draw. However, with a strong education in ethics, novice nurses will draw from that foundation to build and develop competency for professional ethical practice.

There are several essential parts missing from ethics education at all levels, such as the actual bioethical issues, but in my opinion the biggest part glaringly absent at all levels is the theoretical and principled justification for ethical decisions and the associated nursing dialogue. I believe it was Leonardo da Vinci who once said about the theoretical knowledge for drawing and art:

> Those who are in love with practice without knowledge are like the sailor who gets into a ship without a rudder or compass and who never can be certain whether he is going. Practice must always be founded on sound theory, and to this perspective is the guide and the gateway. And without this nothing can be done well in the matter of drawing. (da Vinci, 2005, p. 299)

Leonardo's same thoughts about theory and practice can be applied to nursing ethical theory and practice. Practice without theory is futile. Nursing educators need to integrate ethics-based theoretical and principled justification for ethical decisions.

Dr. Rich: Generally, I do not believe that nursing curricula adequately prepare nurses in theoretical and applied ethics. The fundamental ethical content that I believe is frequently missing from ethics education in nursing is helping nurses to be aware of how often they will confront ethical issues in a place similar to what Schön (1987) called the "swampy lowland" (p. 3). The ethical issues that nurses confront most often are not the big, recognizable issues that people hear about in the media. Instead, they are the day-to-day decisions that nurses must make in their work. One of my favorite ethics quotes says it all for me: "The great ethical danger, I think, is not that when faced with an important decision one makes the wrong choice, but rather that one never realizes that one is facing a decision at all" (Chambliss, 1996, p. 59). Nurses sometimes become so routinized in their everyday relationships with patients that they forget that their work is inherently moral. Opportunities to make ethical decisions are all around them.

Dr. Butts/Dr. Rich: How do you think the domain of ethics should influence the development of the DNP degree?

Dr. Butts: Nurses are taught to treat patients with dignity and human respect in an unbiased, nonjudgmental approach. Educators need to place more detailed ethics content in strategic places and levels within the DNP curriculum so that DNP students can develop complexity in their critical reflection of ethical analysis and decision making. I like what Peirce and Smith (2008) implemented at Columbia University School of Nursing. They have some interesting suggestions regarding integration of ethics in the DNP education. They developed DNP ethical competencies in three of the nine competency domains at that university based on four professional organizations' standards and recommendations: (a) the ANA *Code of Ethics with Interpretive Statements* (2001), (b) the International Council on Ethics *Code of Ethics for Nurses* (2006), (c) the AACN DNP Essentials (2006), and (d) the National Organization of Nurse Practitioner Faculties (NONPF) Competencies (2006). The ethical competencies within the three domains include ethical care based on scientific evidence for patient health and illness and ethical analysis and decision making in the professional role as well as a part of professional accountability.

Dr. Rich: Nursing ethics is grounded in the moral nature of nurse-patient/caregiver relationships. Nurses with a DNP degree should be mentors and role models for other nurses, especially in their relationships with patients and families. These relationships are at the center of nursing practice for DNP graduates who should provide the highest quality of direct nursing care.

Dr. Butts/Dr. Rich: Do you agree that an ethics curriculum should be included in DNP programs? If so, how should this content be integrated in DNP curricula?

Dr. Rich: Of course, I must admit my bias, but I believe that ethics should be taught as a separate course in DNP programs as well as being threaded throughout other courses in the curriculum.

Dr. Butts: Yes I do but do not think enough emphasis has been placed on ethics content for DNP programs. A separate ethics core course and a threading of the ethical content throughout the DNP curriculum is my suggestion, as is Dr. Rich's recommendation. Additionally, I gave an example of one university's development of ethical competencies for its DNP curriculum. I believe that competencies for ethical practice by DNPs need to be created in terms of universal competencies for all DNP programs with specific objectives and strategies for teaching and learning.

Dr. Butts/Dr. Rich: How do you think ethics will affect the future roles that DNP graduates will assume? Is any specific ethics content more essential for future DNP graduates, such as information technology, research, or leadership?

Dr. Rich: I believe that having formal ethics knowledge will be integral to the success of DNP graduates in the future. DNP-educated nurses will be more comfortable in their roles if their feet are on semisolid ground rather than totally in the swampy low ground in terms of ethics. DNP nurses must know an ethics-laden situation when they confront it. They must feel confident in knowing how to make decisions that enhance human flourishing and diminish suffering while practicing according to the nonnegotiable provisions of the American Nurses Association's current *Code of Ethics for Nurses with Interpretive Statements*, which was most recently published in 2001. The specific ethics content that I believe will be more essential for DNP graduates in the future is content related to social justice and population health, nurse entrepreneurship, leadership, and technology.

Dr. Butts: I agree totally with Dr. Rich's summation of the significance of ethics education in DNP programs of study. To Dr. Rich's future essential content list, I also add the ethical theoretical justification component and the translation of ethics research findings to DNP ethical practice.

SUMMARY

- Ethics has been broadly defined as the principles of conduct governing an individual or group. More specifically, Butts and Rich (2008) define ethics as "the study of ideal human behavior and ideal ways of being" (p. 4).

- Morals, on the other hand, are "specific beliefs, behaviors, and ways of being derived from doing ethics" (Butts & Rich, 2008, p. 5).

- A code of ethics describes standards of conduct and states certain principles regarding responsibilities and duties of those professionals to whom they apply (Pozgar, 2010).

- Values have been defined as "ideals, beliefs, customs, modes of conduct, qualities, or goals that are highly prized or preferred by individuals, groups, or societies" (Burkhardt & Nathaniel, 2008, p. 83).

- Reasoning describes the "use of abstract thought processes to think creatively, to answer questions, solve problems, and to formulate strategies for one's actions and desired ways of being" (Butts & Rich, 2008, p. 9).

- Normative ethics involves prescribing values, behaviors, and ways of being that are considered right or wrong when deciding what to do in a specific situation (Butts & Rich, 2008).

- Applied ethics refers to the application of normative ethics to moral problems (Pozgar, 2010).

- Descriptive ethics is more concrete and describes what one thinks about morality or moral behavior (Butts & Rich, 2008).
- Virtue ethics focuses on the inherent character of a person rather than on specific actions (Pozgar, 2010).
- Natural law theory stems from the philosophy of St. Thomas Aquinas. This theory emphasizes that the "law of reason is implanted in the order of nature (usually thought to be implanted by God)" and provides the rules of human nature (Butts & Rich, 2008, p. 21).
- Deontology or "the study of duty" is an ethical theory that focuses on duties and rules.
- Principlism uses principles that serve as rules for conduct dictated by duty.
- Utilitarianism describes actions that are judged by their utility.
- Casuistry describes considering specific situations individually when making ethical decisions
- Narrative ethics is a story-based approach to making ethical decisions and similar to casuistry.
- Critical theory broadly describes "theories and worldviews that address the domination perpetrated by specific powerful groups of people and resulting in the oppression of other specific groups of people" (Butts & Rich, 2008, p. 27).
- Bioethics is defined as "the philosophical study of ethical controversies brought about by advances in biology, research, and medicine" (Pozgar, 2010, p. 403).
- In 1974, Congress passed the National Research Act to regulate studies involving human participants.
- As a result of the National Research Act, a commission was created to define the principles supported for research involving human subjects and a 4-day conference was held at the Belmont Conference Center at the Smithsonian. In 1976, the commission released its report titled "The Belmont Report." This report outlined three principles for all human subject research: respect for persons, beneficence, and justice (National Commission, 1978).
- Personal autonomy has been defined as "self-rule that is free from controlling interference by others and from certain limitations such as inadequate understanding that prevents meaningful choice" (Beauchamp & Childress, 2009, p. 99).
- Informed consent describes the "process by which patients are informed of possible outcomes, alternatives, and risks of treatment, and are required to give their consent freely" (Burkhardt & Nathaniel, 2008, p. 58).
- The principle of beneficence refers to "the moral obligation to act for the benefit of others" (Beauchamp & Childress, 2010, p. 197).
- Paternalism is a form of beneficence and involves individuals or institutions believing they know what is best for the patient/person and thus making decisions for him or her (Pozgar, 2010).

- The principle of nonmaleficence describes the obligation to "do no harm."
- The principle of justice refers to "fairness, treating people equally and without prejudice, and with the equitable distribution of benefits and burdens" (Butts & Rich, 2008, p. 48).
- Nursing ethics has been defined as an extension of bioethics where ethical issues are viewed from a nursing perspective (Butts & Rich, 2008).
- The American Nurses Association (ANA) *Code of Ethics for Nurses with Interpretive Statements* is considered the standard for nurses to refer to as their code for ethical behavior.
- The International Council of Nurses (ICN) *Code of Ethics for Nurses* was initially adopted by the ICN in 1953. The ICN code is based on the four responsibilities of nurses: "to promote health, to prevent illness, to restore health, and alleviate suffering" (ICN, 2006, p. 1).
- Tools for ethical leadership are imperative for the DNP graduate to successfully evaluate ethical scenarios in leadership roles. These tools include traits necessary for ethical leadership, an ethical leadership decision-making tool, and recommendations for avoiding ethical conflicts.
- Ethical scenarios in telehealth may involve many aspects of information technology such as electronic medical records, patients seeking information on the Internet, and social networking issues.
- DNP graduates need not only a grasp of ethical content but also an understanding of information technologies and new developments within telehealth.
- Evaluation of ethical scenarios is importantly a *process* that DNP graduates will need to develop throughout their careers. With experience, understanding of ethical content, and a diligent commitment to upholding the ethical standards of the nursing profession, DNP graduates will become more proficient at this process over time.

REFLECTION QUESTIONS

1. What ethical content do you feel is necessary for DNP graduates to understand to effectively evaluate ethical scenarios?
2. Of the four principles of bioethics, which do you feel influences your decisions when evaluating ethical scenarios?
3. What character traits do you feel are necessary for ethical leadership?
4. Describe some ethical scenarios you are concerned with regarding telehealth. What ethical content would help you to evaluate ethical scenarios related to telehealth?
5. Do you agree that evaluating ethical scenarios is a *process*? Why or why not?
6. What types of ethical scenarios do you think you will encounter as a DNP graduate in your setting?

REFERENCES

American Association of Colleges of Nursing (AACN). (2006). *Essentials of doctoral education for advanced nursing practice.* Washington, DC: Author. Retrieved from http://www.aacn.nche.edu /publications/position/DNPEssentials.pdf

American Association of Colleges of Nursing (AACN). (2008). *Essentials of baccalaureate education for professional nursing practice.* Washington, DC: Author. Retrieved from http://www.aacn.nche.edu /education-resources/BaccEssentials08.pdf

American Association of Colleges of Nursing (AACN). (2011). *Essentials of master's education in nursing.* Washington, DC: Author. Retrieved from http://www.aacn.nche.edu/education-resources/Masters Essentials11.pdf

American Nurses Association (ANA). (2001). *Code of ethics with interpretive statements.* Silver Spring, MD: Author.

American Nurses Association (ANA). (2010a). *Nursing: Scope and standards of practice* (2nd ed., revised). Silver Spring, MD: Author.

American Nurses Association (ANA). (2010b). *Nursing's social policy statement.* Silver Spring, MD: Author.

Beauchamp, T. L., & Childress, J. F. (2009). *Principles of biomedical ethics* (6th ed.). New York: Oxford University Press.

Buell, J. M. (2009, May/June). Ethics and leadership: Setting the right tone and structure can help others in their decision making. *Healthcare Management Ethics,* 54–57.

Burkhardt, M. A., & Nathaniel, A. K. (2008). *Ethics and issues in contemporary nursing* (3rd ed.). Clifton Park, NY: Delmar Cengage Learning.

Butts, J. B., & Rich, K. L. (2008). *Nursing ethics: Across the continuum and into practice* (2nd ed.). Sudbury, MA: Jones and Bartlett.

Centers for Disease Control (CDC). (2011). *The Tuskegee timeline.* Retrieved from http://www.cdc.gov /tuskegee/timeline.htm

Chambliss, D. F. (1996). *Beyond caring: Hospitals, nurses, and the social organization of ethics.* Chicago, IL: University of Chicago Press.

da Vinci, L. (2005). *Leonardo's notebooks* (H. A. Suh, Trans.). New York: Black Dog & Leventhal.

Davis, A. J. (2010). Provision two. In M. D. Fowler (Ed.), *Guide to the code of ethics for nurses: Interpretation and application* (pp. 12–21). Silver Spring, MD: American Nurses Association.

Dayer-Berenson, L. (2011). *Cultural competencies for nurses: Impact on health and illness.* Sudbury, MA: Jones & Bartlett Learning.

Drought, T. S., & Epstein, E. G. (2010). Provision seven. In M. D. Fowler (Ed.) *Guide to the code of ethics for nurses: Interpretation and application* (pp. 90–102). Silver Spring, MD: American Nurse Association.

Facebook. (2011). *Statistics.* Retrieved from http://www.facebook.com/press/info.php?statistics

Fleming, D. A., Edison, K. E., & Pak, H. (2009). Telehealth ethics. *Telemedicine and eHealth, 15*(8), 797–803.

Forman, E. N., & Ladd, R. E. (1991). *Ethical dilemmas in pediatrics: A case study approach.* New York: Springer-Verlag.

Gallagher, A., & Tschudin, V. (2009). Educating for ethical leadership. *Nurse Education Today, 30*(3), 224–227.

Hader, A. L., & Brown, E. D. (2010). Patient privacy and social media. *AANA Journal, 78*(4), 270–273.

Healthcare Coalition. (2010). *Healthcare Coalition eCode.* Retrieved from http://www.ihealthcoalition .org/ehealth-code

Institute of Medicine (IOM). (2010). *The future of nursing: Focus on scope of practice.* Retrieved from http://www.iom.edu/~/media/Files/Report%20Files/2010/The-Future-of-Nursing/Nursing%20 Scope%20of%20Practice%202010%20Brief.pdf

International Council of Nurses (ICN). (2006). *Code of ethics for nurses.* Retrieved from http://www.icn .ch/images/stories/documents/about/icncode_english.pdf

Layman, E. J. (2008). Ethical issues and the electronic health record. *The Health Care Manager, 27*(2), 165–176.

Merriam-Webster. (2011a). *Definition of ethicist.* Retrieved from http://www.merriam-webster.com/dictionary/ethicist

Merriam-Webster. (2011b). *Definition of ethics.* Retrieved from http://www.merriam-webster.com/dictionary/ethics

National Commission for the Protection of Human Subjects of Biomedical and Behavioral Research. (1978). *The Belmont Report.* Washington, DC: U.S. Department of Health, Education, and Welfare. Retrieved from http://videocast.nih.gov/pdf/ohrp_belmont_report.pdf

National Organization of Nurse Practitioners Faculties (NONPF). (2006). *Practice doctorate nurse practitioner entry-level competencies 2006.* Washington, DC: Author. Retrieved from http://www.nonpf.com/associations/10789/files/DNP%20NP%20competenciesApril2006.pdf

National Public Radio (NPR). (2002). *Remembering Tuskegee.* Retrieved from http://www.npr.org/programs/morning/features/2002/jul/tuskegee

Office for Human Research Protections (OHRP). (2005). Retrieved from http://www.hhs.gov/ohrp

Peirce, A. G., & Smith, J. A. (2008). The ethics curriculum for doctor of nursing practice programs. *Journal of Professional Nursing, 24*(5), 270–274.

Piper, L. E. (2007). Ethics: The evidence of leadership. *The Health Care Manager, 26*(3), 249–254.

Phillips, W., & Fleming, D. (2009). Ethical concerns in the use of electronic medical records. *Missouri Medicine, 106*(5), 328–333.

Pozgar, G. D. (2010). *Legal and ethical issues for health professionals* (2nd ed.). Sudbury, MA: Jones & Bartlett Learning.

Sanford, K. (2006). The ethical leader. *Nursing Administration Quarterly, 30*(1), 5–10.

Schön, D. A. (1987). *Educating the reflective practitioner.* San Francisco: Jossey-Bass.

Silva, M. C., & Ludwick, R. (2006). Ethics: Is the doctor of nursing practice ethical? *The Online Journal of Issues in Nursing, 11*(2). Retrieved from http://www.nursingworld.org/MainMenuCategories/ANAMarketplace/ANAPeriodicals/OJIN/Columns/Ethics/DNPEthical.aspx

Simpson, R. L. (2005). E-Ethics: New dilemmas emerge alongside new technologies. *Nursing Administration Quarterly, 29*(2), 179–182.

Skloot, R. (2010). *The immortal life of Henrietta Lacks.* New York: Random House.

U.S. Department of Health and Human Services (2011). *Health Information Protection and Portability Act of 1996.* Retrieved from http://www.hhs.gov/ocr/privacy/hipaa/understanding/summary/privacysummary.pdf

Wocial, L. D., Bledsoe, P., Helft, P. R., & Everett, L. Q. (2010). Nurse ethicist: Innovative resource for nurses. *Journal of Professional Nursing, 26*(5), 287–292.

PART II

Professional Issues Related to the Doctor of Nursing Practice Degree

Part I of this book described the various roles DNP graduates may develop and integrate to meet the demands of today's complex healthcare environment. As these roles are developed, DNP graduates may be faced with unique challenges that result from their distinct educational preparation and goals. These challenges include dealing with issues such as deciding to return to school for a doctorate, using the title "doctor," educating others about their educational preparation, marketing themselves as DNP graduates, and confronting the debate and new concerns regarding this innovative degree.

Doctor of Nursing Practice graduates are charged with the responsibility to lead the way. Indeed, the ways in which DNP graduates manage these issues will shape the future of healthcare delivery and nursing education. The following chapters specifically discuss these issues and provide direction regarding the continued transition for DNP graduates.

CHAPTER 8

So You Want to Go Back to School? Exploring How to Make the Big Decision

■ ELIZABETH JOHNSTON TAYLOR ■

"It is our choices . . . that show what we truly are, far more than our abilities."

—*J. K. Rowling (1965–)*

"Should I? Can I? Should I incur the debt that going back to school would create? Can I really afford a DNP? Should I sacrifice time with my family for the time school would require? Can I really spend less time with my family? Should I forfeit my relatively stress-free lifestyle for the more stressful (albeit temporary) one that going for the DNP would mean? Can I remain healthfully balanced amidst the stress of school? How much are balance and health important to me?" These and myriad other questions inevitably are inherent in the decision about whether to return to graduate school for a DNP.

The purpose of this chapter is to support you as you make this big decision. It is a decision that could be life changing. Indeed, by carefully processing this decision—critically examining how and why you make the decision you make—you may find that your self-awareness and perspective on life are enhanced. Life presents tough decisions (e.g., what career to pursue, whether to discontinue a hurtful relationship, how to spend a large sum of money, whether to have a child). Studious attention to this present decision of whether to go for the DNP or not will improve your ability to make other big choices in life.

Some readers may have uncertainty about whether to get a DNP degree, and others may have already confirmed their decision. This chapter can help the latter type of readers by bringing to their awareness the hows and whys of the decision, allowing them to affirm the decision, and increasing their inner motivation. For some, the process of decision making will end in a choice to pursue the DNP degree, and for others it may lead to a rejection of further advanced practice training (even, perhaps, for some who at the outset may think they want it). This author posits that purposeful deliberation, regardless of outcome, is beneficial; nothing in life is wasted.

After a cursory review of some of the pertinent points for the DNP decision, this chapter reviews some of the decision-making theory and research and presents selected practical decision-making strategies. Because much of this literature is devoid of the spiritual dimension regarding discernment, advice from spiritual giants about how to make a decision is reviewed. The chapter ends with a discussion of how to live with the decision after it is made.

▪ To Be a DNP or Not to Be: Relevant Facts

You may be an undergraduate or graduate nursing student considering what preparation you need for the nursing career you want. Or you may be an advanced practice registered nurse already and are wondering whether to obtain further education. Your question may be whether to be a master's- or doctorally prepared advanced practice registered nurse (APRN). If you want a doctorate, you may be wondering whether to obtain the DNP or PhD degree (or another more research-oriented doctorate).

Most nurses who choose the DNP over the PhD do so because their primary interest is in promoting excellence in clinical practice rather than scholarship (Loomis, Willard, & Cohen, 2007). Others choose the DNP degree because it requires less time; it is impractical for an APRN who is in the last several years of his or her career to invest in a DNP. Some find confirmation of their preference for an advanced practice career when they perceive that PhD professors are occupants of an ivory tower, and they yearn for instruction that enhances their abilities to improve clinical care (Loomis, Willard, & Cohen, 2007).

Grandfathering

For those who are choosing between the DNP and remaining as master's-prepared APRNs, there may be worry that after 2015 they will not be able to continue to practice as APRNs. In their review of the issues surrounding the implementation of the DNP degree, Fulton and Lyon (2005) identified the need to reassure master's-prepared APRNs that they will be "grandfathered," that they will be able to continue to practice without additional education. Subsequently, the American Association of Colleges of Nursing (AACN) mandated a DNP Roadmap Task Force to explore this and other issues in transitioning toward 2015. This task force's report (accepted by the AACN in July 2006) states: "State and national regulatory boards are encouraged to review all statutes and regulations governing advanced or specialty nursing practice and clarify language to require a graduate level degree as minimum preparation for practice as an APN" (p. 21).

However, each state's board of nursing determines the regulations under which APRNs may practice. Portability of state licensure may be a concern. APRNs "must then consider closely their future and decide if mobility is important, as well as how long they wish to practice" (Clinton & Sperhac, 2009). Although licensure may be grandfathered, APRNs must also consider if employers who seek DNP-prepared APRNs will value experience over the DNP degree (Clinton & Sperhac, 2009).

The AACN *Consensus Model for APRN Regulation: Licensure, Accreditation, Certification, Education* (2008) describes the graduate educational requirement for APRN practice as a masters or doctorate degree in nursing. Although future law cannot be guaranteed, it is clearly the intent of the AACN to promote grandfathering. Indeed, historically, grandfathering has been a necessary component of transitions such as this.

■ Decision-Making Research

The study of decision making has advanced substantially over the past few decades. Although it started as a topic for psychologists and economists, decision science now is a very widely encompassing multi- and interdisciplinary field. Researchers are investigating not only the economic, ethical, and sociopsychological aspects of decision making but also the neurobiological processes involved in decision making.

Here is a smattering of findings from recent research (albeit isolated studies) on decision making:

- When an environment feels normal, trustable, and safe, a decision maker with a trusting state of mind will tend to make the decision using routine decision-making strategies and outperform a distrusting decision maker. Conversely, when in an unusual situation that would benefit from nonroutine decision-making strategy, a distrustful stance on the part of the decision maker works best (Schul, Mayo, & Burnstein, 2008).
- Whether information is framed positively or negatively influences a decision maker. For example, when adults were asked whether they would choose resuscitation or comfort care for a premature baby, those who were presented with the baby's survival data were apt to decide on resuscitation, whereas those who were presented with the negativity of mortality data were likely to choose comfort care. Except for the participants who were highly religious, the framing significantly influenced their decision making (Haward, Murphy, & Lorenz, 2008).
- Persons who are indecisive have tunnel vision that limits how they gather information during the process of making a decision. They tend to limit their data collection to data that support what they ultimately choose (Rassin, Muris, Booster, & Kolsloot, 2008).
- A sad mood while making a decision usually prompts people to analyze information very carefully before making a decision, and a happy mood tends to contribute to decisions that are based more on feelings and intuition. When

there is this matchup of mood and decision-making strategy in this regard, the decision maker values the decision outcome more than when there is a mismatch of mood with strategy (de Vries, Holland, & Witteman, 2008).

■ A biologic basis for emotion playing an integral part of decision making has been established (van 't Wout, Kahn, Sanfey, & Aleman, 2006).

Just this bit of psychological research highlights some aspects to consider as you begin your decision making. You may want to think about how you or others are positively framing this decision (and how you frame it for your family). Likewise, this research should stimulate you to consider how you might be using tunnel vision and narrowing your options prematurely or to notice what mood you are in and how that is affecting your decision making.

■ Practical Tools for Decision Making

Several practical strategies have been developed to guide an individual or group in making a decision. These strategies can help managers make business decisions, and they can also help individuals make important personal decisions. Many of these strategies are presented in an easy-to-use format on the MindTools website (http://www.mindtools.com). Because of their simplicity and fit for the decisions surrounding DNP education, the following strategies will be described and illustrated here: Force Field Analysis, Thinking Hats, and Grid Analysis.

Force Field Analysis

Mark Lee, MSN, APRN, is a 33-year-old who is working full time in a public health clinic. He is happily married to Sue, who stays at home with their twin toddlers. Although he is fairly content with his level of clinical knowledge, he is naturally curious and interested in learning more about health policy, research utilization, and ethics. Plus, to be really honest, he would love to be a "doctor." Mark knows that if he could, he would go for the DNP degree. Sue, however, is seriously concerned that his doing so would make their marriage and financial situation suffer. He questions, "Should I get the DNP? Is it appropriate to let my family suffer, even for a few years? Should I ask my wife to go to work and put the kids in day care?"

Force Field Analysis is a decision-making strategy that requires one to specify the desired plan then to identify the forces that support that plan and the forces that are working against it. When this is done, assign a score to each force using a scale of 1 (weak) to 5 (strong). **Figure 8-1** illustrates Force Field Analysis by showing how Mark Lee might weigh the pros and cons of getting a DNP degree.

Mark's analysis suggests that by one point forces favor his pursuing the DNP degree. Given how close the pros and cons balance each other out, however, Mark will want to explore ways that he can minimize the negative forces, especially the strong ones. In this case, for example, he may want to consider how he and his wife

can shore up their marriage before the DNP program starts or receive marriage counseling on how to allow stress to strengthen their marriage. Or, Mark may choose a
DNP program that allows him more time around his twins (i.e., distance and part-
time programs). Likewise, Mark and Sue may decide to downsize their living accommodations to save money. Force Field Analysis leads one to see the changes that could
be implemented to minimize negative forces and promote positive forces.

Thinking Hats

Sarah Brown, BSN, RN, is a 24-year-old intensive care nurse with 2 years of nursing
experience. She realizes that she does not want to work in an acute care setting much
longer and is quite sure she would love to work as an advanced practice registered
nurse in some sort of outpatient clinic. She knows from visiting the AACN website
and talking with the recruiter from a university in her city that getting a DNP degree
is definitely the way to go. She is unmarried and lives near her parents. She still owes
about $30,000 on the loan she got for her BSN degree. Although there is a DNP pro-
gram in her city, she is attracted to the curriculum at a DNP program in a city several
hours away. Sarah is wondering, "Should I get the DNP now or later? Should I get it
from the local university or from the one several hours away? Is it fiscally wise to get
the DNP now?"

Thinking Hats is a decision-making strategy devised by Edward de Bono (http://www
.deBonoConsulting.com). It is a strategy that allows one to systematically look at a
decision from several different perspectives or with different styles of thinking, not just

Forces Supporting Plan	Plan	Forces Against Plan
+1 Wife benefiting from social connectedness at work ⇑	**To get the DNP while minimally stressing himself and his family; wife working part-time while twins are in preschool**	⇓ Less time for wife, −3 marriage stressed
+1 Kids supposedly benefit from part-time preschool ⇑		⇓ Less engaged with −3 kids' development during pivotal years of their lives
+1 Increased income potential after DNP ⇑		⇓ Financial debt for −3 several years
+3 Increased marketability and prestige with DNP ⇑		
+4 Personal benefit of stimulating academic experience ⇑		
+10	*versus*	**−9**

■ **Figure 8-1** Mark Lee's Force Field Analysis.

the habitual way. That is, one puts on each of the following hats during the process of decision making:

- White hat, which encourages intellectual analysis. What do I know from the past that could influence the present situation? What factual information do I yet need to make a good decision? For example, Sarah would calculate the expenses involved in studying full time versus part time and of moving to be near the preferred program versus commuting to it—and check to see if commuting is even possible. She would carefully compare all the curricula of the competing programs. She would project her financial future given her added debts and potential increased income with a DNP degree. She would examine financial aid packages.

- Red hat, which respects intuition and emotional inclinations. For example, Sarah would explore more deeply her gut response to each of the DNP programs that she is considering. She would also do well to listen to her inner energy, to feel out whether it is best to save it up more or spend it now on the DNP program.

- Black hat, which supports a pessimistic stance and thereby allows one to see the fatal flaws or pitfalls and develop contingency plans. For example, Sarah would do well to think about the emotional and financial hardships of doing the DNP program now versus later. (Going to school now might mean feeling the pain of leaving her parents and known community and incurring further debt. Choosing to postpone her education could mean it might be compromised by the distraction of marriage or childbearing.)

- Yellow hat, which encourages positivity, optimism, and a look at what might be the benefits of the options being considered. Sarah might compare the positives of starting a DNP program now versus later (e.g., getting it done while she is unmarried and increased earning potential sooner versus paying off immediate debt and enjoying a less stressful life now). She can also compare the positives of studying locally instead of away from home (e.g., the comfort of being home in contrast with the benefit of cutting the apron strings).

- Green hat, which symbolizes energy for creativity and thinking outside the box about options. For example, Sarah might consider ways to pursue the DNP program while living at home or in inexpensive living accommodations to minimize her debts. She might also consider how she can live near her parents and loved ones and still attend the DNP program that is more distant. Or, she might look elsewhere for long-distance programs or weekend programs that would allow her to continue to work.

- Blue hat, which is the control or process-oriented thinking that decision making requires. For example, if Sarah observes that she is focusing on all the positives, she may realize that putting on the black hat would be helpful; if she senses she is stuck on a problem that she wishes to eliminate, she may put her green hat on.

The Thinking Hats strategy fosters self-awareness about the different perspectives that are all essential to use in a decision-making process. A decision should not be only a rational decision. It must also recognize the value of intuition, thinking outside the box, and even pessimism.

Grid Analysis

Kim Fitzhugh, BS, RN, is a 40-year-old volunteer parish nurse at a large local congregation. She quit the stressful work of staff nursing on an oncology unit when she began suffering from chronic fatigue and fibromyalgia syndromes 2 years ago. She feels that she is recovering and is eager "to do something." The idea of working in an academic setting stirs her passion. Her four children (ages 10–16 years) are all in school, yet she wants to be there for them physically and emotionally when they are home. (To work as an academic would be less physically challenging and would mean flexible work hours and an academic calendar that synchronizes with her children's school year.) Her husband, who is probably eager to see her become "normal" again, is supportive of her returning to school for a DNP degree. The DNP program would pose minimal financial threat to Kim's family. Part- and full-time DNP programs are available to Kim, but she is ambivalent: "Can I really do this? What if it makes me relapse? And then that prevents me from keeping close to the kids! And can I do the DNP without sacrificing the quality of my relationships with my teenagers? Should I really quit the parish nursing? It's been so fulfilling for me, and I am so close to the people of the congregation. And dare I go full time, or should I try part time and take forever to get through? Or should I be content with an MSN degree, which would make me less marketable to a nursing school?"

Grid Analysis (or Decision Matrix Analysis) is an especially helpful strategy when there are several options to choose from and multiple factors to consider. This strategy requires you to list all the possible options being decided (in rows) and then identify all the factors that are important to consider (in columns). Each factor should then be given a weight between 0 (not at all important) and 5 (extremely important). When this grid is established, you can then use the same scoring system to give a score to each option for each of the factors. That is, you can ask, "How does this option allow me to meet or satisfy this factor?" When each factor has been scored, multiply that score by the weight you have already assigned to that factor. Finally, you will add all the scores for each row (i.e., each option). The row/option with the highest score may be the best choice.

This Grid Analysis strategy is illustrated in **Figure 8-2** using Kim Fitzhugh's situation. Of course, more factors could be added, and pursuing the MSN degree full time and part time could have been included as options. Using this strategy, however, shows that Kim's best option is to choose part-time DNP study. This strategy brings to full awareness how much health is a pivotal factor for her decision; she weighted it as 5. Thus, Kim may predetermine some contingency plans in case the part-time DNP study is too stressful for her body. This process may also make plain that dropping

Options	FACTORS (WEIGHTS):					
	Health (5)	Personal fulfillment with further education (2)	Satisfying/ flexible work outside home (3)	Want to please husband (1)	Time with children (4)	Totals (Factor × Option):
DNP full time, quit PN role	1 (5) = 5	5 (2) = 10	5 (3) = 15	3 (1) = 3	3 (4) = 12	45
DNP part time, may need to quit PN role	3 (5) = 15	5 (2) = 10	5 (3) = 15	4 (1) = 4	4 (4) = 16	60
MSN, likely to need to quit PN role	3 (5) = 15	4 (2) = 8	4 (3) = 12	4 (1) = 4	4 (4) = 16	55
Be content with BSN only, keep PN role	5 (5) = 25	0 (2) = 0	2 (3) = 6	2 (1) = 2	5 (4) = 20	53

■ **Figure 8-2** Kim Fitzhugh's Grid Analysis.

the parish nurse role is one way Kim can increase her chances of staying healthy and pursuing her professional goals.

Consulting Others

Although these techniques imply that you will get information from others to make your decision, it is indeed pivotal that you consult others in your close circle of family and friends as you make this decision. Your family members who are significantly affected by the outcome of this decision should be integrally involved in the decision making if mutual respect and harmony are to be maintained in the relationship. Although less important, perhaps, it can be extremely helpful to consult friends who can honestly give you feedback on your decision-making process and on their observations about who you authentically are and how that ought to inform the decision, or they can simply be a sounding board. When discussing your decision with others, try to keep an open or neutral stance toward your decision so that you can more fully hear what your friend or loved one is saying.

■ Spiritual Approaches to Decision Making

Although systematic strategies such as those described above are invaluable for making a big decision, they can fail to respect the spiritual element of decision making. Given that most Americans (Gallup & Jones, 2002; Wuthnow, 1998) and hence, most nurses, describe themselves as at least moderately spiritual (and for many this means religious), it is important to consider spiritual approaches to decision making. Spirituality explains the human quest for purposefulness of work, the need for a reason or mission for living, a desire for inner peace and joy, a desire to connect with and serve others, and a yearning for harmony with others, nature, and an ultimate other (Taylor, 2002). (Given the predominance of the term "God" in American society [Gallup & Jones, 2002], that language will be used subsequently in this discussion.) Decision making that fails to recognize these spiritual yearnings is incomplete and may lead to outcomes that are not congruent with what is ultimately important for the individual. Therefore, for those who experience this spiritual aspect of personhood, it is vital that spiritual approaches and strategies be included in the decision making.

Steps in a Spiritual Approach to Decision Making

Although the following steps are somewhat linear, they are better envisioned as concurrent aspects of a decision-making process. They might also be better thought of as subgoals. The primary goal of a spiritual approach to decisions is that of coorientation, communion, and collaboration with God, or a beckoning to listen to the inner light or inner wisdom. Although sometimes decisions are agonizing, they nevertheless manifest a God whose love means the freedom to choose.

A difficult decision can be viewed as an opportunity to intensely encounter God. In contrast, some might find that making a decision from a spiritual perspective is about trying to maintain control (but attributing the control to "God's will") or about abdicating the decision to God (and the default answer becomes "God's will"). Regardless, how an individual makes a decision will speak volumes about how that person relates to and perceives God.

Step 1: Assuming Humility

Spiritual giants of centuries ago advise that seeking humility is essential as one faces an important decision. Catherine of Siena, for example, stressed how one should assume a stance of respecting the allness and centrality of God in the universe instead of the prideful position of self-centeredness (Schneiders, 1982). Ignatius of Loyola (Backhouse, 1989) wrote that such humility "occurs when I do not find myself desiring riches more than poverty, honour more than dishonour, a long life more than a short one, and feel that the service of our Lord God and the salvation of my soul are equally important" (p. 39). The rationale for such humility is that it is required to be able to take a neutral or indifferent position toward the outcome of the decision-making process.

Step 2: Reaching Neutrality

Having such a neutral position toward the decision will allow the decision maker to recognize and weigh determining factors objectively. This is not to undermine the value of feelings that should inform a decision but to encourage the decision maker to consider the meaning of the feelings while holding them in check. Ideally, the decision maker will arrive at a perch atop a fulcrum where there is a sense that life will be good regardless of which outcome is chosen (Ignatius as cited in Backhouse, 1989).

Step 3: Considering Personal Context: Purpose of Life

When deciding whether to pursue a DNP degree or not, it is beneficial to stage this question in the context of what is the bigger picture: What do you think is the purpose for your existence? For some, the answer may be very specific: "To help find a cure for cancer." For others, it may be broad but nevertheless clear: "To praise, reverence, and serve our Lord God," as Ignatius of Loyola believed (Backhouse, 1989, p. 39). Regardless of what is your life purpose, it is essential that your decision for or against the DNP line up with this life purpose.

When thinking about vocation or purpose in life, it is necessary to think about who we are. That is, who we are authentically. McGraw (2001) describes it this way:

> The authentic self is the you that can be found at your absolute core. It is the part of you that is not defined by your job, or your function, or your role. It is the composite of all your unique gifts, skills, abilities, interests, talents, insights, and wisdom. It is all your strengths and values that are uniquely yours and need expression, versus what you have been programmed to believe that you are "supposed" to be and do. It is the you that flourished, unself-consciously, in those times in your life when you felt happiest and most fulfilled. It is the you that existed before and remains when life's pain, experiences, and expectancies are stripped away. (p. 30)

As one considers whether to become a DNP or not, knowing whether it fits one's life purpose is vital, and one's life purpose will inherently match up with who one is authentically (McGraw, 2001).

Self-exploration to discover or reaffirm one's authentic self is expedient during the decision-making process. Exercises that can help one to become more aware of the authentic self, and hence one's vocation and purpose, include:

- List all the qualities, talents, and personality traits that describe you. Circle the ones that you sense deep down are really you.
- List all your roles. Cross off the ones that do not bring joy because they do not allow you to be you. (Remember that roles are distinct from relationships.)
- Write your obituary. Then write down what you need to do so that the obituary would be realized.

Getting to know your authentic self will not only help you to make a decision regarding your education, but it will also guide you at other times to make choices that are consistent with who you are.

Step 4: Considering Pros and Cons in Light of Life's Purpose

Given your newfound appreciation for who you are and what is your life purpose, proceed to listing the positives and negatives associated with the choices you face.

Follow a strategy such as one previously described. Hold your preferences or biases in check. Consider the options in the context of how they conform to who you are created to be and to what you sense your life's purpose to be. If you share Ignatius's life purpose, then you would ponder the options in terms of which one would most glorify and praise God.

The 19th-century Protestant cleric Oswald Chambers (1992), in his popular devotional book, suggested further reference points for those who are facing decisions. Chambers's (1992) writing suggests that the following guidelines be considered:

- The choice that requires a huge amount of faith and courage, forcing you to lean, trust, depend, and rely on God more, may likely be where God is leading. For this will stretch and challenge you, helping you to grow and become more authentic.
- The choice that is new and frightening, perhaps something that you never thought possible, may well be the way God is leading.
- Usually God's leading involves a steady, quiet persistence in the direction God wills. Your heart is at peace when you consider it.

As Chambers indicates, often what is the best choice is also the hardest choice. Indeed, those decisions in life that are agonizing are often agonizing because we are resisting what seems to us to be the most difficult choice.

A list of questions that can support your decision making is offered in **Table 8-1**. Using these questions as a starting point for prayerful meditation or journal writing may prove to be very informative.

Step 5: Listening After the Decision Is Made

When possible, it is good to allow time to live with a decision before it is made public and action is taken to implement it. A good decision is one that brings consolation or

---

Table 8-1   Questions to Guide a Spiritual Approach to Decision Making

- Which option allows me to live more fully, authentically, more wholly/holy?
- At my deepest level, what do I want? Which option would make me feel most free inside?
- What effect will the choice have on life's meaning?
- What is my body saying?
- What does my "wisest elder" (an internal or external sage) say?
- How do mind/body/spirit line up with an answer? What do my head and heart say when considered in concert?
- Which option do I sense would bring consolation (versus desolation)—a sense of inner peace, a lightness?
- Which option energizes me? Makes me feel at rest inside?
- Which choice would foster greater humility (versus pride)? Which choice would encourage trust and communion with God?
- If I were on my future death bed, what would I advise myself to do today?
- If I were at the Last Judgment (or at an imagined time when your ultimate worth and goodness are calculated), what would I retrospectively choose for now?

that interior movement toward one's Creator and strengthens the soul (versus desolation or an increased slothfulness of heart and inner darkness, as Ignatius described it [Backhouse, 1989]). Listen to your heart (inner wisdom or God) to sense how your choice rests inside. Offer your choice up to God for a blessing. An inner peace may come that affirms your choice. No response may be evident within; God may be stretching you to make a leap of faith.

If a discomfort or doubting about the decision comes, it may indicate you have made the wrong choice. Recognize the source of those feelings; many decisions, for example, inherently mean loss as well as gain. For example, if you have made a decision to move to another city to pursue the DNP degree and sense that your decision is what best praises God, you will undoubtedly also mourn the losses that will occur in the moving on. Recognizing the source of your grief will allow you to make the transition without waffling.

You may notice other indicators of good decisions. In addition to consolation, you will notice that you have patience with the ensuing challenges and chaos that the decision may bring. This patience results from the inner peace of living a congruent and faith-filled life. You may also notice within you more reverence toward all things.

Spiritual Tools for Decision Making

A spiritually sensitive person will find that there are several tools that support the decision-making process. Among these tools are prayer and meditation, journal writing, spiritual direction, and dream reflection.

Prayer and Meditation

One typology of prayer suggests that Americans use petitionary, ritual, conversational, and meditational prayer (Poloma & Gallup, 1991). Although petitionary and ritual prayers are often used during times of crisis, conversational and meditational prayers are more helpful to decision making. Conversational prayer (likely the most common form of prayer in America) is characterized by an individual thinking or verbalizing his or her inner experience for God. Just as human-to-human conversation involves both expression and listening, so does conversation with God. A sense of desolation or getting stuck saying the same things repeatedly are indicators that conversational prayer is one sided.

Meditational prayer, which focuses on listening to God, can ameliorate this condition. Meditational prayer can involve simply spending time in nature or some quiet, sacred space with a heart open toward God. There is no agenda other than to be attentive to whatever may nudge your attention (e.g., a thought, a leaf, the warmth of the sun, a bird's song). Assuming such a receptive and neutral stance allows one to be available to God-sent impressions and insights that are pertinent to the decision.

Journal Writing

Keeping a journal that is private, unstructured, and unedited can allow you to document not only the various analytical strategies (previously discussed) but to record your feelings, thoughts, and informal observations about your inner life and struggle. The journal can also allow you to record your dreams, conversations, reading, and other sources of insight. For some, it is not until these inner processes get concretized in writing that the best insight occurs. Also, rereading the journal can allow you to see recurrent themes that you otherwise might fail to acknowledge.

Spiritual Direction

Spiritual directors or mentors are soul friends or holy listeners. These lay or professionally trained spiritual directors typically have studied spiritual formation and counseling to some degree. Someone who seeks spiritual development intentionally will seek out a spiritual director on a regular basis (e.g., once per month), and an individual amidst the crisis of making a major decision may want biweekly visits with a spiritual director. These sessions (typically 1 hour) will allow the decision maker to explore how to discern God's will, which may lead to discussion about how to encounter God or how God is perceived. A spiritual director can give tips on how to meditate, how to explore one's inner life, and provide support as the directee draws up courage to make a difficult choice. You can find a spiritual director by consulting the Spiritual Directors International website at www.sdiworld.org.

Dream Reflection

Although a discussion of how to analyze and make sense of your dreams is beyond the scope of this chapter, it is valuable to remember that your dreams will provide you with extremely helpful information during your decision-making process. Your dreams may tell you what you are not able to recognize in waking life. They, in a sense, will help you to know your authentic self. A good spiritual director or a trained therapist can assist you, and there are several excellent books on the topic to guide you (e.g., Berne & Savary, 1991; Sanford, 1978).

■ Living with the Decision

Regardless of the option a decision maker chooses, there potentially are ensuing problems or imperfections. Just because a choice leads to seemingly insurmountable challenges does not mean it is the wrong choice. To address such challenges, it is good to keep centered on what prompted the choice in the first place; that is, to remember how this choice lines up with your overall mission in life and allows fulfillment of who you really are. Victor Frankl (1984) was fond of quoting Nietzsche, who posited: "He who has a why to live for can bear almost any how." Indeed, if your decision supports your overall life purpose, you will find it easier to bear the hardships that result from it.

If your decision-making process leads you to choose the DNP degree, there are ways to cope with the stressors of schooling. Some of these include:

- ■ Focusing on what you have yet to do rather than on what you have done to date. According to Koo and Fishbach's (2008) research, this frame of mind is associated with greater goal adherence.

- Simplifying your life. This may require you to think outside the box. Have no more than three foci in your life (e.g., school, family, work). This may require you to resign much-loved roles and forfeit some activities that are wonderful. You might ask yourself, "Would I rather do a few things well or several things poorly?" If living simply means earning a lower income, find the joy in having less money. (Home cooked beans and rice can taste delicious, and old cars may be less likely to be stolen!)
- Delegating some tasks that are not necessary for you to do. Draw together a supportive network of family and friends who can help you with such tasks and support you emotionally.
- Accepting that you may need to be more disciplined than ever now. Just as Lance Armstrong rigidly controls his diet, sleep, and cycling when in training, you may need to restrict your television viewing, eliminate sweets and high-fat foods that make you sluggish or depressed, and exercise and drink water much more to enhance your energy level.
- Appreciating that the best grade for you in courses may be a B (for "Balance"). Although you always want to do your best, your best while maintaining a balanced life may be not to earn top grades.

Such suggestions for coping with the challenges of DNP study require a proactive (rather than reactive) stance.

■ Conclusion

This chapter describes some classic strategies for making a decision. It also emphasizes the importance of considering the underlying spirituality inherent in decisions, such as whether to pursue a DNP degree. Although the outcome of a decision will shape who you become, it is just as true that the process of making a decision will reflect who you are. Thus, this decision presents you with an opportunity to reflect on who you have been and who you want to be.

SUMMARY

- Most people who choose the DNP over the PhD do so because their primary interest is in promoting excellence in clinical practice rather than scholarship (Loomis, Willard, & Cohen, 2007). Others choose the DNP because it requires less time; it is impractical for an APRN to invest in a DNP degree in the last several years of his or her career.
- Although future law cannot be guaranteed, it is clearly the intent of the AACN to promote grandfathering. That is, if you are an APRN now, it is unlikely that you will need a DNP degree to remain an APRN.
- Research about decision making suggests it is important to consider if you are positively or negatively framing the options, what your emotions are that will

influence the decision making, and how you might be using tunnel vision and narrowing your options prematurely.

- Force Field Analysis is a decision-making strategy that requires one to specify the desired plan, then to identify the forces that support that plan and the forces that are working against it (i.e., systematically weigh the pros and cons).
- Thinking Hats analysis allows one to look at a decision from several different perspectives or with different styles of thinking (e.g., intellectual, intuitive, optimistic, pessimistic, outside the box).
- Grid Analysis requires you to list all the possible options being decided (in rows) and then identify all the factors that are important to consider (in columns). Each factor should then be given a weight between 0 (not at all important) and 5 (extremely important). When this grid is established, you can then use the same scoring system to give a score to each option for each of the factors.
- Decision making that fails to recognize spiritual yearnings is incomplete and may lead to outcomes that are not congruent with what is ultimately important for the individual.
- A difficult decision can be viewed as an opportunity to intensely encounter God.
- As one considers whether to become a DNP or not, knowing whether it fits one's life purpose is vital.
- Often what is the best choice (e.g., that which will stretch us, humble us, transform us) is also the hardest choice. The decisions in life that are agonizing are often agonizing because we are resisting what seems to us to be the most difficult choice.
- Tools that the spiritually sensitive decision maker may find helpful include prayer and meditation, journal writing, spiritual direction, and dream reflection.
- Just because a choice leads to seemingly insurmountable challenges does not mean it is the wrong choice. To address such challenges, it is good to keep centered on what prompted the choice in the first place; that is, to remember how this choice lines up with your overall mission in life and allows fulfillment of who you really are.

REFLECTION QUESTIONS

1. What are the reasons for why I want further education? (Go deep, to the most fundamental reasons. For example, you may initially answer with, Because I want to know more. Then ask yourself, Why do I want to know more?)

2. What is the principal purpose for my existence? What is my mission in life? How might getting a DNP degree (or not) contribute to my life vocation or mission?

3. Whose input about this decision do I value? What impressions do they have about my returning to school?

4. How am I relating to this decision? Is it bringing dread? Does it excite me? How will the rest of my life be affected by this decision?

5. Please see Table 8-1 for further reflective questions that are important to the decision-making process.

REFERENCES

American Association of Colleges of Nursing (AACN). (2006). *Doctor of nursing practice roadmap task force report*. Retrieved from http://www.aacn.nche.edu/dnp/roadmapreport.pdf

American Association of Colleges of Nursing (AACN). (2008). *Consensus model for APRN regulation: Licensure, accreditation, certification & education*. Retrieved from http://www.aacn.nche.edu /education-resources/APRNReport.pdf

Backhouse, H. (Ed.). (1989). The spiritual exercises of St. Ignatius Loyola. London: Hodder & Stoughton.

Berne, P. H., & Savary, L. M. (1991). *Dream symbol work: Unlocking the energy from dreams and spiritual experiences*. New York: Paulist Press.

Chambers, O. (1992). *My utmost for his highest: An updated edition in today's language: The Golden book of Oswald Chambers*. Grand Rapids, MI: Discover House.

Clinton, P., & Sperhac, A. M. (2009). The DNP and unintended consequences: An opportunity for dialogue. *Journal of Pediatric Health Care, 23*(5), 348–351.

de Vries, M., Holland, R. W., & Witteman, C. L. M. (2008). Fitting decisions: Mood and intuitive versus deliberative decision strategies. *Cognition & Emotion, 22*(5), 931–943.

Frankl, V. (1984). *Man's search for meaning*. New York: Washington Square Press.

Fulton, J. S., & Lyon, B. L. (2005, November 14). The need for some sense making: Doctor of nursing practice. *Online Journal of Issues in Nursing, 10*(3). Retrieved from http://www.nursingworld.org /MainMenuCategories/ANAMarketplace/ANAPeriodicals/OJIN/TableofContents/Volume102005 /No3Sept05/tpc28_316027.aspx

Gallup, G., Jr., & Jones, T. (2002). *The next American spirituality: Finding God in the twenty-first century*. New York: NexGen.

Haward, M. F., Murphy, R. O., & Lorenz, J. M. (2008). Message framing and perinatal decisions. *Pediatrics, 122*(1), 109–118.

Koo, M., & Fishbach, A. (2008). Dynamics of self-regulation: How (un)accomplished goal actions affect motivation. *Journal of Personality and Social Psychology, 94*(2), 183–195.

Loomis, J. A., Willard, B., & Cohen, J. (2007). Difficult professional choices: Deciding between the PhD and the DNP in nursing. *Online Journal of Issues in Nursing, 12*(1), 6. Retrieved from http://www .nursingworld.org/MainMenuCategories/ANAMarketplace/ANAPeriodicals/OJIN/TableofContents /Volume122007/No1Jan07/ArticlePreviousTopics/tpc28_816033.aspx

McGraw, P. C. (2001). *Self matters: Creating your life from the inside out*. New York: Simon & Schuster.

Poloma, M. M., & Gallup, G. H., Jr. (1991). *Varieties of prayer: A survey report*. Philadelphia: Trinity Press.

Rassin, E., Muris, P., Booster, E., & Kolsloot, I. (2008). Indecisiveness and informational tunnel vision. *Personality and Individual Differences, 45*(1), 96–102.

Sanford, J. A. (1978). *Dreams and healing: A succinct and lively interpretation of dreams*. New York: Paulist Press.

Schneiders, S. M. (1982). Spiritual discernment in The Dialogue of Saint Catherine of Siena. *Horizons, 9*(1), 47–59.

Schul, Y., Mayo, R., & Burnstein, E. (2008). The value of distrust. *Journal of Experimental Social Psychology, 44*(5), 1293–1302.

Taylor, E. J. (2002). *Spiritual care: Nursing theory, research, and practice*. Upper Saddle River, NJ: Prentice Hall.

van 't Wout, M., Kahn, R. S., Sanfey, A. G., & Aleman, A. (2006). Affective state and decision-making in the Ultimatum Game. *Explorations in Brain Research, 169*(4), 564–568.

Wuthnow, R. (1998). *After heaven: Spirituality in America since the 1950s*. Berkeley: University of California Press.

CHAPTER 9

The Dr. Nurse: Overcoming Title Issues

■ LISA ASTALOS CHISM ■

"I never really address myself to any image anybody has of me. That's like fighting with ghosts."

—*Sally Field (1946–)*

With the novelty of being a pioneer, one has the responsibility to lead the way. As more nurses graduate with doctoral degrees, the dilemma of what title to use remains an issue. The dilemma associated with the use of the title "doctor" is not necessarily new in nursing, but it is most definitely now at the forefront due to the advent of the Doctor of Nursing Practice (DNP) degree. Previously, PhD-prepared nurses struggled to be recognized outside of the academic setting for their educational preparation. Most certainly, this issue is not unique to nurses who hold doctorate degrees. All nonphysician health professionals who are prepared at the doctorate level will potentially be faced with this issue. Further, the way in which DNP graduates manage this issue will affect how it develops in the future.

As part of her DNP curriculum, this author attended a leadership seminar in which a panel of DNP graduates was available for questions. The most frequently asked question of the panel was, "Are you referred to as doctor?" The literature also reflects the pertinence of this topic (Klein, 2007; O'Grady, 2007; Reeves, 2008; Royeen & Lavin, 2006). The Institute of Medicine has recommended enhanced educational preparation of healthcare professionals (Greiner & Knebel, 2003). Moreover, parity among multiple healthcare professionals has also instituted an evolution of education preparation to include the doctoral degree (Griffiths & Padilla, 2006; Pierce & Peyton, 1999; Roeser, Thibodeau, & Cokely, 2005). As this evolution unfolds, the use of the title "doctor" by others outside of medicine will continue to be debated. Therefore, a discussion that includes relevant topics, such as the history of the title "doctor," parity among healthcare professionals, review of the states' status regarding title protection, the debate in the literature, and a university's response to this issue is provided in this chapter. An unfortunate case study, along with relevant interviews regarding this issue, are also included. Finally, advice for DNP graduates regarding the most appropriate ways in which to transition to the title "doctor" is reviewed.

■ The History of *Docere*: The First Teachers

The term "doctor," derived from the Latin *docere*, originated in Bologna, Italy during the 12th century (Skinner, 1970). The English translation for *docere* is "to teach," with "doctrine" being what is taught (Skinner, 1970). Merriam-Webster's Online Dictionary (2008) defines the term "doctor" as "a learned or authoritative teacher; a person who has earned one of the highest academic degrees conferred by a university; a person skilled in the healing arts, especially one who holds an advanced degree and a license to practice." Bailey (2003) related that the term "doctor" referred to a religious teacher, scholar, and father of the Christian church; "doctor" also took on the meaning, in the 13th century, "to make to appear right" and "a shower of the way" (p. 490).

The first doctorate was conferred in Bologna and applied to masters who teach (Skinner, 1970). Universities were a community or guild and the doctorate degree was actually a certificate of admission for professors (Marriner-Tomey, 1990). Additionally, licensing men to teach also became the responsibility of clergy as well as professors (Marriner-Tomey, 1990). Eventually, by the second half of the 12th century, the demand for learned men in the community increased and men began earning professional doctorates without the intention to teach (Marriner-Tomey, 1990). As education developed in English universities, the doctorate degree was granted only for law, medicine, and divinity (Skinner, 1970). As universities grew and more men received professional doctorates, those prepared in medicine moved into the communities and among the people. It has been speculated that because of this, the general public began to associate the doctoral degree with medicine (Skinner, 1970). In reality, "doctor" refers to any person with a doctoral degree in any field (Bailey, 2003), not a specific profession. This is an important point for both DNP graduates and other various professionals to remember when questioned regarding their title or educational preparation.

■ Parity Among Healthcare Professionals: One of the DNP Drivers Revisited

It is clear in the literature that one of the drivers of the DNP degree is parity in the healthcare setting (Clinton & Sperhac, 2006; Marion, O'Sullivan, Crabtree, Price, & Fontana, 2005; Newman, 1975; Olshansky, 2004). Arguments for parity have also included the point that current nursing master's degrees already have more requirements than many other professional doctoral degrees (Clinton & Sperhac, 2006). Hence, with the adoption of a doctoral degree, parity with other professionals occurs and nurses finally gain the recognition for their educational accomplishments that they deserve. Olshansky (2004) noted that nurses "who earn a DNP will be on par with our practicing health care colleagues facilitating easier interdisciplinary collaboration on an equal playing field" (p. 211).

As the DNP degree gains momentum, it is interesting to note that other healthcare professions have adopted the doctoral degree as the terminal degree or as entry into practice. Pharmacy was one of the earlier adopters of a doctorate degree for entry into practice (Upvall & Ptachcinski, 2007). Physical therapy also requires a doctorate for entry into practice. Occupational therapy and audiology have followed suit and are moving toward doctoral preparation both as an option and as entry into practice (Griffiths & Padilla, 2006; Pierce & Peyton, 1999; Roeser, et al., 2005). Reviewing other healthcare professions' transition to a doctoral degree, including reasons for adopting doctoral preparation, provides rationale for this evolution and parity across the healthcare team.

Upvall and Ptachcinski (2007) compared pharmacy's transition to doctoral preparation (PharmD) to nursing's adoption of the DNP degree. The PharmD was developed as a response to societal needs for increased clinical services, similar to the need for nursing to increase educational preparation. Pharmacy identified the need for increased preparation in pharmacotherapy in health care and, as a result, parity and advancement of the profession were secondary benefits (Upvall & Ptachcinski, 2007). Further, pharmacy recognized that the 5-year undergraduate degree did not provide a sufficient time frame for the biomedical sciences and clinical component necessary to meet the expectations in practice (Upvall & Ptachcinski, 2007). This is similar to nursing in that a nursing master's degree may not efficiently accommodate the changing needs for preparation of advanced nursing practice (Clinton & Sperhac, 2006). Although this preparation was met with resistance at first (two failed attempts), advocates argued that doctoral preparation in pharmacy met the needs of a changing healthcare environment (Upvall & Ptachcinski, 2007). An evaluation of healthcare outcomes has also shown improvement and a reduction in medical errors as a result of the services from clinical pharmacists (Bond, Raehl, & Franke, 2002). It has also been previously noted that healthcare outcomes are improved by advanced practice registered nurses (Brooten & Naylor, 1995). It would be safe to assume, therefore, that the additional preparation provided by the DNP degree would continually improve healthcare outcomes.

Physical therapy has adopted the doctoral degree for entry into practice and occupational therapy is in the process of adopting doctoral preparation. The incentives for this transition have been cited to parallel pharmacy, medicine, and dentistry in that advanced education, higher standards for entry into practice, and extended clinical experience will provide educational preparation that is necessary to facilitate change (Pierce & Peyton, 1999). Further, these two professions have noted comparable drivers toward doctoral preparation, which include advanced preparation to meet the changing needs of health care as well as parity with other healthcare professionals (Pierce & Peyton, 1999).

Audiology is currently offering doctoral preparation as well, which combines both didactic learning and extensive clinical experiences. Roeser, Thibodeau, and Cokely (2005) described an emerging Doctor of Audiology (AuD) program that combines academic course work, clinical experiences, a research experience, and mentoring. This particular program is 4 years long and offered as a postbaccalaureate degree. The format mirrors that of a postbaccalaureate DNP degree, integrating academic course work, clinical specialization, and research. This degree is yet another example of how the education of healthcare professionals is evolving to meet the demands of society and the healthcare environment.

In summary, understanding the evolution toward doctoral preparation of various healthcare professionals provides further explanation regarding the importance of recognition of all healthcare professionals' educational preparation. The advanced educational preparation of all members of the interprofessional team should be celebrated, not hidden. Indeed, it is this advanced educational preparation that will serve to improve healthcare outcomes and quality of care. Moreover, it is envisioned that someday soon, the entire healthcare team will be doctors. This team of doctors may include pharmacists, physical therapists, occupational therapists, nurses, and physicians who all strive toward the same goal, each with valuable knowledge and expertise that should be acknowledged equally. Diminishing this is any way seems counterproductive to the goals of health care today.

■ Review of "The Pearson Report" Regarding Title Protection

Each year Dr. Linda Pearson publishes a state-by-state national overview of nurse practitioner legislation and healthcare issues. Dr. Pearson has been recapping the latest legislative information from each state's nurse practice act and rules and regulations, along with pertinent government, policy, and reimbursement information, for the past 23 years (Pearson, 2011). A full version of this report is available at http://www.pearsonreport.com.

It is interesting that in recent years Dr. Pearson has included legislation and regulation regarding the use of the title "doctor" by nurses who hold doctoral degrees. Moreover, in the 2008 report, Dr. Pearson included in her "My Impressions" section comments regarding this particular legislation and listed it as "Impression #1." Dr. Pearson specifically states, "We need to legislatively remove NP-degrading discrimination" (Pearson, 2008, p. 10). Dr. Pearson further commented that "NPs must remove any and all statutory restrictions prohibiting those of us with university earned doctorates from being addressed as doctor" (p. 10). In the 2011 Pearson Report, Dr. Pearson noted that several states have legislatively allowed qualified nurse practitioners to be addressed as "doctor" as long as they clarify that they are nurse practitioners (Pearson, 2011). Dr. Pearson related that this is appropriate because nurse practitioners are proud to be nurses and have no interest in being confused with physicians. Unfortunately, five states (Maine, Arkansas, Connecticut, Michigan, and Vermont) currently have restrictions regarding nurses with earned doctorates being addressed as "doctor"

(Pearson, 2011). Dr. Pearson relates that, "a quietly emerging trend in health care [is] likely to have a major effect on who will diagnose and treat illness in the coming years. Rather than a physician, a comprehensive-care provider may very well be a nurse—who also happens to be a doctor" (Pearson, 2008, p. 10). Dr. Pearson's comments and synopsis on this topic are timely and reflect the urgency to protect nurses', as well as other doctoral-prepared healthcare professionals', right to be appropriately recognized for their credentials, knowledge, and expertise.

■ The Debate

A debate previously unfolded in the literature in response to the American Medical Association (AMA) Resolutions, which attempted to restrict the use of the title "doctor" by nurses with doctoral degrees. Nursing organizations have responded to this issue with arguments against such regulations that would restrict nurses from appropriately identifying their credentials. In addition, universities are also responding to this impending issue with ideas for a proactive, solution-based response.

American Medical Association Resolution

The American Medical Association House of Delegates identified Resolution 211 (A-06) in May 2006, titled the "Need to Expose and Counter Nurse Doctoral Programs (NDP) Misrepresentation" (AMA, 2006). This resolution states, "The quality of care rendered by individuals with nurse doctoral degrees is not equivalent to that of a physician" (AMA, 2006). Additionally, this resolution states that "Nurses and other nonphysician providers who hold doctoral degrees and identify themselves as doctors will create confusion, jeopardize patient safety, and erode the trust inherent in the true patient–physician relationship" (AMA, 2006). The resolution further states that "Patients led to believe that they are receiving care from a doctor, who is not a physician, but who is a DNP may put their health at risk" (AMA, 2006). Therefore, the following resolutions were resolved:

- That it shall be the policy of our AMA that institutions offering advance education in the healing arts and professions shall fully and accurately inform applicants and students of the educational programs and degrees offered by an institution and the limitations, if any, on the scope of practice under applicable law for which the program prepares the student; and it be further
- resolved that our AMA work jointly with state attorneys general to identify and prosecute those individuals who misrepresent themselves as physicians to their patients and mislead program applicants as to their future scope of practice; and it be further
- resolved that our AMA pursue all other appropriate legislative, regulatory and legal actions through the Scope of Practice Partnership, as well as actions within hospital staff organizations, to counter misrepresentation by nurse doctoral programs students and graduates, particularly in the clinical setting. (AMA, 2006)

It should be noted when reading these resolutions that if nurses identify themselves appropriately by their earned degree and professional designation, none of these resolutions actually applies. If nurses identify themselves as "Dr. Smith, Nurse–Midwife" or "Dr. Jones, Chief Nursing Officer," it should be quite obvious what discipline these professionals subscribe to. Further, it would be safe to assume that when nurses apply to a Doctor of Nursing Practice program, they are well aware of the discipline in which they are getting their degree. After all, nurses went to college, too.

The Literature

This issue has also been discussed and debated in the literature in response to the AMA's Resolution 211 (A-06). Royeen and Lavin (2007) wrote a commentary on the analysis of healthcare professionals who earn doctorate degrees and responded to the issues regarding the title "doctor." It was acknowledged that the public commonly associates the term "doctor" with physician. However, Royeen and Lavin stated:

> That does not mean that others may not be referred to as doctor when holding a professional degree. It does mean that the nature of the degree needs to be clearly communicated to the public for whom they care and that professionals identify themselves a physicians, nurse practitioners, physical therapists, occupational therapists, and so on instead of using the term doctor as if it were synonymous with one professional group. (p. 102)

Reeves (2008) also responded to the AMA's Resolution 211 (A-06) and highlighted the fact that advanced practice registered nurses do not wish to be confused with physicians, and, in fact, advanced practice registered nurses capitalize on the different type of care they provide. Explaining further, Reeves stated, "It is essential that health care professionals and the public be taught the differences between the disciplines of nursing and medicine. Nurses do not want to misrepresent themselves. We understand that health care often involves working together with an interdisciplinary team to provide optimal patient care" (2008).

O'Grady (2007) shared a similar response to the current debate regarding this issue and reinforced the notion that the public and other healthcare professionals need to be educated regarding this issue. O'Grady (2007) noted that it is the public's right to know who is caring for them and what credentials those individuals hold. "To require health professionals other than physicians to hide their credentials is directly contrary to health care transparency and consumer empowerment" (O'Grady, 2007, p. 8). Moreover, O'Grady (2007) related that "the truth—letting patients know in the clearest possible way who is caring for them—should be the foundation for sound policymaking" (p. 8). Nursing as a whole is responsible to respond to this issue. The belief that the DNP degree results in social good as a consequence of more educated nurses, along with the belief that nurses have power over their practice, means that nurses must work together to be freed from illogical and oppressive policies that force nurses to hide their credentials (O'Grady, 2007).

Nursing's Response

Nursing responded collectively to this issue by addressing the AMA directly. Major nursing organizations drafted a unified statement and published "DNP Talking Points" specific to this issue. In June 2008, the American Nurses Association (ANA) sent a letter to the director of the AMA House of Delegates. This letter specifically addressed protection of the title "doctor." In the letter, Ms. Patton and Ms. Stierle summarized the origin of the title "doctor" and further explained that a doctor is one who has earned a doctoral degree in any field. Ms. Patton and Ms. Stierle also addressed the issue of patient confusion and stated, "If patient confusion is really the concern, the nursing community would welcome the efforts to communicate to patients just who—and what type—of healthcare professionals are examining and treating them" (ANA letter, June 11, 2008, p. 2). Further, the notion of "restraint of trade" was brought to Dr. Lichtman's attention. In previous situations, the U.S. Court of Appeals ruled that the AMA could not "boycott" another's healthcare profession because this would violate the Sherman Antitrust Act. This communication from the ANA to the AMA exemplifies the proactive, united stance that nursing must take when confronted with this issue.

Another example of collectively addressing this issue occurred when several nursing organizations drafted a unified statement regarding nurse practitioner DNP education. This statement was written collaboratively by the American Academy of Nurse Practitioners, the American College of Nurse Practitioners, the National Association of Pediatric Nurse Practitioners, the Association of Faculties of Pediatric Nurse Practitioners, the National Organization of Nurse Practitioner Faculties, the National Conference of Gerontological Nurse Practitioners, and the National Association of Nurse Practitioners in Women's Health, collectively referred to as the Nurse Practitioner Roundtable. This statement addresses certification and titling issues and specifically outlines the utilization of the title "doctor" by nurse practitioners. The recommendations of this statement are as follows:

1. The title doctor represents an academic credential and is not limited to professional programs. Graduate educational programs in colleges and universities in the United States confer academic degrees, which permit graduates to be called doctor. No one discipline owns the title "doctor."
2. In the healthcare field, the term doctor is not limited to medical doctors. Other health professions use their academic title: e.g., Doctor of Osteopathy, Doctor of Pharmacy, Doctor of Podiatry, Doctor of Psychology, Doctor of Physical Therapy, and others.
3. While the titles "Medical Doctor" or "Doctor of Osteopathy" may be protected by statute in a given state, the term "doctor" alone is not.
4. Recognition of the title "doctor" for doctoral-prepared nurse practitioners facilitates parity within the healthcare system. (Nurse Practitioner Roundtable, 2008, p. 2)

Finally, the American Association of Colleges of Nursing (AACN) developed a Talking Points document that describes the rationale for the DNP degree. This document was developed to assist nurse educators and others in responding to questions regarding the DNP degree. These talking points include the following statements:

- The rapid expansion of knowledge underlying practice; increased complexity of patient care; national concerns about the quality of care and patient safety; shortages of nursing personnel, which demands a higher level of preparation for leaders who can design and assess care; shortages of doctorally prepared nursing faculty; and increasing educational expectations for the preparation of other health professionals contribute to the momentum of nursing graduate education (AACN, 2011).
- Many authorities, including the Institute of Medicine, have called for reconceptualizing health professions education to meet the needs of the healthcare delivery system. Nursing is answering that call by moving to prepare APRNs for evolving practice (AACN, 2011).
- "In a 2005 report titled 'Advancing the Nation's Health Needs: NIH Research Training Programs,' the National Academy of Sciences called for nursing to develop a nonresearch clinical doctorate to prepare expert practitioners who can also serve as clinical faculty. The AACN's work to advance the DNP is consistent with this call to action" (AACN, 2011).
- "Nursing is moving in the direction of other health professions in the transition to the DNP. Medicine (MD), Dentistry (DDS), Pharmacy (PharmD), Psychology (PsyD), Physical Therapy (DPT), and Audiology (AudD) all offer practice doctorates" (AACN, 2011).
- "Currently, advanced practice nurses, including nurse practitioners, clinical nurse specialists, nurse–midwives, and nurse anesthetists, are typically prepared in master's degree programs, some of which carry a credit load equivalent to doctoral degrees in the other health professions" (AACN, 2011).
- "Transitioning to the DNP will not alter the current scope of practice for APRNs. State Nurse Practice Acts describe the scope of practice allowed, and these differ from state to state. (These requirements would likely remain unchanged.) The transition to the DNP will better prepare APRNs for their current roles given the calls for new models of education and the growing complexity of health care" (AACN, 2011).
- "The title of doctor is common to many disciplines and is not the domain of any one health profession. Many APRNs currently hold doctoral degrees and are addressed as doctors, which is similar to how clinical psychologists, dentists, podiatrists, and other experts are addressed. Like other providers, DNPs would be expected to display their credentials to insure that patients understand their preparation as a nursing provider" (AACN, 2011).
- "Nursing and medicine are distinct health disciplines that prepare clinicians to assume different roles and meet different practice expectations. DNP programs will prepare nurses for the highest level of nursing practice" (AACN, 2011).

This document can be accessed at http://www.aacn.nche.edu/dnp/talking-points and provides valuable, factual information for DNP graduates, nurses, and other healthcare professionals. DNP graduates may use documents such as these to educate themselves, nurses, and other healthcare professionals in the healthcare environment in an effort to respond to questions and effectively debate title issues.

A University's Response

Oakland University in Rochester, Michigan graduated the first DNP program in the state in December 2007 and May 2008. Twenty-two nurses with DNP degrees returned to their settings, both academic and clinical, and began to proudly display their new credentials. Most were met with support, but unfortunately, as with many pioneers, some graduates were faced with resistance to change in their settings. One case in particular, which will be described later in the chapter, resulted in the DNP graduate being threatened with a misdemeanor charge if she used the title "doctor." Fortunately, Oakland University supported their DNP graduates and responded to this oppressive, irrational behavior. Consequently, Dr. Frances Jackson, Director of Oakland University's DNP program, organized a coalition meeting. This coalition meeting was attended by various university deans, nursing political organizations, Michigan's chief nurse executive, Ms. Jeanette Wrona Klemczak, physical therapy organizations, and various DNP program directors. Dr. Frances Jackson moderated the meeting, and overall the meeting established a unified stance between nursing and physical therapy as an early response to title issues. The minutes for this meeting are reprinted with permission to provide an example of unified support and an early proactive stance against repressive, illogical behaviors toward DNP graduates and other doctoral-prepared healthcare professionals.

Update to American Medical Association Resolution

In June 2008, the AMA House of Delegates officially rejected the resolution that would limit the use of the titles "doctor," "resident," and "residency" to physicians, dentists, and podiatrists. Mason (2008) commented on this in an editorial and stated, "Somehow, the group realized that the term doctor applies to anyone who has earned a doctoral degree" (p. 7). Incidentally, if the resolution would have progressed further, it would have supported making it a felony for a nonphysician to represent her- or himself as a physician by using the title "doctor" (Mason, 2008). It should be noted, however, that despite the rejection of this resolution, states may still individually mandate the use of the title "doctor." These mandates range from prohibiting the use of the title "doctor" by those not specified within the mandate to requiring that the professional designation follow the title "doctor." Nursing has long supported making sure that patients know who is providing their care and will continue to strive to educate the public regarding their educational preparation and professional role.

Coalition Meeting Minutes

The first meeting of the Coalition was held on Monday, June 23, 2008 at Oakland University. The purpose of this meeting was to build support for health professions that award a clinical doctoral degree and who might face opposition from physicians and other healthcare agencies to the use of the title "Dr." Representatives from the following organizations were present:

Oakland University (Nursing and PT)
Grand Valley State University
University of Michigan–Flint
Madonna University
Northern Michigan University
University of Detroit–Mercy
Wayne State University (Nursing and PT)
Michigan Physical Therapy Assn
Michigan Council of Nurse Practitioners
Oakland University School of Nursing DNP Alumnae

The Chief Nurse Executive for the state of Michigan, Ms. Jeanette Wrona Klemczak, was also present.

Consensus was reached on the following:

1. We need a national, coordinated response to physician opposition to the clinical doctoral degrees in nursing and physical therapy.
2. It might be harmful if nursing attempted to become part of Senate Bill 1167 which primarily addresses PT Assistants.
3. There is a need for Nursing, OT, and PT to collaborate to have the Public Health code revised to address the issue of titling.
4. We need to investigate including social work, OT, and pharmacy in the coalition.
5. There is a need to expand data collected about nurses to include the number of nurses who have the DNP in Michigan.
6. We should also include other nursing and PT programs.
7. We should also include Chief Nursing Officers and members of the Michigan Organization of Nurse Executives and PTs in private practice.

Future Plans

1. There is a need to increase the public's knowledge about advanced practice registered nurses.
2. We need a brief paper that introduces the problem of titling and describes what we want to do.
3. The Board of Nursing is opening up the rules on nursing. This might be another way to address the issue of titling.
4. We need to reach out to other professions and see if they want to join us in this coalition.
5. The letter generated by the law firm retained by the Dickinson County Hospital was troubling. We need another opinion on whether their interpretation of the law is accurate.
6. We need to educate our colleagues about this issue.

Coalition Meeting Minutes *(continued)*

---

7. Once we have our one-page, brief paper, we need to approach COMON (Coalition of Michigan Nursing Organizations) to get support for our position.

8. The Michigan Center for Nursing Board conducts a voluntary survey on RNs. We need to add the DNP.

9. Also need to contact the Greater Detroit Health Council and the Regional Area Network for Nursing and get their support for the clinical doctorate.

10. The western part of the state has a similar organization (see #9) and we should approach them as well for support.

Summary of the meeting minutes with suggested next steps (Prepared by Dr. Frances Jackson):

1. Is there a natural division of the above items that would fall into certain categories that would ease the handling of these issues? For example:
   a. Professional Healthcare Organizations (contact, recruit, garner support)
   b. Education (public and professionals)
   c. Policy and Legal (would write the brief synopsis of the issue and what we want; obtain a second legal opinion)
   d. State of Michigan initiatives (Board of Nursing and the rules; Michigan Center for Nursing Board, etc.)

2. Please prioritize the list. It was suggested that rather than numbering items, we might use a system of categories, like Do These First, Do These Next, Long Term, or something of that nature.

3. Form a steering committee that will take a leadership role in keeping our momentum and making sure we don't drop the ball on any of these issues. It is very important to have both PT and Nursing. I would go a step further to say we also need a representative from both MCNP and MPTA. Their knowledge about the state legislators and bills related to health policy, as well as their input from our national organizations is critically important.

Last, considering volunteering for a group once the groups have been identified and named. I look forward to receiving feedback from everyone.

Source: Coalition Meeting Minutes. (2008). *Oakland University coalition meeting minutes.* Rochester, MI: Author. Reprinted with permission.

■ Case Scenario: A Dr. Nurse's Story

Unfortunately, despite the realization that all professionals may earn doctorate degrees as well as use the title associated with an earned doctorate degree, some recent DNP graduates are experiencing significant resistance regarding use of the title "doctor." This case scenario is a true account of a DNP graduate clinician who is a nurse practitioner in rural Michigan. Her interview follows the highlights of her story, which are provided in the case scenario.

Dr. O. was welcomed back after graduation from her DNP program with a congratulatory advertisement in her local newspaper, which addressed her as Dr. O., FNP,

Doctor of Nursing Practice; Family Nurse Practitioner. Shortly after this, the RN Staff Council of her hospital organization received a letter from the hospital's attorney stating that Michigan Public Act 368 of 1978 strictly limits the use of the term "doctor" by anyone licensed under the Public Health Code. It further stated that by specifying the professions licensed under the Public Health Code that are entitled to use the term "doctor," the legislation implicated the limited use of the term to those listed health professionals. The letter surmised that the legislative history suggests that the limitation of the use of the term "doctor" was related to the "high likelihood of confusion among consumers/patients and not an indictment against the degree holder." The letter went on to say that use of the term "doctor" by a health professional not listed in Public Act 368 was a misdemeanor. Dr. O. was notified that the case was apparently discussed with the local prosecuting attorney's office, and they would not take action provided any further use of the designations be in compliance with Public Act 368.

The action from the hospital administration did not change Dr. O.'s title in the clinical setting. The actual clinic did not have any interaction with hospital administration, and Dr. O. has never heard directly from the hospital attorney's office. Therefore, in her practice setting, Dr. O. has continued to use her appropriate title.

Dr. O.'s next actions were very insightful and proactive. She started to write multiple e-mails to hospital administration purporting the benefit of supporting DNPs in the use of the "doctor" title in clinical practice. She also began educating colleagues, patients, and the community regarding the doctorate of nursing practice and the use of the title "doctor" in clinical practice. In an effort to educate her hospital organization directly, Dr. O. personally presented before the RN Staff Council and explained the DNP and title use.

To date, Dr. O. continues to write numerous letters and communicate with multiple nursing organizations regarding the controversial use of the "doctor" title for DNPs. She has also attended state and national meetings to discuss the use of the "doctor" title for DNPs in Michigan and nationally. In addition, she has made personal contacts with the president and president-elect of the nurse practitioner council in Michigan (MICNP). Dr. O. has also been in personal contact with the chief nurse executive of Michigan, Ms. Jeanette Wrona Klemczak. She contacted the legal council for the American Academy of Nurse Practitioners. Dr. O. also gained support from the university from which she earned her DNP degree. In response to her situation, a coalition meeting was organized to begin addressing this issue in Michigan. This meeting demonstrated the support of other professionals regarding this issue. Finally, Dr. O. has become a member of COMON as a representative of MICNP to pursue the issue with nursing organizations throughout Michigan.

Currently, this issue has not been resolved within Dr. O.'s hospital organization. Dr. O. continues to be proactive and use the leadership and interprofessional collaboration skills she garnered in the DNP program to educate others regarding this very controversial and pertinent issue. It should be noted, however, that since this incident, Michigan has been added to the list of states restricting the use of the title "doctor" by nurses.

Interview with a "Doctor Nurse" Champion: Then and Now

Linda Opsahl, DNP, APRN, BC is a family nurse practitioner who works in rural Michigan. Her story was told in the preceding case scenario.

Then . . . 2008

Dr. Opsahl, could you please describe your position?

I am a family nurse practitioner working in the rural Upper Peninsula of Michigan. I work for a hospital organization with several satellite clinics as well as the typical hospital setting. I work in two rural health clinics, and I also fill in for several other clinics on my days off. I am busy. I have a productive and growing practice. I am associated with a physician who is well liked and very knowledgeable. I love being a nurse practitioner. I consider it my calling.

Dr. Opsahl, what was the motivation for you to return to school for a DNP?

What motivated me to spend less time with my family, increase pressures and stressors in my life, and pull all-nighters at the ripe age of 52?

It wasn't that I would gain financially by going back to school. When I told my employer that I would be going back to school, they told me there would be no monetary increase because of the degree. They informed me that the degree would not change the way I practiced in the clinics; therefore, there would be no wage increase. Sadly, I also would not gain financially if I were to become a nursing professor. In fact, I would take a very large pay cut to teach in a university. The wage discrepancy for nursing instructors as compared to other university instructors such as engineers and medical doctors is something our profession must address.

It wasn't that I desired the prestige and recognition that the DNP degree would bring. When I told my physician partner I was going back to school, he told me I should go to medical school rather than obtain a nursing doctorate. Those same thoughts were echoed by family, friends, and patients who wondered just what a nurse doctor was. Many did not have a clear understanding of just what a nurse practitioner was. Some asked, "Will a doctorate in nursing make you equal to a PA?" I was also surprised by the negative responses of some PhD nurses toward the DNP. Their "my degree is better than your degree" attitude is proof that the theory–practice gap in nursing continues to plague our profession.

My motivation was higher education and the opportunities a doctorate degree could bring to my professional practice and the nursing profession in general. I've wanted to be a doctor since I was in grade school. I love the philosophy and foundation of nursing. A nurse doctor fits my personal and professional philosophy of holism and caring as compared to that of a traditional medical doctoral education. I was also motivated by the shortage of nursing instructors and made a personal and professional commitment to help fill that gap in the future.

Dr. Opsahl, how has your role evolved since earning your DNP degree?

My role as a family nurse practitioner has been markedly enhanced by the degree. I use more evidence-based practice. I collect more practice information and study quality indicators more closely. I use the quality indicators to show that nurse practitioners provide quality care with exceptional results. I am much more politically active in regard to healthcare issues affecting nurses, patients, the local community, and the nation. If you asked my employer if my role has changed, they would say no. To most people, the changes in my role are unseen. I think they would not be understood by others unless they were to truly appreciate, understand, and commit to the methods and importance of quality care and patient advocacy in the health of patients.

In the best of worlds, I hope to gain equal standing and respect with other doctorate degrees in health care. In reality, representatives of the administration and medical staff of the hospital where I am employed take a different view. I am told that the doctor designation for a nurse practitioner would be too confusing to the public and therefore should not be associated with the DNP in my current employment.

In my actual clinic sites, patients are proud that I have now become a nurse doctor. Many of them call me "Doctor," and all of them understand that I am a doctor of nursing practice rather than a doctor of medicine. I do not stop them from calling me "Doctor." There are also many patients that continue to call me by my first name. I don't correct them. Many of them have been calling me Linda for over 10 years.

Dr. Opsahl, how have your colleagues in your immediate clinical setting responded to your new degree?

My physician partner and the office staff in my clinical settings have been supportive of the DNP educational process and the new degree. I had no trouble getting time off when needed. I maintained my schedule and actually saw more patients in the one and a half years of the DNP program than in previous years. My physician partner continues to have difficulty understanding why I would choose to be a nurse doctor over a medical doctor. Initially, he felt that physicians held sole rights to the title of "doctor" in the healthcare environment. After I explained the origin and meaning of the word "doctor" as well as described and stated the numerous professions who also hold the title, he understood my reasoning and changed his mind a bit. Professionally, he now introduces me as Dr. Linda Opsahl.

Dr. Opsahl, have you found nursing to be supportive in your clinical setting?

The LPNs in my immediate clinical setting have been supportive. The RNs in my immediate clinical setting have been very supportive. The RNs in the hospital setting and in the community have been very supportive. The office staff in my immediate clinical settings threw me a party at the office and gave me an engraved name pin with the title "Dr." before my name. RNs in the local council of the state nursing organization took out an ad in the local newspaper congratulating me on my accomplishment and recognized me as "Dr. Linda Opsahl, Family Nurse Practitioner." They sent letters of support to the hospital administration for the use of the title "doctor" with nurse practitioners or any nurse achieving a doctorate degree.

Dr. Opsahl, how have you educated your colleagues and patients about your DNP degree?

As a family nurse practitioner, I am very familiar with addressing the question of why I am a nurse practitioner rather than a PA or physician and how my role as a nurse practitioner will affect the care I give to patients. Now I just modify the statement to tell them why I chose to become a nurse doctor. The answer is very similar. I chose to become a nurse practitioner with a doctorate in nursing practice because I love the holistic, caring, all-encompassing philosophy of nursing toward patients, their health, and their environment. As a nurse doctor, I can use the philosophy of nursing to guide my practice and enhance the care I give and patients receive. I tell patients and colleagues that I view multiple issues of a person or patient simultaneously. Each perspective or issue (emotional, financial, personal views, religious views, social, etc.) adds crucial information to the care and treatment plan for that patient. As a nurse, I am a health partner with the patient, developing and providing the necessary information and treatment plan in partnership with each individual.

I tell patients that I have a doctorate degree in nursing, not medicine. I tell them I am a nurse doctor. I combine the philosophy of nursing with the clinical and diagnostic perspective of medicine, integrating both with old and new evidence-based practice for their benefit. I provide the best of both worlds.

Dr. Opsahl, could you describe what happened when the hospital administration realized you were using the title "doctor"?

I was reviewing an article from the public relations department of my organization with regard to my recent DNP degree. The article was wonderful, explaining what a nurse practitioner was and what the new degree entailed. In editing the article, I added the title "Dr." in front of my name. Not only did I deserve the title through my degree acquisition, but I also felt that because this article would be sent to all my patients and other members of the community, it would be respectful and professionally appropriate to use the title. The article then went for review to the physician services department where a nurse manager evaluated the article and, under the direction of administration, removed the title "Dr." from the article. Their rationale was that the designation of "Dr." for a nurse practitioner would be too confusing to the public when associated with a DNP.

Dr. Opsahl, could you describe the legal action that took place as a result of administration restricting your use of the title "doctor"?

When the hospital RN staff council placed a congratulatory advertisement in the paper addressing me as "Dr. Linda Opsahl, FNP; Doctor of Nursing Practice;

Family Nurse Practitioner," the RN staff council received a letter from the hospital attorney stating that Michigan Public Act 368 of 1978 strictly limits the use of the term "doctor" by anyone licensed under the Public Health Code. It further stated that by specifying the professions licensed under the Public Health Code entitled to use the term "doctor," the legislation implicated the limited use of the term to those listed health professionals. The letter surmised that the legislative history suggests that the limitation of the use of the term "doctor" was related to the "high likelihood of confusion among consumers/patients and not an indictment against the degree holder." The letter went on to say that use of the term "doctor" by a health professional not listed in the Public Act 368 was a misdemeanor. The case was apparently discussed with the local prosecuting attorney's office, and they would not take action provided any further use of the designations be in compliance with Public Act 368.

Dr. Opsahl, what has been the reaction in your immediate clinical setting to this?

This issue has not been addressed in my immediate clinical setting. I did not hear directly from the hospital attorney. I have not changed my practice or title in the clinical setting.

Dr. Opsahl, what steps have you taken at this point to be proactive regarding your earned degree title?

I have written multiple e-mails to hospital administration purporting the benefit of supporting DNPs in the use of the "doctor" title in clinical practice. I educate colleagues, patients, and the community regarding the doctorate of nursing practice and the use of the title "doctor" in clinical practice. I explain that there is currently controversy over title use. I went before the RN Staff Council to explain the DNP and title use. I have written numerous letters and communicated with multiple nursing organizations regarding the controversial use of the "doctor" title for DNPs. I attended state and national meetings to discuss the use of the "doctor" title for DNPs in Michigan and nationally. I have made personal contacts with the president and president-elect of the nurse practitioner council in Michigan. I have made personal contact with the chief nurse executive of Michigan. I have made personal contact with legal council for the American Academy of Nurse Practitioners. I have become a member of COMON as a representative of MICNP to pursue the issue with nursing organizations throughout Michigan.

Dr. Opsahl, how do you feel about Oakland University's response and support regarding this issue?

I was very impressed by the response of Oakland University toward the titling issue. Dr. Jackson did an excellent job in bringing nurses across Michigan together to resolve this issue.

Dr. Opsahl, how do you feel this issue should be dealt with by other DNP graduates and healthcare professionals?

I think we are making a mistake by stepping or treading quietly regarding this issue and many issues in nursing. As nurse practitioners in Michigan, we are essentially a very small group. With the current situation in our state nurses' organization (MNA), we are left to fight on our own. Nursing in Michigan, the United States, and internationally must unite for common purpose, one of which is to enhance the profession for all nurses regardless of education. As it sits now, the staff nurses have their group, the nurse practitioners have their group, academia and PhD nurses have their group, and little is being done to bring us all together. By walking softly, there exists a communication gap between nursing organizations. By walking softly, the public is not aware of the controversies between nursing, administration, and medicine that ultimately affect patient care.

We have this attitude in Michigan right now. Nurses are saying that we can't get anything passed or accomplished until so and so is out of office. I don't believe that to be true. I think there are plenty of back doors in many situations. If the public is made aware that their nurse practitioner is being discriminated against, they will also stand up and fight. The DNP titling issue is discrimination. We are being crimped by administrators and the AMA because we are nurses and because we are women, and because we tend to walk softly.

Dr. Opsahl, despite what has occurred regarding your title, do you feel it was a good decision to return to school for a DNP degree?

Oh, yes. I would do it again and again. It was a wonderful opportunity. It has motivated me to become a better practitioner, a better patient advocate. I have become more verbal about important issues in practice because of it. I feel more confident. I feel it has given me the tools to fight discriminatory practice toward nurses.

Now . . . 2011

Dr. Opsahl, we discussed your nursing background and education last time we spoke. Could you please describe your current position?

I continue to work in rural health clinics in the Upper Peninsula of Michigan with the same employer.

Dr. Opsahl, how has your role evolved over the last 4 years since graduating with a DNP degree?

My role is essentially the same. I have been working with the same physician partner in 2 rural health clinics for 15 years. In rural health, a nurse practitioner must fill 50% or more of all open clinic hours. I am often the sole provider in the clinics.

Dr. Opsahl, how has your practice evolved since earning a DNP degree?

Though my role is essentially unchanged, my perception of my role and its philosophical meaning is enhanced. And of course, I am using the knowledge that I learned with the DNP to enhance my practice. I think I give better care with my increased knowledge base. I think I'm a "wiser" person and provider because of the DNP. My patients' perception of my role has also changed as they become more knowledgeable about the DNP degree. I'm proud of the degree and take pride in how I use it in my practice. I think my patients are also proud that their provider has a DNP. I am often introduced by my patients in a local store or social setting with "This is my *doctor* (the word is always emphasized), she's a *nurse doctor . . .* "

Dr. Opsahl, when we last spoke, you had experienced significant resistance regarding using the title "doctor" from a large hospital organization. How has this situation evolved over time?

I suppose I have learned to work around the resistance. I use the title in practice, but the hospital administration has not used the title when I am represented by them in hospital publicity situations. Administration downplays the title (especially during contract negotiations) saying there is no significant difference in my function and role as a nurse practitioner because I have a DNP. I am having difficulty affecting and influencing the antiquated ideas of the current administration. I will just keep working at it. I know what and who I am. My patients and nursing colleagues, as well as many of my physician colleagues, recognize that I am a Doctor of Nursing Practice.

Dr. Opsahl, are you still feeling supported to use the title "doctor" by your colleagues in your immediate clinical setting?

Yes. I am also supported by area nursing staff. But sometimes I feel like I am alone in the "cause." The other DNPs have long since left the employment of this particular institution for more professionally accepting administrations.

Dr. Opsahl, do you use the title "doctor" in your clinical setting? If so, how do you introduce yourself?

Yes and no. I have old and familiar patients who continue to call me "Linda." Many call me "Doctor." I am introduced as "Doctor Opsahl" by my physician partner. To new patients, I generally introduce myself as, "Dr. Linda Opsahl. I am a family nurse practitioner with a doctorate in nursing practice."

Dr. Opsahl, what advice do you have for others graduating with a DNP degree regarding using the title "doctor"?

Be proud of your title and use it. Have a clear understanding of what your role and title mean and how you will explain and defend yourself when needed. Look for supporters. If your nursing organization is slow to help you, call your nursing school. If they are slow to help you, call me or another DNP. There is power in numbers.

Interview with a "Doctor Nurse" Advocate and DNP Program Director—Then and Now

Frances Jackson, PhD, RN is associate professor and director of the Doctor of Nursing Practice program at Oakland University School of Nursing in Rochester, Michigan.

Then . . . 2008

Dr. Jackson, could you please describe your background, including why you pursued a career in nursing?

I came from a family of school teachers, so initially my interest in nursing was met with some resistance. My original interest in nursing stemmed from watching the soap opera *Another World*. I used to like the character Alice; she was a nurse and all she did was visit with friends in the cafeteria, hold patients' hands, wipe their brow. I thought, I could do that. When I started nursing school and experienced my first clinical rotation at Wayne State University School of Nursing, I was in for a big surprise. I thought immediately, "This is fantastic!" I still feel blessed to be in a profession that gives you a front row seat of people's lives—the good, the bad, and the ugly. In nursing, you see people at their best and at their worst. I feel it is a privilege to do so and a privilege to say, "I am a nurse." After graduation from Wayne State University with a bachelor's in the science of nursing, I worked at Harper Hospital in Detroit, Michigan, in substance abuse and home care.

I then returned to graduate school and earned a master's degree in counseling. I worked at Oakland University as a counselor in the School of Nursing. I wanted to give students someone to talk to while they were going through the nursing program. My position was later phased out, and I was faced with a decision. I had an "epiphany conversation" with my dean at the time. She asked me, "Are you a nurse, or a counselor?" If I was a counselor first, she suggested I do that. If I was a nurse first, she said that I needed to return to graduate school. When I asked myself this question, without hesitation, I answered I am a nurse, first, last, and always. I then went back to graduate school at University of Michigan in Ann Arbor, Michigan, and earned a master's in medical–surgical nursing. I worked in hospice care to try to improve end-of-life care and as a medical–surgical clinical nurse specialist. I also began teaching part time at Oakland University. I then returned to Wayne State University and earned a PhD in counseling. During this time I remained on faculty at Oakland University and also worked at Harper Hospital in medical–surgical nursing. I refer to working in med–surg as the "call of the wild" for me. I was successfully able to integrate my nursing background with counseling, and my PhD dissertation was based on the burnout of hospice nurses. Today I am still on faculty at Oakland University. I am the most senior faculty here. I am also the director of the DNP program.

Dr. Jackson, could you please describe your position as the director of the DNP program at Oakland University?

I am responsible for recruitment, understanding how classes work and how they will be scheduled, selection of faculty for the DNP program, interviewing and admission of students, and the DNP student handbook.

Dr. Jackson, do you believe the DNP is gaining momentum in enrollment, and if so, why?

Yes, it is definitely gaining momentum. The role of the advanced practice registered nurse (APRN) has expanded beyond anything we envisioned. Advanced practice registered nurses need other kinds of skills that the master's in nursing does not sufficiently provide. The DNP gives APRNs more skills than the master's degree in nursing and allows APRNs to function more effectively in a 21st century healthcare environment.

Dr. Jackson, could you please describe any challenges you are facing as director of the DNP program?

The challenge is keeping true to the purpose of the degree. People who don't want a PhD but are on faculty at a school of nursing and need a doctorate sometimes feel the DNP is a good degree for them. But this degree is for clinicians. It is not the stepsister of the PhD. Some feel the DNP is a mini-PhD. It is not. It is for nurses whose interest, passion, and priority is patient care.

The second issue I have been surprised about is I did not envision OU's program to be a national program. I am surprised by the enrollment and interest of individuals from all over the country. This is probably due to the delivery of much of the course work being distance-learning oriented. However, even when classes require a student to be on campus, they are making arrangements to be here.

Dr. Jackson, what is your opinion regarding the reaction we are seeing to nurses using the title "doctor"?

I feel the reaction is a smoke screen for the real issues. Advanced practice registered nurses are viewed as competitors and an economic threat to physicians. Hospitals have had problems with nurses using the title "doctor" because doctors have a problem with it. Doctors are considered the hospital's customers and nurses are employees. If doctors were okay with it, hospitals would be okay with it. Look at pharmacy; hospitals and physicians have no problem acknowledging their title when pharmacists have a PharmD. This could be because pharmacists have limited patient contact. Also, pharmacists have an extensive science background. They are identified with science and therefore more respected by the medical community. They are viewed as a resource for physicians and others in health care. Not as one trying to invade physicians' turf.

Dr. Jackson, as a PhD-prepared nurse, how have you dealt with title issues in the past?

I tend to be quite confrontational. I was asked to join a hospital-based hospice committee, and when I attended the first meeting, I noticed only the physicians' credentials were listed in the meeting agenda. I asked immediately, "Is it the culture of this hospital that only physicians went to college?" They responded yes, to which I responded, "Well, aren't you glad I am here to help you change that! I believe it is safe to say that everyone here went to college and therefore, everyone's credentials should be listed." By the next meeting, all of the credentials were listed for all members of the committee. I further explained at this meeting, "I don't mind being 'Frances' if he is 'John,' but if he is 'Dr. Smith,' then I am 'Dr. Jackson.'" This continues to be a problem outside of the academic environment. In the clinical setting, when I have students on a floor in the hospital, the physicians stumble when they read my name badge that clearly displays, "Frances Jackson, RN, PhD, Oakland University School of Nursing." I help them out and say, "Hi, I am Dr. Jackson, professor at Oakland University School of Nursing." Then they struggle less and call me "Dr. Jackson." Let me also say, I always tell patients, physicians, and family members in the clinical setting that I am a nurse. I am proud to be a nurse, and the very last thing I would do is hide that fact.

Dr. Jackson, do you feel this is an issue for all nurses who hold doctoral degrees?

No, not as much so in academia. Those of us in this setting are not an academic threat.

Dr. Jackson, could you describe what the catalyst was for you to call the coalition meeting at Oakland University to bring some leadership to this issue?

Well, Oakland University had the first DNP program in Michigan and the first DNP graduates who graduated from a program in Michigan. My students have been generous in keeping up with me regarding their evolving roles, publications, and reactions to the DNP degree. I was deeply disturbed by the response of Dr. Linda Opsahl's hospital administration. This was a clear attempt to squash any kind of acknowledgement of the accomplishment of the nurses who graduated from our program and went back to practice in this setting. What was really disappointing was so often in nursing we don't celebrate each other's accomplishments. The nurses in this setting were very supportive and wanted to share these students' accomplishments. This is, I am afraid, the tip of the iceberg: the absurdity that nurses being addressed as "doctor" is against the law.

The deeper issue here is that there is a continual assault by physician lobbyists in the state of Michigan on APRNs. Prescriptive authority, limiting what APRNs can do: We know that our doctoral preparation—and the title that comes with this—will be under attack as well. I decided that rather than wait for the attack we would be proactive by having a coalition meeting. Further, we invited physical therapy representation—we will surely not be the only health professionals dealing with this issue.

Dr. Jackson, what do you feel nursing must do to be proactive regarding this issue?

We can't sit back and wait for others. We need to fight our own battles. We need to recruit other professions; there is power in numbers. We can't just sit back and talk about it in nursing, we have to have the numbers. Secondly, we need to ask for help from other organizations with political connections. We need to use the resources we have so we don't create problems. We need to inform and get feedback from our large nursing organizations and garner support from them as well. Third, we need to share successful strategies with other states that are facing similar issues. And fourth, we [need] to respond to threats and answer back, even if it's just a letter to the AMA or to an editor.

Dr. Jackson, do you have any advice for new PhD/DNP graduates who are met with resistance to the title "doctor"?

It is very important to educate yourself about your degree so you can respond appropriately when questioned regarding your title. It is also critically important to educate other nurses. Finally, my advice is don't let other people and their ignorance diminish your accomplishments.

Now . . . 2011

Dr. Jackson, we discussed your nursing background and education last time we spoke. Could you please describe your current position?

I am the Director of Graduate Programs in the School of Nursing. That includes the MSN and DNP programs.

Dr. Jackson, as a DNP program director, could you describe the progress of your program at Oakland University?

It has simply been amazing. As the first DNP program in the State of Michigan, we have enjoyed tremendous success in attracting and graduating DNP students. We have developed a BSN–DNP program and that will be reviewed by the Graduate Council in the fall. We have also developed a DNP track for nurse anesthetists. They will be required to earn the DNP, I believe by 2025, in order to take the certification exam for CRNA.

Dr. Jackson, could you please describe your perception of the progress of the DNP degree in general?

It is clear from the number of new DNP programs listed by the Commission on Collegiate Nursing Education (CCNE) that this degree is enjoying phenomenal success. However, it is also clear that there are many barriers that exist for nurses who earn a terminal degree. The use of the title "doctor" continues to be a source of controversy. One major unresolved issue is whether the organizations that administer the certification exams for nurse practitioners will indeed require the DNP as the credential to take those exams. If they do require the DNP, then the success of the DNP will be assured. Even without it, students see the DNP coursework as value-added for their career plans.

Dr. Jackson, do you think the momentum of enrollment has increased over time? If so, why?

I believe it has increased. Some of the momentum, as stated previously, is directly related to the expectation that the organizations that administer the certification exams will require the DNP in order to take the exam. However, health-care reform is also a driving force behind this degree. Never in my memory have nurse practitioners enjoyed such high employability. Almost every student I interview for admission to our DNP program has an interest in teaching at some point in the future. Most believe that possessing the DNP will enhance their ability to step into that role, even if it's only on a part-time basis.

Dr. Jackson, how has Oakland University benefitted from having a DNP degree program?

As the first DNP program in the state of Michigan, we naturally led the way with implementing this new degree. We also have had a longer time to evaluate what works and what isn't working. There will be some changes to the program starting in 2012. Starting the DNP expanded our visibility in the state but also nationally and even internationally. We have been privileged to attract students from 15 different states and Canada. We are also attracting cohorts as hospitals and other agencies are sending groups of students to our program.

Dr. Jackson, what are some of the new challenges you face as a DNP program director?

We have been approached by nursing programs in foreign countries about offering the DNP abroad. Given the world situation, that is going to require very careful planning. Secondly, I see an increased need for financial aid at a time when the state is cutting back support for public universities.

Dr. Jackson, how do you think the DNP degree has affected nursing education since you became a DNP program director?

CCNE requires that the director of the DNP program is someone who has a DNP. We have several faculty who have a DNP degree, something that was unheard of even 3 years ago. Faculty who are practicing clinicians bring a richness and depth to course work that is unique and special.

Dr. Jackson, do you agree with the AACN's recommended target date of 2015 for the DNP degree as entry into practice for advanced practice registered nurses? If so, how do you recommend we continue to strive toward this goal?

I agree with it. I'm not sure there is much more to be done than what is already being done. Many organizations are working very hard to enhance and support the DNP as the terminal degree for advanced practice registered nurses. If there is one issue on which we must have a united front it is the titling of DNP graduates. We cannot be silent and allow them to be treated as second-class citizens, subject to terrorist tactics by some physicians (not all!) who seem to believe that the title "doctor" is their exclusive domain.

Dr. Jackson, what is your advice to nurses and potential students regarding the DNP degree?

It is very important to understand the differences between the PhD and the DNP. Make sure you are applying for the degree that matches your future plans. If I ask you about your future plans and your response reflects more of a PhD trajectory that could be enough to stop or delay your admission.

Dr. Jackson, do you think nurses have made any progress regarding using the title "doctor"? Why or why not?

If they have, it's not apparent to me. I think the powerful physician lobby has successfully blocked this issue. It's disheartening.

Dr. Jackson, what is your opinion regarding certain states' continued attempts at legislature mandating against nurses using the title "doctor"?

From what I've read, most of those states have forgotten that people like myself, nursing faculty who have an earned PhD, are also entitled to be called "doctor." Nurses have been earning PhDs for decades and there was no legislative push to prohibit the title of "doctor" for nurses with PhDs. However, the amount of time and money physicians have spent on blocking the use of this title for nurses borders on the absurd. Where were these legislators when PharmDs graduated? What about dentists? They also have a professional doctoral degree.

Dr. Jackson, what advice do you now have for nurses graduating with a DNP degree and using the title "doctor" in the clinical setting?

Introduce yourself as "Dr. X," then say "I'm a nurse practitioner," or whatever you are. Make sure they understand your role and the limitations, if any, of your practice. I also think it is important to insist on what you've earned, where appropriate. I'm on several advisory boards, one of which is part of a major medical center. Years ago when we received the minutes of the first meeting, I noted that my credentials were omitted, but not the credentials of the physicians. I told the group that I had 15 years of college and 4 earned degrees, including the PhD, and that I was Dr. Jackson. Either include everyone's credentials, or no one's credentials, but doctors weren't the only people in the room who had been to school. From that day on, everyone's credentials were included. Sometimes it's something as simple as that to make a difference.

■ Tips for Using the Title "Doctor"

First and foremost, DNP graduates, and others, need to be educated about their degree. Royeen and Lavin (2006) noted the need to clear up misconceptions of the practice doctorate and "place the doctorate in context of larger educational change and innovation and share summary judgments about the nature and course of the newer doctoral degrees" (p. 101). Further, these authors predicted that "within less than a generation, the majority of health care practitioners in allied health and advanced practice nursing will be degreed at the level of the clinical doctorate" (p. 105). It is imperative that DNP graduates become familiar with the purpose and goals of their degree, the arguments against their title, the issues associated with their title, the history of the title "doctor," and as Dr. Frances Jackson emphasized, the true meaning of a practice doctorate. Moreover, DNP graduates must have the courage to stand up for their degree, expertise, and accomplishments. During the first day of this author's DNP Advanced Nursing Theory course, Professor Morris Magnan asked the question, "Are you going to stand for something or fall for everything?" This further emphasizes the point made in the beginning of the chapter. As pioneers, DNP graduates have the responsibility to know their degree and role in health care, lead the way, and stand for their educational achievements and value. The value and educational achievements that DNP graduates bring to the healthcare setting should be celebrated and not diminished in any way.

Please refer to **Table 9-1** for a list of tips for using the title "doctor."

My Personal Experiences Using the Title "Doctor"

My experience using the title "doctor" has been a journey of sorts. Upon graduation, I was a proud doctoral-prepared nurse, filled with conviction regarding my title. My previous place of employment was a small private practice environment with a very supportive collaborating physician. He greeted me immediately after graduation and asked if I was going to be "Dr. Chism" or "Dr. Astalos." I had previously practiced under my maiden name (Astalos) but during my DNP program, I began using my married name, Chism. The front desk staff began scheduling patients for Dr. Chism, but had trouble remembering to explain that I was a nurse practitioner. It seemed that others' use of my title had gone to the extreme.

About 2 years after graduation, I began working within a large academic setting in a comprehensive breast center. It is a wonderful, collaborative group of nurse practitioners, a physician assistant, surgeons, medical oncologists, radiologists, radiation oncologists, and pathologists. Some of the providers are also PhD-prepared researchers. Within our group, we all use our first name. In addition, no one in this setting understood or knew what a DNP degree was. Although I was respected as a nurse practitioner, the fact that I had a doctorate was either not noted or understood. Instead of pushing the issue, I followed my colleagues' lead and used my first name and did not use the title "doctor."

I am sure that some of you reading this are surprised; allow me to explain. The skill termed "emotional intelligence" (Goleman, 1995) is useful in any setting and

Table 9-1 Suggested Tips for DNP Graduates Using the Title "Doctor"

- Educate yourself expansively about the history of the title "doctor," including its true meaning and origins.
- Educate yourself about practice doctorates in other fields and become familiar with their issues and title use.
- Take a proactive stance when confronted with these issues and use the literature, comparable practice doctorate patterns with the title "doctor" (PharmD, DPT, PhD), and knowledge about your practice doctorate to support your position.
- Maintain a professional demeanor at all times despite conflicts. The ways in which DNP graduates deal with this issue will set the precedent for others in similar circumstances.
- Form coalitions with other organizations that are possibly confronted with this issue, such as physical therapy, occupational therapy, audiology, and others. A unified stance is always best.
- Educate other nurses and nursing organizations to garner support now and in the future. Our own profession must understand the importance of nursing's evolving academic preparation and the value this has for the entire profession.
- Use every opportunity to educate others about your title and degree, in and out of the practice setting.
- Always and without exception, use the title "doctor" followed by your professional title, such as nurse practitioner, nurse–midwife, nurse educator, or chief nursing officer, to prevent any misrepresentation and advertise that you are a nurse.
- Ease others into the transition if you reenter a practice position where you were referred to differently in the past. Take the time to educate staff members, other nurses, and physicians in your setting regarding your title change, and allow time for adjustment. Be sure to provide resources to others regarding your title and degree preparation to reinforce the importance of the transition.

I used my emotional intelligence to guide me regarding this situation. I knew I was practicing with some of the most accomplished and educated practitioners and researchers in the country, yet no one was concerned with titles. I made a decision to quietly educate others about my degree and lead by example.

After about a year in this setting, I became certified as a menopause practitioner through the North American Menopause Society (NAMS). I then developed a patient education booklet on menopause for patients with and without cancer that is now used throughout the center. Throughout this experience, my credentials became known. Others frequently commented on my degree and preparation. I had used my leadership skills to become certified as a menopause practitioner, develop a patient education booklet that is widely used within a certified cancer center, and develop a menopause consultant role within my practice. I then was selected as Menopause Practitioner of the Year through NAMS in 2011. My emotional intelligence skills had shown me that in this setting, I would become more credible after I had exemplified my DNP skill set through my contributions to patient care and education.

Today, many of my colleagues in this setting refer to me as Dr. Chism when I am introduced. I recently was at a work-related function and a nursing colleague I had not yet met said, "Hello Dr. Chism, it's nice to finally meet you." Many colleagues have also become more aware of my DNP degree after I was inducted as a fellow of the American Academy of Nurse Practitioners. It was in that moment that I realized how important it is that after graduation, we exemplify leadership through our contributions to establish our credibility. Although our title is earned and well deserved, it is through our contributions that we will have an impact on our profession. As DNP graduates' contributions are disseminated, perhaps our title will no longer be questioned.

SUMMARY

- The issues with use of the title "doctor" are not new but are now at the forefront of the debate due to the DNP degree.
- The root of the term "doctor" is *docere*, which is Latin for "to teach" (Skinner, 1970).
- The first doctorate degrees originated in Bologna in the 12th century and were conferred to masters who teach (Skinner, 1970).
- The first doctorally prepared men exposed to the public were physicians, which may explain why the public associates this title with medicine (Skinner, 1970).
- Several other allied health professionals are adopting doctoral preparation, such as pharmacy, physical therapy, occupational therapy, and audiology.
- Doctoral preparation provides parity for nurses within the healthcare setting and places nurses "in an equal playing field" (Olshansky, 2004, p. 211).
- "The Pearson Report" is published each year and provides an update regarding legislative and regulatory issues for advanced practice registered nurses (specifically nurse practitioners). In 2011, Dr. Pearson reported that five states have regulations against the use of the title "doctor" by a nurse, despite academic preparation (Pearson, 2011).
- The AMA introduced Resolution 211 (A-06) in 2006, which suggests that nurses with DNP degrees are at risk for misrepresentation as physicians if they use the title "doctor" (AMA, 2006).
- Nursing responded to Resolution 211 (A-06) with letters to the AMA, responses in the literature, and talking points specifically developed to address this resolution.
- Oakland University responded to Resolution 211 (A-06) by forming a coalition with stakeholders who are taking a proactive stance against restrictive regulation regarding the title "doctor."
- All DNP graduates need to educate themselves regarding the title "doctor," the meaning of a practice doctorate, and their degree to formulate proactive, informed, and professional responses when faced with using the title "doctor."
- All DNP graduates need to educate others, including patients, nurses, and other healthcare professionals, regarding their degree preparation in an effort to effectively and proactively respond to disputes regarding the use of the title "doctor."

REFLECTION QUESTIONS

1. Before reading this chapter, did you know the origin of the title "doctor"? If not, what meaning did you associate with the title?
2. Do you think that DNP graduates, as well as others prepared with practice doctorates, should use the title "doctor"? Why or why not?
3. What is your response to the AMA's Resolution 211 (A-06)? What do you think is really driving this response from the AMA to nurses being prepared at the doctoral level?
4. Do you agree with nursing's proactive stance? What other suggestions do you have to continue to respond to this issue?
5. Upon graduation, how will you refer to yourself in the clinical setting?
6. Do you think you will be intimidated by others with practice doctorates (medical doctors, pharmacists) when you begin to use the title "doctor"? If so, how will you deal with this?
7. If you are met with resistance to your appropriate title, what approach will you take to resolve this issue in your setting?

REFERENCES

American Association of Colleges of Nursing (AACN). (2011). *Talking points.* Retrieved from http://www .aacn.nche.edu/dnp/talking-points

American Medical Association (AMA). (2006). *Resolution 211 (A-06).* Retrieved from http://www.ama-assn .org

Bailey, J. (2003). The story of "doctor," "physician," and "surgeon." *Journal of the National Medical Association, 85*(6), 489–490.

Bond, C., Raehl, C., & Franke, T. (2002). Clinical pharmacy services, hospital staffing and medication errors. *Pharmacotherapy, 22,* 134–147.

Brooten, D., & Naylor, M. (1995). Nurses' effect on changing patient outcomes. *IMAGE: Journal of Nursing Scholarship, 27*(2), 95–99.

Clinton, P., & Sperhac, A. (2006). National agenda for advanced practice nursing: The practice doctorate. *Journal of Professional Nursing, 22*(1), 7–14.

Goleman, D. (1995). *Emotional intelligence: Why it can matter more than IQ.* New York: Bantam Dell.

Greiner, A. C., & Knebel, E. (Eds.). (2003). *Health professions education: A bridge to quality.* Washington, DC: National Academies Press.

Griffiths, Y., & Padilla, R. (2006). National status of the entry-level doctorate in occupational therapy. *American Journal of Occupational Therapy, 60*(5), 540–549.

Klein, T. (2007). *Are nurses with a doctor of nursing practice called "doctor"?* Retrieved from http://www .medscape.com/viewarticle/563176

Marion, L., O'Sullivan, A., Crabtree, K., Price, M., & Fontana, S. (2005). Curriculum models for the practice doctorate in nursing. *Topics in Advanced Practice Nursing eJournal, 5*(1). Retrieved from http://www .medscape.com/viewarticle/500742_print

Marriner-Tomey, A. (1990). Historical development of doctoral programs from the middle-ages to nursing education today. *Nursing and Health Care, 3*(11), 132–137.

Mason, D. (2008). Resolved: The AMA is out of touch. *American Journal of Nursing, 8*(108), 7.

Merriam-Webster's online dictionary. (2008). *Doctor.* Retrieved from http://www.merriam-webster.com /dictionary/doctor

Newman, M. (1975). The professional doctorate in nursing: A position paper. *Nursing Outlook, 23*(11), 704–706.

Nurse Practitioner Roundtable. (2008). *Nurse practitioner DNP education, certification, and titling: A unified statement.* Washington, DC: Author.

O'Grady, E. (2007). Hiding the doctoral degree: Jettison this policy. *Nurse Practitioner World News, 12*(12), 1–8.

Olshansky, E. (2004). Are nurses at the table? A new nursing degree could help. *Journal of Professional Nursing, 20*(4), 211–212.

Pearson, L. (2011). *The Pearson report.* Retrieved from http://www.pearsonreport.com

Pearson, L. (2008). The Pearson report. *American Journal of Nurse Practitioners, 12*(2), 9–80.

Pierce, D., & Peyton, C. (1999). A historical cross-disciplinary perspective on the professional doctorate in occupational therapy. *American Journal of Occupational Therapy, 53*(1), 64–71.

Reeves, K. (2008). *"Doctor" for physicians only?* Retrieved July 6, 2008, from http://findarticles.com/p/articles/mi_m0FSS/is_1_17/ai_n24964200

Roeser, R., Thibodeau, L., & Cokely, C. (2005). The University of Texas at Dallas/Callier Center for Communication Disorders doctor of audiology program. *American Journal of Audiology, 14*(2), 151–160.

Royeen, C., & Lavin, M. (2007). A contextual logical analysis of the clinical doctorate for health practitioners: Dilemma, delusion, or de facto? *Journal of Allied Health, 36*(2), 101–106.

Skinner, H. (1970). *Medical terms* (2nd ed.). New York: Hafner.

Upvall, M., & Ptachcinski, R. (2007). The journey to the DNP program and beyond: What can we learn from pharmacy? *Journal of Professional Nursing, 23*(5), 316–321.

CHAPTER 10

Why Didn't You Just Become a Doctor? Educating Others About the DNP Degree

■ LISA ASTALOS CHISM ■

"Don't compromise yourself. You are all you've got."
—*Janis Joplin (1943–1970)*

It is quite probable that nurses at every level of educational preparation have been asked the question, "Why didn't you just become a doctor?" This question is often posed by patients, family members, friends, and other healthcare professionals. Due to the increasing curiosity toward the DNP degree, this question may be posed by others, including nurses, even more frequently than in the past. Therefore, developing a well-formulated, knowledgeable, and accurate response to this question has become the responsibility of all DNP graduates. Further, the responses provided to these types of questions will have implications for the continual education of all who may inquire about the DNP degree.

To provide appropriate responses to these types of questions, those representing nursing, especially those with a DNP degree, need to be very clear about their professional and educational preparation. Often the water becomes muddied by titles, roles, and other factors that may make it difficult to quickly respond when asked about one's profession or degree. Hence, this chapter reviews the definitions of nursing, nursing practice, advanced practice nursing, medicine, physician, and doctor. Easily accessible definitions of these terms are provided in an effort to maintain consistency. The practice doctorate and the DNP degree are also discussed in an effort to provide clarity and enable nurses to develop the well-formulated, knowledgeable, and accurate responses necessary to effectively educate others about the DNP degree. This chapter also provides tips for educating patients, nurses, and healthcare professionals about the DNP degree. Finally, recommendations for speaking publicly about the degree are reviewed. As pioneers, DNP graduates will likely be expected to speak publicly about the degree. Expertise in this area will further promote the degree and nursing as a whole.

■ Definitions Revisited: Know Who You Are

The ability to educate others about the Doctor of Nursing Practice (DNP) degree is largely dependent on DNP graduates' ability to define their profession and degree. It is therefore pertinent to develop a clear understanding of nursing and of the DNP degree. The following information is provided to enable DNP graduates to efficiently and accurately educate others about their degree.

Nursing

Nursing has been defined as the "autonomous and collaborative care of individuals of all ages, families, groups and communities, sick or well and in all settings. Nursing includes the promotion of health, prevention of illness, and the care of ill, disabled and dying people. Advocacy, promotion of a safe environment, research, participation in shaping health policy and in patient and health systems management, and education are also key nursing roles" (ICN, n.d.). According to the American Nurses Association (1995), nursing is "the diagnosis and treatment of human responses to actual or potential health problems" (p. 6). It should also be mentioned that nursing is an "essential part of the society from which it has grown and within which it continues to evolve" (American Nurses Association [ANA], 1995, p. 2). Further, nursing is dynamic rather than static and continues to reflect the changing needs of society (ANA, 1995). To summarize, nursing continually evolves to meet the societal needs of others by caring for individuals, families, and communities in an effort to maintain their health and well-being in various states of health and illness.

Nursing Practice

Nursing practice describes what nurses do when they provide nursing care (Bryant-Lukosius, DiCenso, Browne, & Pinelli, 2004). Nursing practice "includes direct care giving and evaluation of its impact, advocating for patients and for health, supervising and delegating to others, leading, managing, teaching, undertaking research and developing health policy for health care systems" (ICN, 1998). Hence, nursing practice includes both the act of caring for individuals, families, and communities in an effort to promote health and well-being as well as the relationship that develops between nurse and patient.

To further elaborate, the American Nurses Association (1995) asserted that "nursing is a scientific discipline as well as a profession" (p. 7). Hence, to further develop the scope of nursing practice and "expand the knowledge base of the discipline of nursing, nurses generate and utilize theories and research findings that are relevant to nursing practice and fit with nursing's values about health and illness" (p. 7). It is therefore pertinent for nurses and DNP graduates to understand that nursing is a discipline, science, and profession. Nursing practice is derived from the science and discipline of nursing. In other words, the profession of nursing includes a knowledge base (discipline) and reproducible modes of inquiry (science) that purport to explain how, why, and what nurses do when providing care (nursing practice).

Advanced Practice Nursing

Advanced practice nursing describes the "whole field of a specific type of advanced nursing practice" (Bryant-Lukosius, et al., 2004). Advanced practice nursing may include several specialty roles in which nurses function at an advanced level of practice (ANA, 1995; Brown, 1998). The advanced practice registered nurse "acquires specialized knowledge and skills through study and supervised practice at the master's or doctoral level in nursing" (ANA, 1995, p. 14). Advanced practice registered nurses incorporate their advanced knowledge and skills within their specialty roles to care for individuals, families, and communities.

Medicine

Medicine is defined as "the science or practice of the diagnosis, treatment, and prevention of disease" (Medicine, 2007). Medicine has been further defined as the "science and art of dealing with the maintenance of health and prevention, alleviation, or cure of disease" (Merriam-Webster, 2008a). Hence, medicine is focused on the diagnosis, treatment, and alleviation of disease and disease states.

Physician

The term "physician" is thought to have originated in ancient Greece. A group of philosophers called *physicos* were known for garnering their knowledge of nature from firsthand experience as opposed to studying from books (Bailey, 2003). From these experiences, these philosophers derived what they learned firsthand in nature as biology and medicine. These philosophers "taught" and hence were referred to as "doctors"; their students were referred to as *physicos*, which later evolved to the term "physician." The modern definition of "physician" includes "a person skilled in the art of healing; educated, clinically experienced, and licensed to practice medicine" (Merriam-Webster, 2008b).

Doctor

The relevant history of this term includes its origination in the 12th century in Bologna (Bailey, 2003; Marriner-Tomey, 1990; Skinner, 1970). The term "doctor" is derived from *docere* in Latin, which is translated as "to teach" (Skinner, 1970). Although medicine was included in early doctoral professional degrees, along with divinity and law (Marriner-Tomey, 1990), the actual term refers to one who holds the highest degree awarded by a graduate school (Encyclopedia.com, 2008). Bailey (2003) agreed that "today, the term 'doctor' is applied to both a person with a doctoral degree in nonmedical subjects, as well as physicians and surgeons" (p. 490).

Practice Doctorate

The terms "professional doctorate," "clinical doctorate," and "practice doctorate" have all been used somewhat interchangeably when referring to the highest or terminal degree in a field or profession (AACN, 2006a; Marriner-Tomey, 1990; Montoya & Kimball, 2006; Royeen & Lavin, 2007). For clarification, "practice doctorate" has been adopted as the term to describe the terminal degree in nursing (AACN, 2006a). A practice doctorate can be generally defined as an entry into practice degree, such as physical therapy or pharmacy (Griffiths & Padilla, 2006; Upvall & Ptachcinski, 2007), or the terminal degree awarded within a particular profession, such as nursing and occupational therapy (AACN, 2006a; Griffiths & Padilla, 2006). It should be mentioned, however, that the practice doctorate in nursing (DNP) has been adopted as both the terminal degree for nursing practice as well as the entry-level degree for advanced practice nursing (AACN, 2006a). A practice doctorate differs from a research doctorate, or Doctor of Philosophy degree (PhD), in that the PhD degree is a research-focused degree with an emphasis on the development of new knowledge, and the practice doctorate is a practice-focused degree with an emphasis on the skills and expertise necessary for a particular discipline (Montoya & Kimball, 2006; Newman, 1975).

Doctor of Nursing Practice Degree

The Doctor of Nursing Practice (DNP) degree is a practice-focused doctorate and the terminal practice degree for nursing. The DNP degree is designed to prepare nurses to meet the changing demands of health care and healthcare delivery systems. The DNP degree curriculum is focused on, although not limited to, evidence-based practice, scholarship to advance the profession, organizational and systems leadership, information technology, healthcare policy and advocacy, interprofessional collaboration across disciplines of health care, and advanced nursing practice (AACN, 2006b). The DNP degree is currently offered as a post-master's degree, with the intent that it will be offered as a postbachelor's degree in the future. The AACN projects that the DNP degree will replace master's degree programs, which prepare advanced practice registered nurses, by 2015 (AACN, 2006a).

■ Current DNP Trends: A DNP, LLC/DNPPD Outcome Study

DNP students and graduates should also familiarize themselves with current trends related to various types of DNP programs, DNP student demographics, and specifics regarding DNP graduate practice. Doctors of Nursing Practice, LLC/Doctors of Nursing Practice Professional Development, Inc. developed and conducted an outcome study related to these current trends (DNP, LLC, 2010). The following is a summary of the data from this study.

Genesis of the DNP Outcome Survey

- Planned and developed by DNP, LLC/DNP, PD, Inc.
- The goal is to determine the "state of the practice" of DNP graduates on an annual basis.
- The initial plan was to disseminate findings at the 2010 annual DNP conference and annually thereafter.
- Another "arm" of this survey is an analysis of current DNP university programs (to compare curricula, hours, track emphasis, and other features).
- A contextual logical analysis of the clinical doctorate for health practitioners: The survey was open through August 31, 2010.

Development Team Members

- Stephanie Ahmed, DNP, FNP-BC
- Catherine S. Bishop, DNP, NP, AOCNP
- Karen Crowley, DNP, APRN-BC, WHNP, ANP
- Donald Grimes, DNP, RN
- Star Evangelista Hoffman, DNP, MEd, CNL
- David G. O'Dell, DNP, FNP-BC
- Marie G. Young, DNP, MSN, MPH, FNP, PMHNP

DNP University/College Program Comparison: 131 Programs

- 44% have BSN-DNP entry
- 66% MSN-DNP entry
- APRN requirements
  - 73.3% nurse practitioner entry
  - 51% clinical nurse specialist entry
  - 40.5% certified nurse–midwife entry
  - 36.6% certified registered nurse anesthetist entry
- Role concentration
  - 29.5% no specific role concentration
  - 29.7% nurse executive
  - 14.5% educator
  - 0.05% health policy
  - 0.05% informatics
  - Others: scientist, clinical nurse leader, public health, clinical research management
- Credit hours
  - BSN-DNP average: 97
  - MSN-DNP average: 41
- Clinical Hours
  - BSN-DNP: up to 1260
  - MSN-DNP: up to 1125

A survey of DNP graduates revealed the following:

Total number of DNP graduate respondents to the survey: 292 *(n = 292)*

Demographics:

Age:
25–30: 1%
31–35: 7%
36–40: 8%
40–45: 14%
46–50: 22%
51–55: 31%
55–60: 12%
60–65: 4%

Gender:
Female: 88%
Male: 12%

Practice area:
APRN: 78%
Nurse executive: 9%
Nurse educator in an academic setting: 31%
Policy/legislation: 3%
Researcher: 3%
Other: 7%

Work environment:
Primary care: 39%
Acute care: 30%
Long-term care: 3%
Rehabilitation: 2%
Community-based care: 11%
Public health: 5%
Academia: 38%
Other: 18%

Percentage of DNP-prepared nurse educators in an academic setting: 47% are NPs (family nurse practitioner, adult nurse practitioner, certified nurse–midwife, certified registered nurse anesthetist, clinical nurse specialist)

Universities that have a tenure track (reported by DNP-prepared academics): 22%

Since earning the DNP degree, has your practice *area* changed?
Yes: 34%
No: 66%

Since earning the DNP degree, has your practice *setting* changed?
Yes: 26%
No: 74%

The reason why I pursued a DNP degree:
Job requirement: 9%
Personal goal: 88%
Peer pressure: < 1%
Professional advancement: 76%
Other: 5%

Income/salary:
Since earning the DNP degree, salary has:
Increased: 30%
Remained the same: 66%
Decreased: 3%

Survey responses that correlate with the Eight Essentials:
AACN Essential II: Organizational and System Leadership
30% function as an administrator
29% develop, implement, and evaluate business plans
23% have initiated a program to address disparities
20% have a leadership role in a specialty nursing organization
16% have a leadership role in a national nursing organization
20% have a leadership role in a state nursing organization
10% are currently involved in a nationwide policy
29% are currently involved in a statewide policy

AACN Essential III: Clinical Scholarship and Analytical Methods of Evidence-Based Practice (EBP)
86% utilize EBP skills more
75% translate and disseminate relevant research into practice
70% utilize EBP skills to develop/translate practice guidelines
67% are able to translate research to identify gaps
45% actively translate EBP skills outside of their practice

AACN Essential IV: Information Systems/Technology
24% develop, implement, and evaluate information systems
52% utilized available technology to promote a change in practice

AACN Essential V: Healthcare Policy
42% are actively involved in health policy issues
23% initiated a program addressing health disparities
53% are active members in a specialty nursing organization
75% are active members in a national nursing organization

AACN Essential VI: Interprofessional Collaboration
60% lead and participate in an interdisciplinary team
66% are able to implement practice changes
61% actively participate in interprofessional activities
55% pursue practice change initiatives

AACN Essential VII: Clinical Prevention and Health Promotion
74% incorporate health promotion and disease prevention
23% initiated a program addressing health disparities
58% are more aware of the impact of culture in their practice
55% utilize their understanding of cultural differences

AACN Essential VIII: Advanced Nursing Practice
62% develop, implement, and evaluate practice initiative
51% have increased the scope of their practice
61% function to the fullest capacity for their role

Source: Study summary reprinted with permission from DNP, LLC/DNPPD, Inc. (www.Doctors ofNursingPractice.org).

■ Go Forth and Teach

Once graduates develop an understanding of the DNP degree, it is their responsibility to go forth and educate others about the degree. Discussion regarding others' perceptions of the DNP degree is limited. Therefore, the literature regarding what is known about others' perceptions of advanced practice registered nurses is reviewed. This information may be used to guide DNP graduates when educating others about the DNP degree.

Educating Patients: The Literature

To date, little is known regarding patients' perceptions of DNP graduates. However, discussion regarding patients' perceptions of advanced practice registered nurses was noted in the literature and may be appraised to provide insights for DNP graduates. Although not all DNP graduates may be in advanced practice nursing roles, understanding patients' perceptions of advanced practice registered nurses will enable DNP graduates to develop strategies to educate patients about the DNP degree.

It is interesting that patient awareness regarding nursing was studied as early as the 1970s. Levine, Orr, Sheatsley, Lohr, and Brodie (1978) examined patient satisfaction and comfort level with nurse practitioners. This study found that patients were "generally satisfied with nurse practitioners and felt comfortable being treated by them" (Levine, Orr, Sheatsley, Lohr, & Brodie, 1978, p. 253). Further, patients who participated in this study "formulated highly complimentary opinions of nurse practitioners" (Levine, et al., 1978, p. 253). Notably, 57% of the pediatric patients and 70.9% of the adult patients formulated highly complimentary opinions after seeing a nurse practitioner for the first time (Levine, et al., 1978).

Whitemore and Jaffe (1996) evaluated patients' perceptions of nurse practitioners through surveys. The results were summarized, and it was found that "most of the respondents generally had knowledge about the scope and practice of nurse practitioners" (Whitemore & Jaffe, 1996, p. 19). Further, the majority of these respondents described their quality of care to be excellent. It was related that these respondents felt that the nurse practitioner's care was "more thorough, more attentive, spent more time with them, and was a better educator" (Whitemore & Jaffe, 1996, p. 19). Patients' comfort levels were also noted to be high in all but two of the respondents ($n = 16$). Overall, the patients who were surveyed felt their quality of care was at least equal to that of other healthcare providers (Whitemore & Jaffe, 1996).

Mitchell, Dixon, Freeman, and Grindrod (2001) surveyed 277 patients regarding their perceptions of nurse practitioners. The authors found that most patients (91.9%) were agreeable to nurse practitioners treating their illnesses. It was also noted that patients with higher education levels were more familiar with the nurse practitioner role. This would suggest that familiarity with nurse practitioners could be fostered with increased education regarding nurse practitioners and their role (Mitchell, Dixon, Freeman, & Grindrod, 2001). Further, the majority of the respondents in this study were from an academic clinical setting where patients were familiar with comprehensive, high-quality care from nurse practitioners. This may also lend support to the notion that with increased education and familiarity with nurse practitioners, the level of satisfaction is increased (Mitchell, et al., 2001).

Brown (2007) studied consumer perspectives of nurse practitioners in independent practice. A large majority of this sample (90%) indicated that they were familiar with the role of a nurse practitioner and had seen a nurse practitioner for care (Brown, 2007). This study also provided support that previous experience with an advanced practice registered nurse (nurse practitioner) resulted in an increased intention to use a nurse practitioner's services as well as increased satisfaction with these services.

Sheer (1994) also agreed with the notion that the patient's perceptions of nurse practitioners were directly related to their exposure to nurse practitioners. Conversely, those patients who have not had exposure to the nurse practitioner role may not have favorable perceptions of nurse practitioners. Sheer suggested that socialization of the nursing role must take place early on to enable nurses and nurse practitioners to influence public opinion and "take their place as equal and autonomous providers of health care" (Sheer, 1994, p. 216). Sheer (1994) related that through the socialization of nurses and nurse practitioners to be independent, strong leaders in health care, they will become empowered to impact the public's perceptions and act as strong role models for the profession.

Edmunds (1988) discussed visibility of the nurse practitioner role and noted that the multiple titles used by nurses who practice in an expanded role may lead to patients' confusion about the role of the nurse practitioner. This lack of unity within nursing has hurt the profession's recognition in the healthcare setting. Edmunds further related that nurse practitioners remain largely unknown to many prospective patients and stated that "not enough people in the United States are aware of nurse practitioners' unique contributions to health care" (p. 53). In an effort to change this, Edmunds offered some strategies to increase patient awareness about nurse practitioners. These strategies included using the media to gain visibility, such as calling local radio or television stations to volunteer for interviews, prepare public service announcements, or write health information spots (Edmunds, 1988). Additional strategies suggested by Edmunds included utilizing nurse practitioners' political power effectively to garner support from legislators as well as establishing relationships within their professional communities. This strategy would include personally visiting local hospitals, nursing homes, retirement communities, and charity organizations in an effort to increase visibility of their unique role (Edmunds, 1988). Finally, an increased effort to educate the patients was mentioned. This could be done in the form of brochures or pamphlets distributed locally and kept in offices or exam rooms (Edmunds, 1988). Overall, Edmunds reinforced that nurse practitioners should never miss an opportunity to hand out business cards and explain who they are and what they do. Similar strategies could be employed by DNP graduates to increase their visibility and educate patients regarding the DNP degree.

Educating Patients: Seize Your Moment

Although the literature primarily discusses patients' awareness and perceptions of advanced practice registered nurses, this information provides useful insights regarding educating patients about the DNP degree. First and foremost, it is supported by the literature that patients who are cared for by advanced practice registered nurses (even through one experience) have favorable perceptions of advanced practice registered nurses (Brown, 2007; Levine et al., 1978; Mitchell et al., 2001; Sheer, 1994). DNP graduates have likely already established trusting relationships with their patients and established patient comfort and satisfaction. Therefore, patients are likely to be receptive to DNP graduates introducing the concept of a practice doctorate in nursing and what this means. The rapport DNP graduates have established with patients will enable the open communication necessary to seize the moment during patient visits and share with patients what a DNP degree is and the impact that DNP graduates have on an ever-changing, complex healthcare environment.

For patients who are new to either a practice setting or advanced practice registered nurses, or who may have limited knowledge regarding nursing in general, the research has shown that even limited experience with advanced practice registered nurses usually results in patients having a favorable perception of them (Brown, 2007; Levine et al., 1978; Mitchell et al., 2001). Therefore, DNP graduates should use every opportunity with patients, regardless of the length or context of the relationship, to educate them about advanced practice registered nurses' preparation, including defining for patients what a DNP degree is. This author has found that patients who are new to the practice setting are often eager to learn what it means to have a DNP degree and are impressed at the level of preparation DNP graduates have.

Finally, DNP graduates should utilize their knowledge base regarding nursing. What better time to promote nursing and educate patients about what nursing actually is? DNP graduates should also familiarize themselves with the terms presented in the beginning of the chapter. It seems the pertinent issues include clearly defining for patients the terms "nursing," "nursing practice," "medicine," "doctor," "physician," "practice doctorate," and "Doctor of Nursing Practice." This author has found that patients are receptive and appreciative when a DNP graduate takes the time to explain his or her educational preparation, role, and degree. **Table 10-1** lists some tips for educating patients about the DNP degree.

Educating Nurses: The Literature

Nurses' perceptions of the DNP degree have not yet been studied extensively. However, the attitudes of nurses toward advanced practice registered nurses were studied. Gooden and Jackson (2004) noted that nurses' attitudes toward nurse practitioners in the healthcare environment could affect the patient's attitude toward the nurse practitioner and have an impact on healthcare outcomes. The same may be implied

Table 10-1 Tips for Educating Patients About the DNP Degree

- Educate yourself and your patients regarding the meaning of "nursing," "nursing practice," and "advanced practice nursing."
- Educate yourself and your patients regarding the meaning and origins of the terms "physician," "doctor," and "medicine."
- Seize every opportunity with patients to distinctly explain that you are a nurse with a doctorate in nursing practice.
- If a patient questions the term "doctor," explain that you are a doctor and a nurse; you are a Doctor of Nursing Practice.
- Use consistent language with patients when describing the DNP degree (e.g., use the terms "Doctor of Nursing Practice" or "DNP"). Consistency will prevent patient confusion and promote unity (Edmunds, 1988).
- Develop a brochure or pamphlet explaining your role and degree preparation and leave it in your practice setting lobby and exam rooms.
- Clearly display your degree and title on your nametag.
- Educate the staff in your practice setting to ensure that your preparation is appropriately communicated (e.g., "Dr. Smith has a doctorate in nursing practice").
- Educate receptionists that when making patient appointments, your appropriate degree and title should be used (e.g., Dr. Smith, Nurse Practitioner).
- Volunteer to provide in-service training to the staff and patients regarding your degree and preparation.
- Volunteer to provide patient education presentations with a quick introduction regarding your title and your educational preparation.
- DNP graduates in the nurse educator role, including those who precept students in the clinical setting, should begin socializing students (in all nursing degree programs) to be strong, autonomous, independent practitioners of nursing practice. This will encourage empowerment when communicating with patients regarding their roles as nurses, advanced practice registered nurses, and DNP graduates (Sheer, 1994).
- Educate your family members and friends regarding your degree and the defined terms as well. They are often patients too at some time in their life.

regarding nurses' attitudes toward DNP graduates. Gooden and Jackson (2004) found that, overall, nurses had positive attitudes about nurse practitioners. Specifically, these authors found that nurses agreed that "nurse practitioners made a positive impact on health care" (Gooden & Jackson, 2004, p. 363). Further, Gooden and Jackson related that nurses considered the role of nurse practitioners to be valuable, necessary, and helpful. Participants in this study had exposure to nurse practitioners in multiple settings and possessed a clear understanding of the scope of nurse practitioner practice. The nurse participants also expressed confidence in the care provided by nurse practitioners. It is important to note that the nurse participants also felt that nurse practitioners were a valuable resource for advice as well as receptive to suggestions regarding patient care (Gooden & Jackson, 2004). DNP graduates may also be looked to as a resource for nursing within the healthcare setting. Continuing to be a resource, while exhibiting receptiveness to nursing's suggestions to improve quality of care, will promote credibility and trust toward DNP graduates.

Although positive attitudes toward advanced practice registered nurses have been noted, Richmond and Becker (2005) note that these attitudes need to be cultivated by advanced practice registered nurses. These authors suggest specific characteristics that promote an "advanced practice nurse–friendly culture" (Richmond & Becker, 2005, p. 58). These characteristics may also be helpful in promoting credibility and trust toward DNP graduates. Credibility and trust will facilitate receptiveness by nurses as well as increase credibility of the DNP degree. Richmond and Becker's (2005) characteristics of an advanced practice registered nurse–friendly culture are as follows:

- Clarity of visions, values, and role in an effort to align the advanced practice registered nurse with the rest of the nurses
- Commitment to practice, the nursing profession, and to continued professional development
- Communication with patients and families, with the healthcare team, within the medical record, and through professional presentations and publications
- Collaboration that is clearly defined, occurs across disciplines, and within nursing
- Credibility through credentialing, clinical experience, and by securing payment for services
- Contributions to patient outcomes and to the organization
- Confidence in oneself and as a change agent
- Complexity to become solution oriented while conveying professional serenity

Educating Nurses: An Opportunity to Role Model

DNP graduates can employ Richmond and Becker's (2005) characteristics to establish trust and credibility with nursing. When credibility and trust are established, nurses will be more receptive to understanding the DNP degree. Furthermore, to successfully educate other nurses about the degree, it is essential that DNP graduates set an exceptional example. What better way to educate other nurses and promote the DNP degree than to be a role model? DNP graduates garner leadership and interprofessional collaboration skills that can be employed to facilitate role modeling for other nurses. Additionally, many of the explanations and tips provided regarding educating patients about the DNP degree may also be employed when educating nurses about the DNP degree. Please refer to **Table 10-2** for a list of tips for educating nurses about the DNP degree.

Educating Other Healthcare Professionals: The Literature

The literature related to healthcare professionals' attitudes and perceptions regarding the nursing profession focused primarily on physicians' attitudes toward nurse practitioners. Fottler, Gibson, and Pinchoff (1978) specifically examined physician receptivity of nurse practitioners. Only approximately one-third (29%) of physicians questioned were willing to employ a nurse practitioner in their practice. Further, approximately one-half (49%) of physicians questioned expressed negative attitudes regarding working with nurse practitioners. The reasons for this were evaluated, and the highest reported response was a lack of incentive for physicians to work with nurse practitioners. The second most reported response was physician satisfaction with the traditional roles and relationships of nurses and physicians. The authors speculated that this may be due to physicians' tendency to "prefer certainty over

Table 10-2 Tips for Educating Nurses About the DNP Degree

- Educate yourself and other nurses regarding the meaning of "nursing," "nursing practice," and "advanced practice nursing."
- Educate yourself and other nurses regarding the meaning and origins of the terms "physician," "doctor," and "medicine."
- Develop trust and credibility with other nurses in an effort to increase receptiveness regarding the DNP degree.
- Develop trust and credibility with other nurses in an effort to promote credibility of the DNP degree.
- Lead by example and be a role model for other nurses.
- Provide in-service training for other nurses regarding the DNP degree.
- Promote professional development by presenting at conferences and providing information regarding the DNP degree.
- Join and volunteer to present at professional nursing organizations to garner nursing support of the DNP degree.
- DNP nurse educators, including those who precept students, have an opportunity to serve as role models. Those in the nurse educator role may also provide a detailed description of the DNP degree to students in every nursing program.

uncertainty, known over unknown and current practices over innovative practices" (Fottler, Gibson, & Pinchoff, 1978). It was noted that physicians' attitudes are not static. Rather, the authors asserted that increased experience working with nurse practitioners resulted in more positive attitudes from physicians.

More recent research has in fact shown that physicians' attitudes become more positive with increased experience working with nurse practitioners. Aquilino et al. (1999) found that, overall, physicians had supportive attitudes about nurse practitioners. Not surprisingly, this study also found that experience with nurse practitioners led to more positive attitudes about nurse practitioners. The authors related that this finding had implications for the training of physicians and nurse practitioners regarding interdisciplinary care (Aquilino, Damiano, Williard, Momany, & Levy, 1999). Further, Aquilino et al. stated that, "the results of this study support initiatives to encourage interdisciplinary training as an effective way to begin the process of mutual understanding and respect between professionals that can continue throughout their practice careers" (p. 227). This is reflective of the Institute of Medicine's (IOM) recommendation that all healthcare professionals be formally educated to integrate interprofessional care into healthcare delivery to adequately provide health care in the 21st century (Greiner & Knebel, 2003).

Educating Other Healthcare Professionals: Education Through Demonstration

Patients', nurses', and other healthcare professionals' perceptions of advanced practice nursing roles have largely been influenced by previous experience with the high-quality care that is provided by advanced practice registered nurses (Aquilino et al., 1999; Brown, 2007; Gooden & Jackson, 2004; Levine et al., 1978; Mitchell et al., 2001; Sheer, 1994). It may therefore be safe to assume that effectively educating other healthcare professionals depends on DNP graduates consistently demonstrating the value and expertise they bring to the delivery of health care. Other healthcare professionals, such as physicians, pharmacists, and physical therapists, will be more receptive to understanding the DNP degree if patient care outcomes are shown to improve. Additionally, many of the explanations and tips provided regarding educating patients and nurses about the DNP degree may also be employed when educating other healthcare professionals about the DNP degree. Please refer to **Table 10-3** for a list of tips for educating other healthcare professionals about the DNP degree.

■ Speaking Publicly About the DNP Degree

Stephen Covey (2004) asserted that communication is the most important skill in life, with the four basic forms of communication being reading, writing, speaking, and listening. Of these, speaking and listening have a synergistic effect. When one

Table 10-3 **Tips for Educating Other Healthcare Professionals About the DNP Degree**

- Educate yourself and other healthcare professionals regarding the meaning of "nursing," "nursing practice," and "advanced practice nursing."
- Educate yourself and other healthcare professionals regarding the meaning and origins of the terms "physician," "doctor," and "medicine."
- Develop trust and credibility with other healthcare professionals in an effort to increase receptiveness regarding the DNP degree.
- Develop trust and credibility with other healthcare professionals in an effort to promote credibility of the DNP degree.
- Provide in-service training for other healthcare professionals regarding the DNP degree.
- Develop clinical projects/practice guidelines that demonstrate the use of leadership, evidence-based practice, information technology, and interprofessional collaboration.
- Make an effort to collaborate consistently with other healthcare professionals and highlight the benefits of interdisciplinary/interprofessional patient care.
- Nurse educators, including those who precept students, have an opportunity to teach students and demonstrate the importance of interprofessional collaboration with other healthcare professionals. Through demonstration, the value of interprofessional collaboration will be reinforced for both students and healthcare professionals.

listens as well as speaks, communication is improved. Moreover, Covey (2004) expressed that understanding others, through empathic listening, is essential to being understood.

Empathic listening is defined as listening with the intent to understand (Covey, 2004). Through empathic listening, one understands another's "frame of reference" (Covey, 2004, p. 240). Empathic listening is facilitated by listening and evaluating first before offering a response. When a response is offered, it should be clear, specific, and in the context of the understanding of the other's frame of reference (Covey, 2004).

Speaking publicly about the DNP degree requires DNP graduates to first understand their audience. The literature pertaining to the perceptions of advanced practice registered nurses was provided to give DNP graduates and others a sense of patients', nurses', and other healthcare professionals' frames of reference. When speaking to others publicly about the DNP degree, DNP graduates can first develop an understanding of others' perceptions regarding nursing and health care and employ empathic listening to communicate effectively and be understood.

Kravitz (2007) also related that when speaking publicly, one should know the concerns, interests, and beliefs of the audience. It was noted that understanding the perceptions of the audience would influence speaking strategies (Kravitz, 2007). Additional pointers regarding speaking publicly included knowing the essence of the presentation, showing enthusiasm toward those you are speaking to, expressing passion about the topic, practicing your material, daring to be different yet professional, and making a memorable impression (Kravitz, 2007).

With regard to speaking publicly, it would be remiss not to mention the work of Dale Carnegie, who was a pioneer in teaching others the art of public speaking. In a revised version of his work titled *Public Speaking for Success*, he shares an essential point: "When speakers have a real message in their head and heart—an inner urge to speak—they are almost sure to do themselves credit" (Carnegie & Pell, 2005, p. 41). The definitions in the beginning of the chapter were provided to ensure that DNP graduates develop a clear understanding regarding who they are and what they contribute to nursing, the delivery of health care, and society—in essence, their message. This author has often found that when speaking about the DNP degree, the passion and enthusiasm expressed are contagious. Even others who are not in health care can sense the excitement and are therefore receptive to learning about the DNP degree. Carnegie and Carnegie Hill (2007) agreed and stated, "When you become intensely interested in your talk, you will forget your fears, you will gain self-confidence, and your enthusiasm will carry the crowd with you" (p. 41). Additionally, this author has found that the sincerity expressed when speaking publicly leaves an impression on the audience: "If you speak with a deep sincerity and whole-heartedness, your hearers will be imbued by your spirit" (Carnegie & Carnegie Hill, 2007, p. 41). Whether formally to a large audience or informally in a small group, DNP graduates are expected to lead, have an inner urge to speak, and share their message about their innovative and unique degree. Please refer to **Table 10-4** for a list of tips for speaking publicly about the DNP degree.

Table 10-4 **Tips for Speaking Publicly About the DNP Degree**

- Know your audience's perceptions, interests, and beliefs regarding nursing and health care.
- Express an understanding of your audience's frame of reference and utilize empathic listening when presenting (Covey, 2004).
- Express a clear understanding of your topic (the DNP degree) and know your material.
- Be unique and make an impression.
- Use the leadership skills you have garnered and be fearless.
- Share personal anecdotal stories that are relevant to your audience and/or topic.
- Express sincerity and interest when speaking to an audience.
- Review the AACN's DNP talking points, which are available at http://www.aacn.nche.edu /dnp/talking-points.
- Express passion and enthusiasm about the DNP degree with every audience—it will be contagious!

Interview with a Co-Founder of DNP, LLC: Then and Now

David O'Dell, DNP, FNP, BC is the founder of D. G. O'Dell, Inc. and co-founder of Doctors of Nursing Practice, LLC.

Then . . . 2008

Dr. O'Dell, could you please describe your current position, including your nursing background?

I've been an RN since the age of 19, first with an associate's degree in nursing, later earning my BSN, and evolving into an MSN and NP licensure. I soon realized that to have a strong voice for change a terminal degree was needed and made an easy transition into the DNP educational route.

I currently work part-time jobs as an independent contractor with several medical groups, including internal medicine physicians, neurologists (my clinical interest is neurocognitive disorders), and also physical medicine and rehab. I have been teaching nursing students part time since 2002 and will soon accept a full-time faculty position in a local university school of nursing for undergraduate, graduate, and DNP students.

Dr. O'Dell, could you please describe what motivated you to return to school for a DNP degree?

This is a great question. After working as an NP for a few years, I realized that my role had evolved into being an extension of the physician and physician group. I was generating several hundred thousand dollars in revenue for the practice, and when I shared this information requesting an increase in salary, I was turned down. I knew my contribution was not adequately recognized, so I had to make plans for change. Returning to school was my next best step.

I realized that the bigger world of health care had greater needs and greater opportunities beyond the tasks I had grown into. I also knew I had to earn a terminal degree in order to be effective in promoting change. I looked at several PhD programs, but none felt right. When I heard about the DNP program, there were only five universities with this option. After reading what the AACN had proposed, and reviewing as many articles as I could find on this degree option, I knew that this was right for me for several reasons. First, earning a practice degree fit well with my concept of being a clinician first. The DNP degree spoke to this goal better than any other degree. Additionally, as this degree was evolving, I saw an opportunity to catch the first wave in order to be a part of a growth shift in our profession. I'm amazed daily at how the DNP degree is promoting change (sometimes through controversy). I will invest the rest of my professional career as a DNP trying to positively influence the healthcare delivery system and promote the growth of advanced nursing practice. My evolution into being a DNP was right on time for me.

Dr. O'Dell, could you please describe how earning your DNP degree has influenced your nursing practice?

My nursing practice in terms of patient care has become much easier now that I better understand the larger picture of the healthcare system and more clearly see my role as a clinician. I'm more confident in all patient interactions and know that I can incorporate sound judgment based on evidence in my decisions. The clinical hours required for my residency were more than most DNP programs require now, but I don't regret the extra experience and hands-on learning. I'm much better for the experience.

My nursing practice has taken on a much different tone since my MSN days. I'm more intrigued and capable to make change and provide leadership to whatever group that I choose to belong. I've seen more opportunity to contribute.

Dr. O'Dell, could you please describe the history of DNP, LLC, including how you became involved with this venture?

Like many good things in life, sometimes events evolve through serendipity. In the first semester of the DNP program at the University of Tennessee Health Science Center College of Nursing, one of the core classes was philosophy of science. We had several projects to develop, and the online chats between and among classmates were amazing. Even though we didn't see each other face to face often, the daily (and sometimes several times per day) conversations online built a bond that will always be with us. One of the conversations spun off into comments that there was no publication of DNP literature (because the degree was so new) and that there was no mechanism to communicate among other DNPs and DNP students. Someone mentioned the need for creating such an organization, and others chimed in agreeing to the idea, but we put it aside as we were not in a position to act on these notions.

About a year later in an advanced leadership course, our assignments were to develop either a grant application or a business plan. A few of us picked up on the idea of forming an organization from the online conversation about a year earlier, and we moved it forward. By the end of that semester we had a business plan. Before that semester was complete we had incorporated and began our website that opened within 4 months of incorporation. We're very fortunate to have put into place many of our business plan ideas and have modified others as the environment and culture of DNP education and communication needs have changed.

Dr. O'Dell, what are the mission and purpose of DNP, LLC?

That's easy to share as this has been discussed in detail while developing our business plan, and we have revisited it several times since our inception.

The mission of Doctors of Nursing Practice, LLC is to create a forum for the communication of information, ideas, and innovations to promote the growth and development of the practice doctorate degree.

The purpose (or vision) is grounded in the following principles:

a. Dedication to providing accurate and timely information
b. Support, develop, and disseminate professional practice innovations

   c. Professional collaboration that demonstrates universal respect for others, honesty, and integrity in communications

   d. Responsive and open discussions and dialogues that promote the evolution of advanced nursing practice and the growth of the DNP degree

You may be interested to know that as a result of this mission and purpose statement, we have created a subsidiary organization, Doctors of Nursing Practice Professional Development, Inc. This is a nonprofit organization dedicated to the educational needs of advanced practice registered nurses. One of our first group efforts is the First National Doctors of Nursing Practice Conference: Transforming Care Through Scholarly Education and Practice. This conference will take place in October of 2008 in Memphis, Tennessee (the birthplace of our organization). Future conferences are already being planned. We invite all interested to visit our sites at www.apn-dnp.com and/or www.DoctorsofNursingPractice.org.

Another big step for DNP, LLC as an organization is the development of a professional membership-driven organization for and by DNPs. As you know, there are many issues and controversies surrounding our degree and practice. I've spoken with DNPs throughout the United States and other countries and see that the need for communication and collaboration is more important now than ever and no doubt will continue to be important in the future.

The inception, growth, and evolution of DNP, LLC and its subsidiaries and efforts are directly related to the needs of this unique and growing community. I'm very proud and honored to be a part of this process and look forward to continuing to support our collective evolution.

Dr. O'Dell, what do you feel is your role to educate patients, nurses, and others about the DNP degree?

That's a tough question to answer. I see my role as being the best clinician possible in my chosen discipline and continue to support the health of individuals and communities. This is accomplished through growth of organizations and systems designed to meet these needs. At this point in the evolution of the DNP degree, I must explain again and again what a practice degree in nursing is all about to patients and colleagues. In the future I hope that the DNP will be better understood and won't require repetitive explanations. Time will tell on that front. The message I try to convey consistently is that the DNP is exactly what it says it is: a doctor (meaning the highest level of achievement in a discipline—a teacher or guide) of nursing practice, which is a demonstration that this degree is all about the discipline of nursing. I'm amazed and sometimes concerned that others in health care (particularly physicians) do not see the forest for the trees. We are not trying to practice as physicians; rather we are well-educated and capable nursing clinicians who can meet the needs of most every patient who is likely to walk into a practice. I'm raising the bar on my game and expect other disciplines to do the same rather than trying to downgrade, discount, or obstruct professional growth. The most confident and secure physicians I've worked with had no issue with my doctorate degree.

Dr. O'Dell, what role do you envision DNP, LLC having with regard to the education of others about the DNP degree?

Doctors of Nursing Practice, LLC is an organization that promotes and enhances. If I had to put our product or service into one word, it would be "information." With that in mind, we have the opportunity to consistently share the past, present, and future of the DNP for anyone that may be curious. Education is about exchange, not just dissemination of data. In order for individuals or groups to grow and evolve in any venture, an exchange of thoughts is essential. We have established a venue for this purpose and have made definitive plans to continue this effort in the future.

The first national conference will be our first collaborative effort to demonstrate what DNPs are doing in practice and education. I look forward to seeing what will happen in the future compared to these simple times of 2008.

Dr. O'Dell, what is your advice to other DNP graduates regarding educating patients, other nurses, and other healthcare professionals about the DNP degree?

I've seen many discussions about the title of "doctor" and the consternation that it is causing. Even though I'm smart enough to understand human nature and motivations for actions, I'm still surprised that some have challenged the title of "doctor," especially when our degree and title are so clear. We are doctors of nursing practice. This is easy to convey to patients, other nurses, and any other healthcare professional. I don't have to explain what I am not. Rather, I try to consistently point out the title and what it means.

I had an interaction with a patient a few days ago that illustrates the insignificance of title. I introduced myself as a nurse practitioner with a doctor in nursing practice degree and then went on to relay some of my background before exploring his needs and goals for that particular visit. He asked me, "Are you a doctor?" I replied that I'm a nurse practitioner with a doctorate degree. He then asked me a pointed question and made this ironic statement, "Why don't other doctors tell me what they can do like you just did? I don't have any idea why they are there or what they know. A doctor doesn't mean much to me other than someone that can help me." He didn't care that I was not a physician; he just wanted to know that I could help with his problem. That reinforced my approach to anyone I talk with regarding the DNP. I'm there to help with the skills and education at the highest level of my discipline. That's all that matters to my patients.

We are prepared through our education to evaluate and manage organizations and systems. I'm proud to be associated with DNPs that are influencing huge systems, even entire countries, through their practice. We are truly an international breed of professionals that can (and do) make a difference as a result of our education and skills. Our title reflects who we are and what we do. Staying true to that title is the best way to be consistent regarding the education of our patients and colleagues.

Dr. O'Dell, do you believe there is increased awareness among patients, nurses, and other healthcare professionals regarding the DNP degree?

I think there is most definitely more awareness among all the groups you mentioned regarding the DNP degree compared to a few years ago, but I'm not naïve [enough] to think that awareness means acceptance. The dialogue about the DNP and its implications for all parties is just beginning. I don't think that even DNPs realize the potential of our future practices (clinical, leadership, educators, and researchers). As we move closer to 2015, and more DNP graduates enter the field, we'll have greater awareness and hopefully acceptance. We are in an early phase of a paradigm shift for our nursing discipline. Our entire healthcare delivery system—our industry—is changing too. We will no doubt be a large part of this shift as nursing is such an essential player in this process. The discussion about whether or not the DNP should exist is irrelevant. We are here. The discipline and number of graduates are growing exponentially. We will not disappear. Awareness and acceptance will be an evolutionary process. This is inevitable.

Dr. O'Dell, what impact do you expect DNP graduates will have on health care in the future?

This is a great question, and many folks are watching and waiting to see what the DNP will do to or for health care. I can speculate, but certainly cannot predict, what will happen to health care in general as a result of the DNP. I think that the degree will catalyze change rather than be the specific agent of change alone. The presence of a practice doctorate in nursing has already initiated dialogue and expectation for change. Those wheels are now in motion. The mere presence of the DNP has changed the way we educate nurses and how advanced practice nursing (in all of its forms) will be integrated into our current system of patient care. As more DNPs confer and compare how practice is changing, and as we grow in our experiences collectively, we will impact the future of health care. These are indeed exciting times. I'm proud to help direct the trajectory of our discipline just a little by working to create systems for communication and growth specific to advanced practice nursing and the DNP degree.

Now . . . 2011

Dr. O'Dell, we discussed your nursing background and education last time we spoke. Could you please describe your current position?

Since being a part of your book development my career has taken some interesting turns. My clinical experiences have decreased yet have become more focused, and my academic roles have increased and become broader in scope. Currently I'm the Graduate Nursing Program Director at the West Palm Beach Campus of South University while working part-time with a group of local physicians.

Dr. O'Dell, how has your position evolved since earning your DNP degree?

My position has evolved as the need for nurse educators has grown. Advanced practice nursing is at an interesting place in history and the need to contribute to the growth of the profession in order to meet the needs of our patients is very high. I'm honored to be a part of this process on my specific level using my past experiences and education to address these dynamics.

Dr. O'Dell, how has your practice evolved since earning your DNP degree?

My practice has become more refined and specific. Tapping into my DNP education, I am better able to manage my patients in terms of efficiency and with a higher clinical expertise. Experiences from these last several years have renewed my commitment to the growth of our discipline through practice, education, and support of colleagues in their efforts to evolve professionally.

Dr. O'Dell, could you describe the progress and growth of DNP, LLC?

We are proud to share that Doctors of Nursing Practice, LLC has grown reflecting the evolving needs of nursing professionals. The website now has hundreds of visits daily and the online community continues to grow at a rate of about 100–125 members per month. Searchable databases of pertinent information such as a bibliography, listing of DNP programs, and listing of DNP student projects have also grown. An archive of the 2008, 2009, and 2010 national conferences is also available on the site. Information about each annual national conference is available along with easy registration. The networking and community growth as a result of the online forums and blogs continue to contribute to the development of the DNP nursing professional. In essence, the DNP website has matured to better meet the needs of DNP graduates, students, and faculty.

Dr. O'Dell, when we last spoke, we talked about the role of DNP, LLC in educating others about the DNP degree. To date, what impact do you think DNP, LLC has had on informing others about the DNP degree?

The impact of the DNP, LLC organization on educating others about the DNP degree has been significant, but is difficult to quantify. We can relay the increased numbers of website visitors and growing numbers of members in the online community, but these are only part of the picture of education and professional growth. The national conferences are another significant element of growth for all in our discipline and also for the general knowledge of anyone interested in this degree. It has been gratifying seeing nurses with diverse backgrounds discuss issues about elevating the expectations of nursing education and practice. It's also been satisfying to have nonnurses join some of the conversations to share their perspectives about practice and expectations of the practice doctorate degree.

Dr. O'Dell, what new methods/venues has DNP, LLC developed to educate others about the DNP degree?

The current venues of the website, including an online community and several searchable databases, have shown a good response. The national conferences also continue to grow in size and caliber of content. The inaugural conference in 2008 had about 145 attendees. The 2010 conference had over 220 and we expect the 2011 and future conferences to draw close to 300 registrants. We are also exploring the possibilities of producing webinars and enduring continuing education events to be provided online. The future is looking bright with all of the possibilities to expand and help the discipline of nursing grow specific to the practice doctorate degree.

Dr. O'Dell, how do you suggest DNP graduates continue to educate others about the DNP degree?

This is a very good question. As you know, education never stops, and it only briefly takes place in the classroom. Educating others (including nursing colleagues, healthcare professionals in other disciplines, the general public, and policy makers) is an ongoing process. I hope that those involved in practicing nursing at the top of their capabilities never miss an opportunity to share with others what can be done to enhance patient outcomes. After all, improved health and outcomes is the bottom line for all of our efforts.

Specifically, the evolution of improved patient outcomes includes changes in policies that address access to patient care services. An expansion of advanced nursing practice roles is essential to providing services, maximizing the educational abilities of these nursing professionals.

Dr. O'Dell, what advice do you have in general for DNP graduates regarding educating others about the DNP degree?

General advice I have for DNP graduates is to educate by demonstration. I hope that we all perform our respective tasks to the best of our abilities and document our skills and talents in any way possible (case studies, literature reviews, published articles reflecting the application of research to practice). As we know in the undergraduate nursing field, the award of the Bachelor of Science in Nursing degree and earning the registered nurse license reflects a license to provide safe care—and above all to learn and grow professionally. The growth of the DNP-prepared nurse also begins again after earning the degree. The contributions to our patients' outcomes are paramount, and include many approaches. In our respective practices as clinicians, administrators, researchers, or educators, we all have a responsibility to provide the best we have to offer. I hope that new DNP graduates recognize that upon graduation the work really begins.

SUMMARY

- Educating patients, nurses, and other healthcare professionals about the DNP degree is the responsibility of all DNP graduates.
- It is necessary that DNP graduates have a clear understanding of the terms "nursing," "nursing practice," "advanced practice nursing," "medicine," "physician," "doctor," "practice doctorate," and "Doctor of Nursing Practice."
- Overall, the literature has shown patients to have favorable attitudes and perceptions of advanced practice registered nurses (Brown, 2007; Levine, et al., 1978; Mitchell, et al., 2001; Sheer, 1994). This information provides insights for DNP graduates to develop strategies when educating patients about the DNP graduate's role and educational preparation.
- The literature has shown that nurses look to advanced practice registered nurses as a resource and value their contribution to health care (Gooden & Jackson, 2004). DNP graduates can also be a resource for nursing and act as role models for nurses. This will increase DNP graduates' credibility and nurses' receptiveness toward the DNP degree.
- Physicians' attitudes toward nurse practitioners have evolved. Research has shown that physicians' attitudes improve when physicians work with nurse practitioners (Aquilino et al., 1999). Therefore, in an effort to effectively educate healthcare professionals about the DNP degree, DNP graduates should continue to collaborate with other healthcare professionals and provide interdisciplinary care. This will also demonstrate improvement in patient care outcomes.
- Empathic listening, or listening with the intent to understand (Covey, 2004), can enable the DNP graduate to understand the audience's frame of reference, which will allow the audience to understand the DNP graduate's message.
- When preparing to speak publicly about their educational preparation, DNP graduates should be very clear about their message.
- DNP graduates should always convey sincerity and enthusiasm to their audience when presenting information about their educational preparation.

REFLECTION QUESTIONS

1. Do you have a clear understanding of nursing as a discipline, science, and profession?
2. Do you have a clear understanding of the differences between nursing and medicine?
3. How do you think patients perceive nursing? Advanced practice nursing? The DNP degree?
4. What can be done to increase patients' understanding of nursing and the DNP degree?
5. Do you think other nurses have a clear understanding of the DNP degree, including the rationale for a practice doctorate in nursing?

6. If not, what do you think can be done to increase nursing's understanding of the DNP degree?

7. How do you think other healthcare professionals perceive nursing and the DNP degree?

8. What can be done to increase other healthcare professionals' understanding of nursing and the DNP degree?

9. Do you agree that it is every DNP graduate's responsibility to educate others about the DNP degree?

10. What strategies do you think DNP graduates can use to increase overall awareness and understanding of the DNP degree?

REFERENCES

American Association of Colleges of Nursing (AACN). (2006a). *Doctor of nursing practice roadmap task force report*. Retrieved from http://www.aacn.nche.edu/dnp/roadmapreport.pdf

American Association of Colleges of Nursing (AACN). (2006b). *Essentials of doctoral education for advanced nursing practice*. Retrieved from www.aacn.nche.edu/publications/position/DNPEssentials.pdf

American Nurses Association (ANA). (1995). *Nursing's social policy statement*. Washington, DC: Author.

Aquilino, M., Damiano, P., Williard, J., Momany, E., & Levy, B. (1999). Primary care physician perceptions of the nurse practitioner in the 1990s. *Archives of Family Medicine, 8*(3), 224–227.

Bailey, J. (2003). The story of "doctor, " "physician, " and "surgeon. " *Journal of the National Medical Association, 85*(6), 489–490.

Brown, D. (2007). Consumer perspectives on nurse practitioners and independent practice. *Journal of the American Academy of Nurse Practitioners, 19*(10), 523–529.

Brown, S. (1998). A framework for advanced practice nursing. *Journal of Professional Nursing, 14*(3), 157–164.

Bryant-Lukosius, D., DiCenso, A., Browne, G., & Pinelli, J. (2004). Advanced practice nursing roles: Development, implementation, and evaluation. *Nursing and Health Care Management and Policy, 48*(5), 519–529.

Carnegie, D., & Pell, A. (2005). *Public speaking for success: Revised and updated version*. New York: Penguin.

Carnegie, D., & Carnegie Hill, M. (2007). *Tips for public speaking*. Sausalito, CA: E & E.

Covey, S. R. (2004). *The 7 habits of highly effective people*. New York: Free Press.

DNP, LLC. (2010). Doctors of Nursing Practice, LLC/Doctors of Nursing Practice Professional Development, Inc. outcomes study. Jupiter, FL: Author.

Edmunds, M. (1988). Promoting visibility for the nurse practitioner role. *Nurse Practitioner, 13*(3), 53–55.

Encyclopedia.com. (2008). *Doctorate*. Retrieved from http://www.encyclopedia.com/searchresults.aspx?q=doctorate

Fottler, M., Gibson, G., & Pinchoff, D. (1978). Physician attitudes toward the nurse practitioner. *Journal of Health and Social Behavior, 19*(3), 303–311.

Gooden, J., & Jackson, E. (2004). Attitudes of registered nurses toward nurse practitioners. *Journal of American Academy of Nurse Practitioners, 16*(8), 360–364.

Greiner, A. C., & Knebel, E. (Eds.). (2003). *Health professions education: A bridge to quality*. Washington, DC: National Academies Press.

Griffiths, Y., & Padilla, R. (2006). National status of the entry-level doctorate in occupational therapy. *American Journal of Occupational Therapy, 60*(5), 540–549.

International Council of Nurses (ICN). (n.d.). *The ICN definition of nursing*. Retrieved from http://www.icn.ch/about-icn/icn-definition-of-nursing

International Council of Nurses (ICN). (1998). *Position statement: Scope of nursing practice*. Retrieved from http://www.icn.ch/images/stories/documents/publications/position_statements/B07_Scope_Nsg_Practice.pdf

Kravitz, L. (2007, January). Public speaking 101. *IDEA Fitness Journal*, 108–109.

Levine, J., Orr, S., Sheatsley, D., Lohr, J., & Brodie, B. (1978). The nurse practitioner: Role, physician utilization, patient acceptance. *Nursing Research*, 27(4), 245–254.

Marriner-Tomey, A. (1990). Historical development of doctoral programs from the middle-ages to nursing education today. *Nursing and Health Care*, 3(11), 132–137.

Medicine. (2007). In *New Oxford American Dictionary* (2nd ed.) [Computer software]. Cupertino, CA: Apple, Inc.

Merriam-Webster's Online Dictionary. (2008a). *Medicine*. Retrieved from http://www.merriam-webster .com/dictionary/medicine

Merriam-Webster's Online Dictionary. (2008b). *Physician*. Retrieved July 18, 2008, from http://www .merriam-webster.com/dictionary/physician

Mitchell, J., Dixon, H., Freeman, T., & Grindrod, A. (2001). Public perceptions of and comfort level with nurse practitioners in family practice. *Canadian Nurse*, 97(8), 20–26.

Montoya, I., & Kimball, O. (2006). Marketing clinical doctorate programs. *Journal of Allied Health*, 36(2), 107–112.

Newman, M. (1975). The professional doctorate in nursing: A position paper. *Nursing Outlook*, 23(11), 704–706.

Richmond, T., & Becker, D. (2005). Creating an advanced practice nurse–friendly culture: A marathon not a sprint. *AACN Clinical Issues*, 16(1), 58–66.

Royeen, C., & Lavin, M. (2006). A contextual logical analysis of the clinical doctorate for health practitioners: Dilemma, delusion, or de facto? *Journal of Allied Health*, 36(2), 101–106.

Sheer, B. (1994). Reshaping the nurse practitioner image through socialization. *Nurse Practitioner Forum*, 5(4), 215–219.

Skinner, H. (1970). *Medical terms* (2nd ed.). New York: Hafner.

Upvall, M., & Ptachcinski, R. (2007). The journey to the DNP program and beyond: What can we learn from pharmacy? *Journal of Professional Nursing*, 23(5), 316–321.

Whitemore, S., & Jaffe, L. (1996). Public perceptions of nurse practitioners. *Nurse Practitioner*, 21(2), 19–20.

CHAPTER 11

Shaping Your Brand: Marketing Yourself as a DNP Graduate

■ LISA ASTALOS CHISM ■

"Success can make you go one of two ways; it can make you a prima donna, or it can smooth out the edges, take the insecurities away, and let the nice things come out."

—*Barbara Walters* (1931–)

The number of students enrolled in a DNP program continues to increase. From 2008 to 2009, the number of students enrolled in DNP programs increased from 3,415 to 5,165 and the number of DNP graduates increased from 361 to 660 (AACN, 2011b). Despite these increasing numbers, the DNP degree is still new to many outside of and within the nursing profession. It is therefore likely that the DNP degree will be new to potential employers of DNP graduates. DNP graduates have a responsibility not only to educate others about the DNP degree but also to develop unique strategies to market themselves as DNP graduates.

Many DNP graduates may not have a background in marketing; therefore, some basic marketing concepts are reviewed in this chapter. These concepts include the definition of marketing and branding, becoming a "marketpreneur" (Mackey & Estala, 2008), and creating a mission and vision statement unique to DNP graduates. Also, general marketing strategies are discussed in relation to the DNP graduate. Finally, unique marketing strategies for the DNP graduate are reviewed with specific suggestions that this author has used to market herself as a DNP graduate.

■ Marketing vs. Branding

Marketing has been defined by the American Marketing Association as "an organizational function and a set of processes for creating, communicating, and delivering value to customers and for managing customer relationships in ways that benefit the organization and its stakeholders" (AMA, 2011). Marketing also describes various concepts, such as business development, through advertising, brand and logo design, making sales calls, and designing websites, brochures, packaging, and business cards (Haim, 2005). Beals (2008) describes a more in-depth definition of marketing as a *"process,* from planning to execution, which identifies consumers for a specific product or service, communicates how the product satisfies consumer wants and needs and spurs the consumer to make a purchase" (p. 7).

Conversely, Putman (1990) describes three functions that are not inclusive of marketing, but rather are various functions of marketing. Advertising is noted to be one function of marketing, but not equivalent to marketing. Promotion, or making potential clients aware of your business, is also noted to be a function of marketing but not inclusive of marketing. Finally, sales may or may not be a part of marketing (Putman, 1990). Sales generally involves interactions with potential clients to explain the benefits of products or goods (Dayhoff & Moore, 2004).

Branding, a component of marketing, is an essential marketing strategy. A brand consists of a "trademark, a distinctive name, and a combination of images that creates associations and expectations in the minds of consumers" (Beals, 2008). Beals related that "in your lifelong self-marketing campaign, *you* are the 'brand' . . . the work you do and the value you add are your *product*" (Beals, 2008, p. 8).

Why develop a brand for yourself? Despite the fact that DNP graduates practice within the healthcare or academic arena, the world continues to become a more competitive place. According to Beals (2008), one may develop a brand for the following reasons:

- To benefit your career
- To increase personal recognition
- To improve your reputation
- To promote your employer's business
- To obtain new clients/patients
- To advance your own social beliefs or cause

DNP graduates may develop a brand to share what unique talents, skills, and knowledge they bring to their career environment. A DNP graduate's brand may be unique to the role or setting in which he or she is practicing. A DNP graduate in the academic setting may develop a brand based on a curriculum he or she develops or his or her area of expertise. A DNP graduate in a clinical setting may develop his or her brand based on his or her specialty such as an additional certification he or she has earned.

For example, one of this author's colleagues, Ms. Christine Rymal, MSN, ANP, BC, CLT, practices in a breast health setting and holds additional certification as a lymphedema specialist (CLT). Ms. Rymal has created a brand and has a unique niche within her setting as a lymphedema specialist. Because of her brand, Ms. Rymal is regularly consulted by multiple providers within her setting and has developed a successful practice (personal communication, March 10, 2011). Developing a brand is one method DNP graduates can employ to market their unique product.

■ DNP Graduates as "Marketpreneurs"

Mackey and Estala (2008) describe "marketpreneurship" as employing leadership and innovation when marketing. Specifically, these authors refer to nurse practitioners as "marketpreneurs" who "use their imagination to build relationships and focus on target markets" (Mackey & Estala, 2008, p. 14). As innovators and leaders, marketpreneurs have a "vision they can articulate and sell this vision to others" (Mackey & Estala, 2008, p. 14). Additionally, a marketpreneur has "desire, determination, dedication/ commitment, and a focus on success" (Mackey & Estala, 2008, p. 14).

DNP graduates are charged to become "marketpreneurs." The DNP degree is an innovative degree that emphasizes leadership in practice. DNP graduates may develop a mission and a vision and apply these when developing their brand. The innovative contributions to improving practice and leadership skills that DNP graduates embody will foster their success as "marketpreneurs."

■ Mission Statement

A mission statement has been defined as "a sentence describing a company's function, markets and competitive advantages; a short written statement of your business goals and philosophies" (Entrepreneur, 2011). Further, "a mission statement defines what an organization is, why it exists, its reason for being" (Entrepreneur, 2011). DNP graduates may develop their own mission statement based on their setting or specialty. For example, this author has a clinical practice and specializes in breast and menopausal health. The following is her mission statement:

> "To provide expertise, empathy, and compassion while evaluating and caring for patients' breast and menopause health issues."

Developing a mission statement enables DNP graduates to define exactly what they bring to their setting and decide how their unique talents and skills may be marketed. A mission statement will also help DNP graduates define their focus and channel their efforts to achieve their mission.

■ Vision Statement

A vision statement has been defined as an "aspirational description of what an organization would like to achieve or accomplish in the mid-term or long-term future" (Business Dictionary, 2011). DNP graduates may also develop their own vision statement when they graduate to guide them toward their long-term goals. This author's vision statement is as follows:

> "Develop expertise regarding the DNP degree and serve as a consultant providing pedagogical materials nationally and internationally while maintaining a clinical practice specializing in caring for patients' breast and menopause health issues."

By developing a vision statement, DNP graduates will begin to actualize their goals and as well as develop their new roles within their setting.

■ Marketing Strategies

The marketing literature offers several marketing strategies. Specifics of each strategy will depend on your setting or practice site (Mackey & Estala, 2008). The following marketing strategies offer insight for DNP graduates to begin developing their own marketing strategies that are most appropriate for their setting.

Rogers's Diffusion Theory

Dr. Everett Rogers is widely known as the creator of the Diffusion of Innovation Theory. His work stems from his personal interest in understanding why farmers in Iowa (including his father) resisted using new inventions in their fields. Instead, these farmers adopted innovations over a period of time. Dr. Rogers earned a degree in agriculture followed by a PhD in sociology and statistics from Iowa State University and wrote the book *Diffusion of Innovations* in 1962.

Diffusion is defined as "the process in which an innovation is communicated through certain channels over time among the members of a social system" (Rogers, 2003, p. 5). An innovation is defined by Rogers (2003) as "an idea, practice, or project that is perceived as new by an individual or other unit of adoption" (p. 12). According to Rogers (2003), Diffusion of Innovation occurs when consequences are shared with all parties, in other words, the advantages and disadvantages must be shared to reduce uncertainty regarding an innovation. Second, communication must take place between parties regarding the innovation. Rogers (2003) defines communication as "a process in which participants create and share information with one another in order to reach a mutual understanding" (p. 5).

In summary, Rogers (2003) describes the Diffusion of Innovations process as "an information-seeking and information-processing activity, where an individual is motivated to reduce uncertainty about the advantages and disadvantages of an innovation" (p. 172). This process involves five steps: (1) knowledge, (2) persuasion, (3) decision, (4) implementation, and (5) confirmation (Rogers, 2003). This process has been used to explain the "tipping point," or the time when an idea or innovation catches fire and spreads throughout a population (Orr, 2003). The idea of the DNP degree is an example of the Diffusion of Innovation Theory in action. At one point, the degree was an idea, or innovation, and has now been adopted as the educational preparation of APRNs with over 153 programs now offered nationwide and 160 in development (AACN, 2011b). DNP graduates may have followed this theory while deciding whether or not to adopt this degree as their own academic preparation, weighing the advantages and disadvantages and communicating with others to make their decision. DNP graduates may have employed knowledge, persuasion (with their families and colleagues), decision making, implementation, and finally confirmation when making the decision to return to graduate school. DNP graduates may employ this process when marketing themselves to new employers or others.

The Four Ps

The literature also discusses the Four Ps as a marketing strategy. Landrum (1998) relates the Four Ps to Rogers's (2003) work and describes the Four Ps as **p**roduct, **p**rice, **p**lace, and **p**romotion. Landrum (1998) describes the product as the advanced practice registered nurse, the price as the cash flow involved, the place as the setting of the practice, and the promotion as advertising to promote the services provided by the advanced practice registered nurse. Haim (2005) also describes these Four Ps in the literature. Product is described as the service offered by the advanced practice registered nurse, price is described as how much is charged for the service, place is described as the location of the practice, and promotion is described as the process of presenting your practice to the target markets (Haim, 2005).

DNP graduates may adapt this strategy to their own practice setting or career environment. They may consider themselves or their services as the product, their contribution or cash flow as the price, their practice setting as the place, and their promotion as the process of communicating the benefits and advantages of adding a DNP-prepared advanced practice registered nurse to a particular organization.

Beals's Rules

Beals (2008) relates self-marketing to playing a game. As with any game, there are basic "rules" to self-marketing. These rules include positive thinking, develop an expertise, be prepared, have the right attitude, everyone counts, realize you are being watched, embrace professionalism, and communicate clearly (Beals).

Beals (2008) describes "positive thinking" as believing "you are a strong, talented person who has something worth marketing" (p. 17). DNP graduates should adopt a positive attitude when marketing themselves. They should also realize that a positive outlook will have an impact on their success and become contagious.

"Developing an expertise" is a given for many DNP graduates because advanced practice registered nurses are already experts in their field. DNP graduates are challenged to not be shy about their expertise and "beat their own drum" regarding this expertise. This would include becoming active as a speaker or writing articles, columns, or blogging professionally. By drawing attention to their area of expertise, DNP graduates become known as experts in their field.

"Being prepared" involves always being ready to embrace an opportunity for self-marketing (Beals, 2008). DNP graduates may embrace this rule whenever in networking situations. This would include conferences or meet and greet opportunities when there are opportunities to market themselves.

The rule "everyone counts" refers not only to attempting to impress those who appear to be influential (Beals, 2008). Everyone in professional settings "counts" when DNP graduates are marketing themselves. It is important for DNP graduates to make a positive impression on everyone they encounter, especially when in professional settings.

Beals (2008) relates the rule "you are being watched" to the dramatic arts when actors stay in character: "As a professional trying to market yourself, you must always stay in your professional 'character'" (Beals, 2008, p. 26). Beals (2008) further points out that what one does or says when no one is watching may hurt your career. DNP graduates should heed this rule and always maintain professionalism, even when they think no one is paying attention. It is very difficult to undo unprofessional behavior and repair one's reputation and legitimacy once the damage is done.

"Embrace professionalism" emphasizes that "behavior and image are critical parts of self-marketing" (Beals, 2008, p. 27). In addition, how one treats others will reflect professionalism. Although assertive behavior may be necessary to succeed, aggressive behavior may have a long-term negative effect on your career. "A truly professional person is nice, sincerely nice, and consistently nice" (Beals, 2008, p. 28). This rule is excellent advice for DNP graduates. After graduation, others may be waiting to see how DNP graduates assimilate into their roles. It would be easy for others to develop a negative perception of DNP graduates if they are aggressive in their behavior.

"Communicating clearly" refers to thinking about what one is going to say before anything is said (Beals, 2008). DNP graduates should employ this rule whenever speaking publicly, especially about their degree. Further, many DNP graduates will be in leadership roles and what they say will be listened to. DNP graduates have a responsibility to make sure what they say is accurate, concise, and clear.

■ Unique Strategies for DNP Graduates

The preceding section of the chapter reviewed marketing strategies that may apply to any professional. These strategies are adaptable to any setting in many career choices. The following section reviews unique strategies this author has found effective in marketing one's self as a DNP graduate after graduation and beyond.

The Introduction

Throughout the previous chapter, educating others about the DNP degree and speaking publicly about the DNP degree were discussed. It is indeed imperative that DNP graduates know who they are and are able to describe their degree. Knowing who they are and being able to describe their degree will enable DNP graduates to develop a concise introduction. The introduction is essential to communicating to others the value that a DNP-prepared advanced practice registered nurse adds to the practice, academic, or organizational setting.

The introduction has sometimes been referred to as the "elevator pitch" (Beals, 2008; Mackey & Estala, 2008). The elevator pitch is a brief introduction that takes 60 seconds or less to introduce someone to who you are, why you are unique, and what your expertise is. The elevator pitch "gets to the point and places an image in the listener's mind . . . it should be brief, descriptive, and paint an interesting picture" (Beals, 2008, p. 29). DNP graduates should base their elevator pitch on the DNP degree and their setting/or expertise. This author has used the following "elevator pitch":

> "I am a nurse practitioner specializing in breast health, menopause, and related health issues. My background includes caring for geriatric and women's health populations in various settings. I currently practice in an academic, multidisciplinary, comprehensive breast center. My educational preparation includes a Doctor of Nursing Practice degree, which has prepared me as a nurse leader and given me additional skills in information technology, evidence-based practice, and healthcare policy, which in turn enables me to address the challenges of a complex healthcare environment."

In addition, this author has an "elevator pitch" to explain *why* a DNP was pursued. When asked "Why a DNP? What are you going to do with that?" this author responds,

> "The Institute of Medicine has called for higher education in all health professions, including nursing. Also, the National Academy of Sciences has endorsed nurses earning practice doctorates. Personally, earning a DNP was about personal and professional growth. I am a nurse leader charged to improve nursing practice through the additional skills I have acquired. I am committed to the advancement of the nursing profession and the promotion of the nurse practitioner role."

The Interview

Most DNP graduates have already had experience interviewing for positions either in the practice or academic setting. However, interviewing as a DNP graduate will be a unique experience for DNP graduates. A few key pointers are worth mentioning.

Kathleen D. Pagana, PhD, RN, wrote a very informative book titled *The Nurse's Etiquette Advantage* (2008). Dr. Pagana offers many pearls of wisdom regarding etiquette that DNP graduates can use as a guide when marketing themselves. Throughout an interview, Pagana (2008) recommends the following discussion points:

- What experiences do you have that qualify you for the position?
- What distinguishes you from other candidates?
- What are your strengths?
- What are your weaknesses?
- What are your long-term goals?
- What experiences have you had working with others in teams?

These discussion points were included because of their pertinence to what DNP graduates may offer in any setting. DNP graduates may tailor their responses based on their experiences and how these experiences may enhance the position they are applying for. Also, the additional skills acquired in a DNP program may be added as additional strengths a DNP may highlight throughout the interview.

Appearances

Appearances matter when marketing one's self as a DNP graduate, especially while the DNP degree is still relatively new to others. "No matter what people say, you are judged by the way you dress" (Pagana, 2008, p. 43). Further, Pagana (2008) states "whether you are interviewing for a job, giving a presentation, or asking for a promotion, the way you dress is important to your overall presentation" (p. 42).

Generally, underdressing may cause embarrassment and overdressing may cause intimidation. Sloppy or inappropriate attire may imply that one does not value one's appearance or care that appearance may affect the overall organization. DNP graduates may pay attention to what others are wearing in the organization they wish to be a part of. If one is seeking an academic position, notice what type of attire seems appropriate in that setting (Pagana, 2008). If one is seeking an organizational leadership position, note what others are wearing in that setting.

Most advanced practice registered nurses in a practice setting will wear a lab coat over their professional clothes. One way to make sure DNP graduates are marketing themselves is to include "DNP" after their name. This author has taken this a step further by spelling out "Doctor of Nursing Practice" under her name on her lab coat. This is done in an effort to further explain and point out the DNP degree and what the initials stand for. Even this subtle effort explains to others in the elevator, in the hallway, or in line to get coffee, what the "DNP" after her name means.

Networking

Some additional guidance is offered here that may assist DNP graduates when networking. The following recommendations refer to conversing with others at networking events.

When engaging in initial small talk at a networking event, Pagana (2008) suggested using the acronym OAR to aid conversation. "O" stands for observation—make a comment about the event in general; "A" stands for ask a question, such as "Have you been here before?"; and "R" stands for revealing something personal, such as "This is my first time at this event" (Pagana, 2008). This acronym may help when one is a bit nervous and in an unfamiliar group.

Also, when talking with many different professionals at a networking event, a good rule of thumb is to be courteous, respectful, and considerate of others feelings. "Good manners are for good business and bad manners may mean no business" (Pagana, 2008, p. 22). DNP graduates should also avoid going from person to person, handing out business cards and shaking hands with as many people as possible. This may convey insincerity and lack of interest in folks as individuals (Pagana, 2008). In addition, DNP graduates should avoid monopolizing conversations with others. This is when the elevator pitch comes in handy, especially if others ask about the DNP degree. DNP graduates may quickly and concisely explain their degree and not monopolize the conversation unless asked further specific questions about the degree. Finally, DNP graduates should employ good listening skills when networking. "A good listener can make a person feel as if they are the only person in the room" (Pagana, 2008, p. 27).

Becoming a Voice in the Community and Professionally

Marketing one's self as a DNP graduate involves exposing one's self to the public. The following recommendations refer to self-marketing by becoming active in the community and professionally.

DNP graduates should become active speakers in various settings. This may include joining a speaker's bureau related to one's specialty. DNP graduates may demonstrate their expertise as well as educate others about their degree. This will also promote one as an expert and facilitate creating a brand.

DNP graduates may also volunteer to speak at community events to the lay public. This too will share their expertise and educate others about their degree. Additionally, volunteering to speak at community events may lead to other volunteer activities in the community that may create opportunities to promote DNP graduates' expertise. One of this author's colleagues, Ms. Catherine Nichols, MSN, ANP, BC, is a DNP student and speaks regularly in her community. Ms. Nichols has spoken about breast health at Girl Scout events as well as educational talks within her church (personal communication, March 14, 2011).

Another way for DNP graduates to market themselves includes writing for a local newspaper, journal, or professional organization. DNP graduates may write about topics related to their specific expertise or about the DNP degree. This will also promote DNP graduates' expertise and facilitate developing a brand. This author joined a professional journal's blog as an expert on the DNP degree. After blogging successfully on topics related to the DNP degree, this author offered to write a regular column related to the DNP degree. As a blog expert, columnist, and author of DNP-related topics, this author is developing a brand as a DNP expert.

Finally, DNP graduates should maintain membership and become active in professional organizations. This affiliation promotes the DNP graduate's professionalism and provides numerous networking opportunities. By becoming active in various professional organizations, the DNP graduate is also able to promote the DNP degree.

Involvement in Policy

Health policy is included in the AACN's *Essentials of Doctoral Education for Advanced Nursing Practice* (AACN, 2006) and is a part of DNP curricula. Health policy defines many aspects of advanced practice nursing and DNP graduates are charged to become involved in health policy. This involvement also fosters promotion of the DNP degree. Hall (2000) related that "educating legislators, corporate executives, and the public about NPs is the key to success in both advancing and marketing the profession" (p. 323). DNP graduates should heed these words and remember that educating legislators is also essential to promoting and marketing the DNP degree. The nursing profession, including DNP graduates, will benefit from our policy makers knowing about and understanding the DNP degree.

Specific Marketing Tools

DNP graduates may have already developed various marketing tools to promote their practice, academic appointment, or position within an organization. However, once a DNP graduate returns to the workplace or applies for a new position, these tools should be modified. The following section discusses a few relevant marketing suggestions for DNP graduates.

Most DNP graduates will already have business cards with their prior degree and title displayed. Upon graduation, the DNP graduates should develop new business cards with a few pertinent changes. First, their new degree should be included as part of their credentials. This is sometimes referred to as the "alphabet soup" that appears after an advanced practice registered nurse's name. Regardless, it is necessary that "DNP" be added after one's name. Generally, the highest degree is listed as the first credential (likely DNP) followed by advanced practice designation/certification, any additional certifications, and then membership as a fellow of a professional organization, if applicable. For example, this author has a DNP degree, is a board certified gerontological nurse practitioner, certified as a menopause practitioner, and was inducted as a fellow of the American Academy of Nurse Practitioners in 2011. Therefore the credentials are as follows: Lisa Astalos Chism, DNP, GNP, BC, NCMP, FAANP. Although one's credentials may be extensive, it is still important to display them proudly. One adjustment this author added is explanations on her business cards under her name and credentials.

For example:

Lisa Astalos Chism, DNP, GNP, BC, NCMP, FAANP
Doctor of Nursing Practice
Gerontological Nurse Practitioner
Certified Menopause Practitioner

This gives patients, colleagues, and others an explanation of the credentials listed. Finally, when adding DNP after one's name, it is not necessary or appropriate to add "Dr." in front of one's name even if using the title "Dr." "Dr." is a title, not a credential.

Sometime after graduating with a DNP degree, this author applied for a new position. As part of her marketing tools, this author developed a pamphlet describing the DNP-prepared nurse practitioner. The pamphlet is included as a chapter appendix.

The pamphlet describes what makes the DNP-prepared nurse practitioner unique and includes brief details about the DNP degree. The pamphlet has been a valuable marketing tool especially during a time when the DNP degree was very new (2007). DNP graduates may develop their own pamphlet as part of their marketing tools to describe their specialties and the DNP degree.

Pagana (2008) recommended the use of thank-you notes after an interview or pertinent meeting. This author also found it useful to design and order stationery with her new credentials listed with her name. It is recommended that the stationery be generic and therefore may be used for any occasion, professionally or personally. The stationery is a professional yet warm way to communicate with others, especially when a more personal form of communication is warranted.

Finally, as technology advances, many advanced practice registered nurses with their own businesses, practices, or pedagogical materials have a website. This marketing tool may be helpful for DNP graduates to create, especially if developing a consulting business or their own practice. DNP graduates may devote a section of the website to explain the DNP degree and use the opportunity to market themselves as being DNP-prepared consultants, providers, or educators.

A summary of tips for marketing yourself as a DNP graduate can be found in **Table 11-1**.

Table 11-1   **Tips for Marketing Yourself as a DNP Graduate**

- Develop your brand based on your specialty and setting. Engage in activities that will help develop your brand, such as writing and speaking on topics related to your expertise.
- Develop an "elevator pitch" (Mackey & Estala, 2008) to briefly explain yourself including the DNP degree.
- Dress for success and model your attire after those in positions you aspire to.
- Add "DNP" to your credentials on your lab coat if in the clinical setting.
- While conversing at networking events, be courteous, respectful, and considerate of others' feelings. Also, do not monopolize conversations and remember to be a good listener.
- Get involved speaking about your expertise or the DNP degree in your community and professionally.
- Start writing in your community or for professional journals. Examples include local newspaper articles, blogging, columns, and professional manuscripts.
- Get involved in health policy by staying current regarding issues or contacting/volunteering for your local legislator and educating him or her about the DNP degree.
- Customize your business cards to include DNP and possibly "Doctor of Nursing Practice" under your name to explain what DNP means to others.
- Develop a pamphlet to explain your expertise/specialty including what the DNP degree is.
- Order personalized stationery with your name and credentials after graduation. Stationery may be used to send a thank you or communicate with others in a professional yet warm way.
- Create a website to explain your business, practice, or pedagogical materials including an explanation of the DNP degree.

Interview with Dr. Margaret Fitzgerald, Owner, Fitzgerald Health Associates

Dr. Fitzgerald, could you please describe your current practice and educational background?

1993–2006: Case Western Reserve University, Cleveland, OH, Frances Payne Bolton School of Nursing, Doctor of Nursing Practice, GPA 4.0

1984–1986: University of Lowell, Lowell, MA, Master of Science in Nursing, Family and Community Health, Family Nurse Practitioner Role Preparation, Honors GPA

1977–1983: Salem State College, Salem, MA, Division of Continuing Education, Bachelor of Science in Nursing, with Honors

1968–1970: Northern Essex Community College, Haverhill, MA, Associate Degree in Science, Nursing Major

Family Nurse Practitioner: Greater Lawrence Family Health Center, Lawrence, MA. Primary healthcare provider in a family-centered healthcare center serving an ethnically diverse, inner-city population. Clinical practice includes obstetric, infant, child, and adult primary healthcare and same-day urgent care. Clinical preceptor for nurse practitioner and medical students. Adjunct faculty with Family Practice Physician Residency Program, the only NP to hold such an appointment, sponsored by the health center (primarily responsible for teaching psychopharmacology).

Founder, President, Principal Lecturer: Fitzgerald Health Education Associates, Inc. (FHEA), an NP-owned company dedicated to helping nurse practitioners and advanced practice registered nurses achieve certification and maintain professional competence by providing live continuing education seminars including NP Certification Exam Review to more than 60,000 NPs throughout North America. Additional programs include Pharmacology Updates, Clinical Skills Workshops, Speakers School, web- and computer-based learning courses, audio/video learning modules, and books. Developed and taught pharmacology and laboratory assessment program used in six universities. Responsible for product development, program planning, speaker development and mentorship, and liaison with NP profession.

Publisher, Fitzgerald Health Education Associates' News: A monthly e-mail newsletter; responsible for editorial oversight of a publication on healthcare issues received by more than 40,000 NPs in North America and abroad.

Dr. Fitzgerald, could you please describe your company including what gave you the idea to start your company and the steps you took to develop it?

The earliest days of Fitzgerald Health Education Associates, Inc. (FHEA) evolved from an opportunity to provide certification review for a small group of

NPs who approached me to help them out. The state nursing association had for years provided such a course but was not going to do so that year due to relocating their headquarters. This helped to create the opportunity, as NPs had no local review option. This humble start, with six people around my dining room table, marked the beginnings of the company that is the industry leader and the largest company of its kind in the world.

Dr. Fitzgerald, how did you market your company in the beginning?

Early marketing was largely word of mouth, but word traveled fast! That first year, I ended up giving the course a second time, since word traveled throughout the eastern Massachusetts area. Given that this was pre-Internet, before wide use of e-mail, and the number of NPs was quite low nationwide, relatively few options existed for getting information out about our programs. However, by the early 1990s, we were exhibiting at most major NP meetings and advertising in the major NP journals. Our earliest adverting was done largely on a barter basis. Indeed, we continue to barter for select services in exchange for disturbing promotional materials at our courses.

Dr. Fitzgerald, how has your marketing plan changed over time as your company has grown?

By 1998, we had a website and store, only 4 years after Amazon. By the early 2000s, we had an e-mail newsletter, a point that distinguishes FHEA from the competition and is currently the most widely distributed NP-focused monthly newsletter, with more than 45,000 subscribers. We maintain a presence in print ads, online, focused e-mail promotion, a print and online product and conference catalog, and exhibiting at most major state, regional, and national NP meetings. We also maintain an active presence with the National Organization of Nurse Practitioner Faculties through a variety of activities. Our Facebook page has thousands of followers and we are branching into Twitter.

The FHEA faculty are featured speakers at numerous NP meetings across the country. Personally, I speak about 100 times a year, both for FHEA and other organizations. This helps maintain a high profile in the relatively small market that comprises the NP population in North America.

Dr. Fitzgerald, what do you believe are the successful ingredients for a great marketing plan?

In this digital age, the adage "be everywhere all the time" still holds. But the consumer can be simply bombarded with information. Focusing promotion is critical.

Dr. Fitzgerald, do you believe DNP graduates should market themselves as well as the DNP degree?

All nurses need to market themselves, period. Those of us who have earned the DNP date are pioneers in this educational preparation and need to have a strong understanding of the significance of the shift in the education of advanced practice registered nurses. We need to be able to say what it is we do, how we do it, and what are our outcomes.

Dr. Fitzgerald, what advice do you have for DNP graduates to market themselves and the DNP degree?

Truly understand the significance of being in the earliest cohorts earning the degree. Soon, all newly graduating APRNs will follow. Setting the DNP as the entry into advanced practice nursing helps recognize the rigor of current master's-level education in nursing while providing a venue for the APRN student to study areas not currently included, or presented in a less formal fashion, in the current programs; this includes but is not limited to education in evidence-based practice, quality improvement, and systems leadership. The DNP also offers an alternative to research-focused doctoral programs. DNP-prepared nurses can facilitate the implementation of the science developed by researchers prepared in PhD and other research-focused doctorates.

Another important factor is the need for APRNs to achieve educational parity with other professions including law, dentistry, social work, pharmacy, medicine, and physical therapy that have established the practice doctorate as entry into practice. This parity is critically important to NP advancement in the area of healthcare policy and leadership. The NP profession has survived and thrived since the transition from the certificate to master's level as entry into practice. I believe the transition to the DNP will yield similar results.

Over the years, requirements for the profession of nursing have evolved, consistent with needs of the healthcare environment. Nurses prepared at the doctoral level with a blend of clinical, organizational, economic, and leadership skills are most likely to be able to critique nursing and other clinical scientific findings and design programs of care delivery that are locally acceptable and economically feasible, and that have a significant impact on healthcare outcomes. This will help advance the NP profession beyond its current considerable reach.

SUMMARY

- DNP graduates have a responsibility not only to educate others about the DNP degree but also to develop unique strategies to market themselves as DNP graduates.
- Marketing has been defined by the American Marketing Association as "an organizational function and a set of processes for creating, communicating, and delivering value to customers and for managing customer relationships in ways that benefit the organization and its stakeholders" (AMA, 2011).
- Marketing is also defined as a *"process,* from planning to execution, which identifies consumers for a specific product or service, communicates how the product satisfies consumer wants and needs and spurs the consumer to make a purchase" (Beals, 2008, p. 7).

- Branding, a component of marketing, is an essential marketing strategy. A brand consists of a "trademark, a distinctive name, and a combination of images that creates associations and expectations in the minds of consumers" (Beals, 2008).
- DNP graduates may develop a brand to share what unique talents, skills, and knowledge they bring to their career environment.
- "Marketpreneurship" is employing leadership and innovation when marketing (Mackey & Estala, 2008).
- A mission statement has been defined as "a sentence describing a company's function, markets and competitive advantages; a short written statement of your business goals and philosophies" (Entrepreneur, 2011).
- Developing a mission statement enables DNP graduates to define exactly what they bring to their setting and decide how their unique talents and skills may be marketed.
- A vision statement has been defined as an "aspirational description of what an organization would like to achieve or accomplish in the mid-term or long-term future" (Business Dictionary, 2011).
- DNP graduates may also develop their own vision statement when they graduate to guide them toward their long-term goals.
- Diffusion of Innovations process is described as "an information-seeking and information-processing activity, where an individual is motivated to reduce uncertainty about the advantages and disadvantages of an innovation (Rogers, 2003, p. 172).
- The Four Ps, a marketing strategy, are described as product, price, place, and promotion (Landrum, 1998; Haim, 2005).
- Beals (2008) describes the eight rules of self-marketing as positive thinking, develop an expertise, be prepared, have the right attitude, everyone counts, realize you are being watched, embrace professionalism, and communicate clearly.
- The elevator pitch is a brief introduction that takes 60 seconds or less to introduce someone to who you are, why you are unique, and what your expertise is.
- When talking with many different professionals at a networking event, a good rule of thumb is to be courteous, respectful, and considerate of others' feelings.
- DNP graduates should become active speakers in various settings as part of self-marketing.
- Health policy defines many aspects of advanced practice nursing, and DNP graduates are charged to become involved in health policy as part of their marketing strategy.
- DNP graduates may have already developed various marketing tools to promote their practice, academic appointment, or position within an organization. Once a DNP graduate returns to the workplace or applies for a new position, these tools (business cards, pamphlets, stationery, website) should be adapted to include the DNP degree.

REFLECTION QUESTIONS

1. What marketing strategies/tools have you used in the past to market yourself?
2. Do you feel it is important for DNP graduates to market themselves differently after graduating with a DNP degree?
3. What will your mission statement be after graduation?
4. What will your vision statement be after graduation?
5. How do you think Dr. Rogers's "Diffusion of Innovation" theory applies to the momentum of the DNP degree?
6. Do you agree with Beals's eight rules of self-marketing? How would you apply these rules to marketing yourself after you graduate with a DNP degree?
7. What is your elevator pitch going to be?
8. Do you agree that involvement in health policy is important to marketing the DNP degree?
9. What types of marketing strategies/tools will you use after graduating with a DNP degree?

REFERENCES

American Association of Colleges of Nursing (AACN). (2006). *Essentials of doctoral education for advanced nursing practice*. Retrieved from http://www.aacn.nche.edu/publications/position/DNPEssentials.pdf

American Association of Colleges of Nursing. (2011a). *DNP program schools*. Retrieved from http://www.aacn.nche.edu/dnp/program-schools

American Association of Colleges of Nursing (AACN). (2011b). *Fact sheet: The doctor of nursing practice*. Retrieved from http://www.aacn.nche.edu/media-relations/fact-sheets/dnp

American Marketing Association (AMA). (2011). *Dictionary*. Retrieved from http://www.marketingpower.com/_layouts/Dictionary.aspx?dLetter=M

Beals, J. (2008). *Self marketing power: Branding yourself as a business of one*. Omaha, Nebraska: Keynote Publishing.

Business Dictionary. (2011). *Definition of vision statement*. Retrieved from http://www.businessdictionary.com/definition/vision-statement.html

Dayhoff, N. E., & Moore, P. S. (2004). CNS entrepreneurship: Marketing 101. *Clinical Nurse Specialist, 18*(3), 123–125.

Entrepreneur. (2011). *Homepage*. Retrieved from http://www.entrepreneur.com

Haim, A. (2005). *Marketing kit for dummies* (2nd ed.). Indianapolis, IN: Wiley.

Hall, R. A. (2000). Marketing nurse practitioners is the key to lobbying. *Journal of Pediatric Health Care, (14)*6, 321–323.

Landrum, B. (1998). Marketing innovations to nurses, part 2: Marketing's role in the adoptions of innovations. *Journal of Wound, Ostomy, and Continence Nursing, 25*(5), 227–232.

Mackey, T. A., & Estala, S. (2008). Marketing your nurse-managed practice: Become a "marketpreneur." *Clinical Scholars Review, 1*(1), 13–17.

Orr, G. (2003). *Diffusion of innovations by Everett Rogers (1995)*. Retrieved from http://www.stanford.edu/class/symbsys205/Diffusion%20of%20Innovations.htm

Pagana, K. D. (2008). *The nurse's etiquette advantage*. Indianapolis, IN: Sigma Theta Tau International.

Putnam, A. O. (1990). *Marketing your services*. New York: Wiley.

Rogers, E. M. (2003). *Diffusions of innovations* (5th ed.). New York: Free Press.

Sample Marketing Pamphlet Describing the DNP-Prepared Nurse Practitioner

The Doctor *of*
Nursing Practice
(DNP)

Quality Healthcare and
Compassion Combined

The Doctor of
Nursing Practice

Nursing's Response to the
Institute of Medicine's Call
for Higher Standards in
Healthcare Professionals'
Educational Preparation

What is a Doctor of Nursing Practice?

A board-certified advanced practice nurse (nurse practitioner, nurse midwife, or nurse anesthetist) with a Doctor of Nursing Practice degree.

What can a Doctor of Nursing Practice do for you?

Provide high quality healthcare including:

❧ Diagnose and treat acute and chronic illness

❧ Order, perform, and interpret diagnostics test such as labs and X-rays

❧ Prescribe medications and other treatments

❧ Provide regular health maintenance for disease detection and prevention

❧ Provide expert patient education and health counseling

❧ Help patients understand how their health related behaviors affect their health and well-being

Why are Doctors of Nursing Practice Unique?

Doctors of Nursing Practice are advanced practice nurses who have developed expertise in research-based practice, information technology, healthcare policy and advocacy, and leadership and collaboration.

"These additional skills collectively improve healthcare delivery by enabling Doctors of Nursing Practice to navigate through complex information sources, shape healthcare policy, advocate on behalf of their patients, and provide high quality, collaborative healthcare."

Dr. Lisa Chism
Doctor of Nursing Practice,
Board Certified Nurse Practitioner
Author and Editor
"The Doctor of Nursing Practice: A Guidebook for Role Development and Professional Issues"

CHAPTER 12

Where Do We Go from Here? The Future of the DNP Degree

■ LISA ASTALOS CHISM ■

"The way I see it, if you want the rainbow, you gotta put up with the rain."
                                                —*Dolly Parton (1946–)*

"We are the music-makers, and we are the dreamers of dreams . . ."
                        —*Arthur William Edgar O'Shaughnessy (1844–1881)*

The rapid evolution toward a practice doctorate in nursing has truly been astonishing. However, this evolution has not been without much debate in the literature. Early discussions seemed to focus on the advantages and disadvantages of a practice doctorate in nursing, and current literature reflects the accelerated growth of DNP degree programs across the country, as well as implications of the DNP degree. The impact of the Doctor of Nursing Practice (DNP) degree on the future of nursing education remains to be seen; however, one can speculate that as a practice doctorate becomes accepted as the terminal degree in nursing practice, the profession of nursing is likely to benefit from the increased standards of educational preparation as well as the recognition of nursing's expertise in healthcare delivery.

A discussion of the debate regarding the DNP degree provides interesting dialogue when considering the future of nursing education. Therefore, highlights of this debate are reviewed in this chapter. The future of the DNP degree is influenced by the growth of the DNP degree, faculty availability, program development, and student enrollment. Additional factors influencing the future of the DNP degree such as "nurse residencies" and an update from the AACN are also discussed. Finally, it is proposed that DNP graduates will shape the future by meeting societal needs. This chapter concludes with comments regarding the role DNP graduates will fulfill in meeting the societal needs evident within this challenging healthcare environment.

■ Nursing's Debate Regarding the DNP Degree

Early publications regarding the DNP degree reflect the position that it was largely unknown whether a practice doctorate in nursing would be accepted. The practice doctorate in nursing was mentioned in the 1970s (Newman, 1975), but earlier attempts to implement such a degree failed. A review of early arguments related to the DNP degree may provide insights regarding why a practice degree in nursing seems to have finally taken root. Current literature related to the role of the DNP graduate in research is also reviewed to provide insight regarding more recent dialogue related to the DNP degree.

An editorial by Dracup and Bryan-Brown (2005), with response from Burman, Hart, and McCabe (2005), pointedly illustrated key early issues and rebuttal regarding the DNP degree. Dracup and Bryan-Brown's article titled "Doctor of Nursing Practice—MRI or Total Body Scan?" has been cited numerous times when arguments against the DNP degree were presented. Dracup and Bryan-Brown discussed the following key issues:

- "A new nursing degree will add to the public's confusion about educational requirements in nursing" (p. 279).
- Practice doctorates "will threaten the already tenuous supply of nurses who pursue a PhD" (p. 279).
- The DNP degree will "enlarge the gap that already exists between academic and clinical nursing and increase discord within the profession" (p. 280).

This editorial presented an opportunity for Burman, Hart, and McCabe (2005) to respond with these counterpoints:

- The DNP degree will not enlarge the gap that exists between academic and clinical nursing but will instead do the opposite. In fact, this degree will "bridge the practice–research chasm that has haunted nurses professionally" (p. 463). Further, this degree may "bring together the spectral ends of the continuum of professional life: The academician researcher and the clinician" (p. 463).
- The DNP degree will not force nurses to choose between a research doctorate and a practice doctorate. This choice already occurs frequently, and claims that this will worsen with a practice doctorate are unsubstantiated. "Nurse educators should be able to be clinicians, at the highest degreed level, with or without a mantle of research layered over their shoulders" (p. 463).
- "The DNP gives nursing the opportunity to reconceptualize what advanced practice nursing is and should be to develop the core sciences of true advanced nursing practice" (p. 464).

Sperhac and Clinton (2004) also thoroughly presented some of the pertinent challenges and advantages related to the DNP degree. One challenge noted was the dissemination of accurate information about the DNP degree and entry into practice.

Currently, the master's degree is still required for entry into practice for advanced practice registered nurses. However, the DNP degree has sparked concern among advanced practice registered nurses regarding eligibility to practice. If and when the DNP degree is mandated for entry into practice, individual state boards will have to reflect these standards (Sperhac & Clinton, 2004).

Another challenge presented by Sperhac and Clinton (2004) is the confusion regarding titles. The ND, DNS, DrNP, DNP, and DNSc degrees have all been referred to as practice doctorates in the past. However, the American Association of Colleges of Nursing (AACN, 2006b) has recommended that one title, the Doctor of Nursing Practice, be used. Further, the Nursing Doctorate (ND) will be phased out. In the future, two degrees will represent the highest level of education in nursing: the DNP and the PhD (Sperhac & Clinton, 2004).

The question of higher compensation for additional education was also presented by these authors. Although patient outcomes have been shown to improve with care provided by advanced practice registered nurses (APRNs), increased compensation should not be an expectation of those seeking a DNP degree. Rather, "market forces shall prevail and incomes may commensurate with demographic characteristics, geographic areas, and the rules of supply and demand" (Sperhac & Clinton, 2004).

An advantage of the DNP degree was presented as increased educational preparation that will meet the needs of a complex healthcare environment, which requires a knowledge base that integrates a growing set of skills and level of expertise. Most master's degree programs that prepare APRNs are increasing in length to meet these needs. Frequently, many master's degrees in nursing are found to be lengthier than practice doctorates in many other fields, such as pharmacy, audiology, or physical therapy (Sperhac & Clinton, 2004). The DNP degree accommodates the increased preparation required to meet the demands of a complex healthcare system and provides nursing with parity among other healthcare professionals (Sperhac & Clinton, 2004).

Finally, Sperhac and Clinton suggest that increasing educational preparation of APRNs to the doctorate level will convey a level of competence to legislators and facilitate increased scope of practice and privileges. "The public, legislators, and other stakeholders understand the significance of a doctorate and what this represents in other disciplines" (Sperhac & Clinton, 2004, p. 293). It is therefore speculated that a practice doctorate will increase parity with other disciplines with regard to legislative regulations. To date, however, the DNP degree has not changed the scope of practice of APRNs on a federal or state level.

Chase and Pruitt (2006) discussed the DNP movement as "innovation or disruption" and asked the question, "Does the DNP movement provide an innovation that solves a problem of complexity by providing a simpler solution to problems or does it add increasing complexity and enhance the position of key stakeholders?" (p. 156). In an attempt to answer this question, the authors posited several issues related to the adoption of the DNP degree.

First, the point was made that the nursing professoriate has finally achieved senior ranks in academia in leading universities. The AACN has stated that additional education is needed for DNP graduates to pursue roles in education. Chase and Pruitt (2006) asserted that "by preparing graduates whose credentials will not prepare them for full preparation in the academic community, the DNP degree disrupts the flow of graduates to a single terminal degree" (p. 157).

Chase and Pruitt (2006) also related concerns regarding titling and licensure. It was noted that although the DNP is an academic degree, it remains unclear how certifying bodies will credential DNP graduates. The point was also made that if there is no change in the scope of practice of DNP graduates, how will health care delivered by DNP graduates differ from that delivered by APRNs without a DNP degree (Chase & Pruitt, 2006)?

Issues related to curriculum development were also described by Chase and Pruitt (2006). The lack of course work devoted to the development of the discipline of nursing was mentioned as a concern. The variance that exists among current DNP degree curricula and outcomes was noted by these authors. Finally, a concern regarding the addition of nurse residency programs to the DNP degree course work was raised. "The idea that a doctoral program would have a training mentality with a residency attached does not move doctoral education forward; it looks backward and borrows from other professions" (Chase & Pruitt, 2006, p. 159).

Hathaway, Jacob, Stegbauer, Thompson, and Graff (2006) specifically addressed Chase and Pruitt's (2006) concerns. It was explained that the practice doctorate in nursing is both innovation and disruption, not either/or. It was noted that the movement of the DNP degree is "predictable" given that "DNP programs enable nurses to move competently upmarket in today's complex practice environment" (Hathaway, et al., 2006, p. 488) in an effort to fulfill unmet needs of a changing market. Further, Hathaway et al. purport that any change causes disruption, but indeed that should not prevent innovation from occurring. Moreover, it will undeniably take time to validate the contributions of DNP graduates to health care. Hathaway et al. further asserted that "society must recognize that world changing innovations cannot always be built around quantitative science" (Hathaway et al., 2006, p. 488).

The number of nurses pursuing doctoral study has been an issue for nursing. With the adoption of the DNP degree, there has been an increase in the number of nurses returning to school for doctoral work. Hathaway et al. (2006) pointed out that this includes PhD enrollment as well. Nurses enrolled in doctoral programs have increased the number of nurses discussing doctoral study, which has increased the number of nurses pursuing PhD degrees as well (Hathaway et al., 2006). The increased number of nurses pursuing doctoral degrees is fulfilling a previously unmet need and is therefore an advantage of the DNP degree.

Chase and Pruitt (2006) criticized the addition of a practice doctorate in nursing by stating, "To now support a degree that allows graduates to be recognized as doctoral prepared when the same level of rigor in their preparation has not been required risks dismantling the hard work of doctoral educators over the past 50 years" (p. 159). Hathaway et al. (2006) responded to this criticism by stating, "This claim discredits all individuals who hold professional degrees" (p. 490). Hathaway et al. (2006) further asserted that, "the discipline of nursing, like other health science disciplines needs both research scientists and practice-scientists" (p. 490). Additionally, the DNP degree fosters the theory–research–practice feedback loop, which has been a goal of nursing for years (Hathaway et al., 2006). Moreover, nursing science will advance more rapidly to continue to build the discipline of nursing by having experts in both the research and practice realms (Hathaway et al., 2006).

More recent literature discussed concerns regarding DNP graduates and research. Florczak (2011) published an essay related to the DNP graduate conducting research. This essay described the concerns of a PhD-prepared nurse named "Katie." "Katie" appeared disturbed by the idea of DNP graduates and PhD-prepared nurses working together and voiced concerns about being in a consultant role to the DNP graduate. Further, Florczak (2011) related that "Katie's anxiety began to intensify as she read some of the studies conducted by nurses without research experience" (p. 17).

"Katie" seemed threatened by the DNP graduate, yet the literature clearly states that a partnership should exist between the PhD-prepared nurse and the DNP graduate. Edwardson (2010) related that PhD-prepared researchers and DNP graduates should work interdependently, each drawing from the other's expertise. "Rather than obsessing about the relative proportion of PhD faculty members, the more cogent issue may be how can the practice expertise of the DNP faculty complement and supplement the research and scholarship of the PhD prepared faculty" (Edwardson, 2010, p. 138).

Others also related that the PhD researcher and DNP graduate should complement each other when engaged in research endeavors. Vincent, Johnson, Velasquez, and Rigney (2010) related that "as practitioner-researchers, DNP prepared nurses are uniquely qualified to reduce the research-to-practice gap" (p. 28). These authors also stated that "DNP prepared nurses transform knowledge generated in research into feasible studies and application" (Vincent, Johnson, Velasquez, & Rigney, 2010, p. 30).

Summary

A review of the arguments related to the DNP degree provides insights regarding the issues that have shaped the progression of this innovative degree. It is interesting that it would seem that each time a concern related to the adoption of a practice doctorate was argued, a thoughtful and valid response was formulated. Newer concerns related to the role of the DNP graduate's role in research also seem unfounded as the PhD and DNP graduate actually have been found to complement each other. Issues related to the DNP degree will likely continue to provide interesting debate in the literature in the future.

▪ The Future of the DNP Degree

The future of the DNP degree may be influenced by various factors such as the growth of DNP programs, faculty availability, program development, and student enrollment. These factors are fluid and continue to shift as the momentum of this degree continues. Additional future developments such as "nurse residencies" are discussed, and an update from the AACN regarding the recommendation to adopt the DNP degree as entry for advanced nursing practice by 2015 is provided.

The Growth of DNP Programs

It seems the number of DNP programs continues to grow at an astounding rate. The AACN maintains an updated program list of all approved DNP programs across the country. This list is frequently updated and reflects the addition of new programs as well as developing programs. The DNP program list may be accessed at http://www .aacn.nche.edu/dnp/program-schools. At the time of this writing, 153 programs existed, and 160 programs were in development. Programs will vary regarding clinical content; however, the *Essentials of Doctoral Education for Advanced Nursing Practice* (AACN, 2006a) described by the AACN should be used as a guide for program content. Prospective students are encouraged to research DNP degree programs when deciding which program most accurately fulfills their needs. Additionally, prospective students will be able to assess specific program curricula by visiting the website of each school's DNP program using the program list on the website previously provided.

Faculty Availability

Although DNP program availability seems to be abundant, the incredible growth of this degree may present new issues related to faculty availability. Faculty availability has been a pervasive problem for schools of nursing and is a valid concern. The AACN reported that schools of nursing turned away 67,563 applicants across the country in 2010 (AACN, 2011). The reasons cited included insufficient numbers of faculty, insufficient numbers of clinical sites, limited classroom space, limited preceptors, and budget constraints (AACN, 2011). Additionally, a survey reported by the AACN in 2010–2011 noted that out of 603 schools of nursing, there were over 1,088 vacancies for faculty positions (AACN, 2011). Ideally, the influx of new DNP graduates will help to meet the need for clinical faculty positions. Who better to teach nursing than those who are currently practicing? Nursing is a practice discipline, and although a need will always exist for nursing scientists to broaden nursing's knowledge base, expert clinicians clearly have a role in nursing education.

The development of numerous DNP programs across the country presents a similar dilemma: As these new programs are developed, who will educate DNP students? Should DNP graduates teach future DNP graduates? This notion may require paradigm shifts for both universities and nursing faculties. Acceptance of nursing faculty members with practice-focused doctorates has been varied. Until parity between the two doctorates (PhD and DNP) is established, this will continue to be a controversial concern among universities and nursing faculty. While this particular paradigm shift evolves, DNP graduates can shape the future by continuing to combine nursing scholarship and practice.

Program Development

DNP curricula are guided by the *Essentials of Doctoral Education for Advanced Nursing Practice* outlined by the AACN (2006a). In an effort to decrease ambiguity regarding nurse practitioner curriculum development, the National Organization of Nurse Practitioner Faculties (NONPF) has designed curriculum templates for DNP programs to help guide course development. These templates may be accessed at http://www.nonpf.com/associations/10789/files/DNP-NPCurricTemplates0907.pdf. The National Association of Clinical Nurse Specialists (NACNS) has developed *Core Practice Doctorate Clinical Nurse Specialist Competencies* that may also help guide curriculum development for CNS-focused DNP programs (NACNS, 2009).

It is important to note that although there may be variations among programs with regard to length, clinical components, and course structure, the content and length of programs should be somewhat unified for DNP programs to establish credibility. Moreover, a concern has been noted that programs may become too research intensive, which would result in the DNP degree becoming more similar to a PhD degree, much like what happened to the DNS degree. DNP program lengths should also remain unified. Current master's degree programs in nursing have traditionally become longer with regard to credit hours. DNP programs should maintain consistency regarding credit hours and length. This will also increase the likelihood that the content of DNP programs is consistent.

Student Enrollment

Finally, student recruitment does not seem to be an issue thus far; however, this author has noted that many APRNs are still cautious about the DNP degree. Through a professional online blog that specifically addresses concerns related to the DNP degree (Advance for NPs and PAs, available at http://nurse-practitioners-and-physician-assistants.advanceweb.com), this author has noted that APRNs are concerned about the time commitment, cost, and marketability of a DNP degree. Many APRNs inquiring about the DNP expressed a lack of understanding regarding how the DNP degree will improve their practice.

Despite the concerns voiced, current enrollment has increased with 5,165 students enrolled in DNP programs in 2009 (AACN, 2010b). The DNP graduates who were interviewed for this book shared that their motivation for returning to school was to pursue a practice-focused doctorate. Nursing had been discussing a practice-focused doctorate for decades. Many DNP graduates and prospective students expressed to this author that they had been waiting for a practice-focused doctorate to meet their practice needs and professional goals. The practice-focused doctorate seems to have filled a niche within nursing, especially among advanced practice registered nurses who aspire to pursue additional educational preparation but also wish to maintain a practice-oriented career.

The success, productivity, and enthusiasm of current DNP graduates will also help to determine whether others continue to pursue this degree. It is imperative that DNP graduates publish their doctoral work after graduation to share their contributions to nursing from a practice-oriented perspective. It is also important that DNP graduates continue to stay involved in nursing scholarship by maintaining interests in clinical research projects and pursuing leadership and educational opportunities (formal or informal). The enthusiasm regarding a practice-focused doctorate seems to have only grown over the past decade. This will also contribute to the momentum of future enrollment in DNP programs. DNP graduates should continue to be proactive about their degree by maintaining their enthusiasm and contributions to the nursing profession and society.

■ A Word About Nurse Residencies

Many DNP programs offer a "residency" or clinical experience within their programs. The National Organization of Nurse Practitioner Faculties addressed the number of clinical hours required in DNP programs, post-master's degrees, and postbachelor's degrees. NONPF published a document titled *Clinical Education Issues in Preparing Nurse Practitioner Students for Independent Practice: A Series of Ongoing Papers* (NONPF, 2010). NONPF has recommended a minimum of 500 hours post-BSN for nurse practitioner students. However, it is acknowledged that additional clinical hours will be required to achieve the DNP Competencies outlined by NONPF. Therefore, many DNP programs have integrated "residencies" or "role immersion" experiences that focus specifically on the skills outlined by the NONPF Competencies and the AACN's *Essentials of Doctoral Education for Advanced Nursing Practice*. Clinton and Sperhac (2009) related that "generally these residencies provide the student with a mentored experience that is intended to assist them in acquiring the DNP competencies" (p. 349). To review each program's requirements for residencies or clinical hours, prospective students may go to the AACN DNP program list (http://www .aacn.nche.edu/dnp/program-schools) and click on the school name to visit each DNP program's website.

■ An Update from the AACN

In 2010, the American Association of Colleges of Nursing published *The Doctor of Nursing Practice: A Report on Progress*. This report confirmed that 2015 remained the target date for adoption of the DNP degree as entry into advanced nursing practice. It was also acknowledged that great progress toward the 2015 goal had been made, with significant program growth and student enrollment. The report also summarized a survey done in 2009 that evaluated the progress of the DNP degree. Overall, 72% of schools with APRN programs were offering or planning a DNP degree program and 62% of schools were offering or planning a postbachelor's option of the DNP degree (AACN, 2010b). Additionally, when asked what the greatest challenges were to opening a DNP degree program, responses included insufficient faculty, limited financial resources, state regulations, and lack of faculty support (AACN, 2010b). Within the report, the AACN offered resources to schools of nursing and committed to continue to identify challenges and address the issues of importance during transition to the DNP (AACN, 2010b).

■ The DNP Degree and Societal Needs

Societal needs have historically affected the development of healthcare innovations. The nurse practitioner movement in the 1970s occurred as a result of societal needs for more primary care providers, especially in underserved, impoverished areas. Although this movement was initially met with opposition, nurse practitioners have consistently been proven to be high-quality healthcare providers (Mundinger, et al., 2000).

The DNP movement may be compared to the nurse practitioner movement in that societal needs were noted, and nursing responded by increasing "nursing's capacity to lead and improve the health of the nation" (Brown et al., 2006, p. 132). The Institute of Medicine (Greiner & Knebel, 2003; IOM, 2010) has recommended that healthcare professionals' educational preparation focus on specific needs in health care such as expertise in leadership, information technology, interprofessional collaboration, and evidence-based practice. The *Essentials of Doctoral Education for Advanced Nursing Practice* outlined by the AACN (2006a), which guides the curriculum of DNP programs, specifically addresses these topics. Additionally, a complex and chronically ill population has driven the need for increased preparation of healthcare professionals. Caring for this type of population requires expert healthcare providers who can "work across disciplines, mobilize resources, and coordinate care interventions" (Brown et al., 2006, p. 132).

Societal needs also require that healthcare professionals develop an awareness of the health disparities that exist in health care today. DNP programs "will enable graduates to apply a social justice framework to guide leadership efforts in multiple arenas" (Brown et al., 2006, p. 132) and address the unique needs associated with healthcare disparities. DNP graduates' "enhanced ability to integrate multicultural awareness and knowledge into their healthcare practices and programs will encourage them to challenge social, cultural, economic and political inequities as major determinants of health" (Brown et al., 2006, p. 132). Caring for individuals and communities with health disparities continues to be a prominent and growing need in health care and society. DNP graduates have an opportunity to improve the care of these populations through expertise in leadership, the development of health policies, and the use of evidence-based practice measures to design healthcare delivery specific to these populations' needs.

Over the past several decades, societal needs have influenced the necessity for nursing to deliver safe, effective, high-quality health care. It is therefore prudent to reflect on nursing's social policy statement, which describes the goals and purpose of nursing in relation to societal needs. The practice of nursing is "based on a social contract that acknowledges professional rights and responsibilities as well as mechanisms for public accountability" (American Nurses Association [ANA], 1995, p. 3). Further, "Professional nursing's scope of practice is dynamic and continually evolving, characterized by a flexible boundary responsive to the changing needs of society and the expanding knowledge base of applicable theoretical and scientific domains" (ANA, 2010, pp. 16–17). Through the knowledge and expertise garnered in a DNP program, graduates expand their knowledge base to meet the changing needs of society. DNP graduates' preparation enables them to utilize information technologies, provide evidence-based practice, develop healthcare policies, and provide leadership in an effort to meet the societal needs of a multicultural, complex healthcare environment. Whether fulfilling roles as leaders, clinicians, researchers, health policy advocates, educators, or an integration of these roles, DNP graduates are on the cutting edge of shaping the future of healthcare delivery.

Interview with an Innovative DNP Program Director: Then and Now

Nancy O'Connor, PhD, APRN, BC is professor and chair of Nursing Graduate Programs and director of the Nurse Practitioner Program at Madonna University in Livonia, Michigan.

Then . . . 2008

Dr. O'Connor, could you please describe your nursing background, including your current position?

I graduated from Henry Ford Hospital's School of Nursing diploma program in Detroit, Michigan in 1974. My first nursing position was in the coronary care unit. I had an interest in developing long-term relationships with patients, so I pursued a position in cardiac rehab. This allowed me to see patients over time and become more involved in health prevention. I completed my bachelor's degree at Madonna University in Livonia, Michigan, which proved to be a wonderful experience. I received credit for my previous experience as an RN and was able to build on this foundation. I then began a master's in nursing program at Wayne State University in Detroit, Michigan. At that time, the program was a health nurse clinician program, which led me to become a nurse practitioner. I graduated with an MSN from Wayne State University in 1980. During my master's program, I approached the director of the program and suggested that due to the length and intensity of the program (52 credits), it should actually be a clinical doctorate program. Even then I felt that the current master's degrees in nursing were beyond the scope of other master's degrees because of the theoretic and clinical content required to fulfill the role of a nurse practitioner.

I then pursued a career as an adult primary care nurse practitioner and held various positions, including working on a grant-funded project as an NP in chronic disease care, and eventually ran three outpatient NP clinics in Detroit, Michigan. This led me back to Wayne State University, where I began teaching in a nurse practitioner program. I was able to combine teaching and practice in a primary care nursing services program at Detroit Receiving Hospital in a joint practice–faculty appointment. Eventually, my interest in teaching led me to pursue graduate school once again, and I began doctoral study at Wayne State University in 1989.

During my doctoral study I became interested in exploring what made NP practice unique and why NPs made such a difference in health care. I developed a theory inductively through my practice experiences, which is linked to Orem's self-care deficit theory. My theory focused on self-care enhancement strategies for patients. While attempting to develop this theory, I independently studied qualitative research methods but found that the intensive research focus took me further away from patient care. While pursuing my doctorate in nursing at Wayne State University, I also taught in an adult health nurse practitioner program at Oakland University in Rochester, Michigan.

I graduated in 1995 with a PhD in nursing and was faced with a common dilemma: I felt I could not adequately balance teaching, research, and practice while attending to all three in an ethical way. Because of my strong desire to teach, I accepted a faculty position at Madonna University in 2000. I helped to develop additional NP programs at Madonna and became the chair of Nursing Graduate Programs and program director of Nurse Practitioner Programs. Since I joined as NP program director, we have added the acute care nurse practitioner track and the palliative care nurse practitioner track. I am also very excited that in May 2009 we will be starting our new Doctor of Nursing Practice program. This is the first doctoral program in any field here at Madonna. We were officially approved last March by the North Central Higher Learning Commission and became an accredited program. Eventually, we will be phasing out the nurse practitioner master's degree programs, and the program will be offered as a post-baccalaureate degree.

Dr. O'Connor, could you please share how you think nursing education has evolved over the years?

We are getting better about responding to the needs nursing can fill and also getting more realistic about meeting those needs. This is evidenced by the second degree nursing programs; we are capturing those interested in nursing with a former skill set and still able to bring them into nursing. On a graduate level, we have done well with our master's degrees in nursing. We have created a generation of highly educated, master's-prepared nurses who are doing amazing things in health care. These individuals are the folks who will return to graduate school for a DNP degree. These nurses will want the additional skill set the DNP offers: additional knowledge in applied research and leadership. These nurses will also want recognition for their level of education and expertise in healthcare delivery. We have sensibly created a degree that is doable and value added to the experience master's-prepared nurses already have. Madonna's DNP program is innovative in that each student will have the opportunity to pursue their degree in an individualized way. Also, students will have the opportunity to work interprofessionally with others, such as physical therapy students, occupational therapy students, and pharmacy students. With the experiences of learning together with other professionals, the DNP graduate is poised to lead and become more system savvy. We hope to promote more PhD–DNP relationships as well through our program. This way, more research in nursing will get done by the PhDs and DNPs working in teams. This seems to be the perfect model.

I also feel that the American Association of Colleges of Nursing (AACN) made a powerful decision with the DNP target date of 2015. By taking a stand, the AACN has empowered nursing to move forward. We may not have solved all of the problems related to entry into practice, but at least we can move forward with the DNP degree. Nurses are responding to this empowerment by applying and graduating from DNP programs across the country.

Dr. O'Connor, what do you think was the impetus for the development of the DNP degree?

The need for a practice-based terminal degree in nursing compared to having only a research-based terminal degree. Both degrees are needed for nursing to be full spectrum.

Dr. O'Connor, could you please describe why Madonna University's School of Nursing has adopted a DNP program?

We wanted to remain on the cutting edge of graduate education in nursing. We have established a program of excellent nurse practitioner faculty as well as faculty for nursing administration. This represents a certain depth and skill set of healthcare expertise. It is exciting to offer a program so closely integrated in practice. We also want to be on the forefront of the theory–practice interface. The DNP program is aligned with Madonna's mission to provide a practical, yet doctoral-level degree to serve the vulnerable and underserved populations in health care.

Dr. O'Connor, could you please describe the process involved in developing a new DNP program at Madonna University?

First, a task force was formed within the school of nursing faculty. We spent about a year and a half developing the curriculum, attending conferences relate[d] to the DNP degree, and meeting with others who were developing a DNP degree program. The program had to be approved by Madonna's governance process, college university board of trustees, and finally the North Central Higher Learning Commission. This process was completed in March 2008.

Dr. O'Connor, what were some of the challenges you experienced regarding the adoption and development of a DNP program at Madonna University?

People questioned whether nurses should be encouraged to get a DNP degree when we currently need more BSN-prepared nurses at the bedside, especially with the shortage of nursing faculty. Some felt that this was a misguided use of resources. However, most have moved forward in their thinking. People realized that you can't just offer nurses a BSN without career mobility as an option. It's not about an either/or option; nurses are needed at all levels. We reviewed our resources (faculty and library) and made sure we had the infrastructure to support doctoral study.

Dr. O'Connor, what are some of the benefits of developing a DNP degree at Madonna University?

It has been exciting work and a great teamwork opportunity for all of us. We wouldn't have followed the DNP movement so closely if we weren't developing a DNP program. Also, the DNP program offers the university recognition through the addition of the first doctoral program at Madonna University. This program also enabled us to educate our professional colleagues about what nursing is doing at all levels. Others now know about the capabilities and possibilities of nursing.

Dr. O'Connor, what do you think are the future challenges related to the adoption of multiple DNP programs across the country?

Mostly faculty shortages and the right mix of faculty. We will need enough PhD and DNP faculty to really teach at all levels. At Madonna, we are attempting to solve this resource problem by collaborating with other universities to share faculty. This will also ensure that DNP students have exposure to a wide variety of faculty. We are also providing students with a role immersion experience where they participate in a practicum experience within a healthcare system. This will bring DNP students close to the healthcare system as well as provide mentorships through leadership and policy experience. A practicum experience will also teach DNP students how to work in teams.

Dr. O'Connor, how do you think the DNP degree will affect nursing education?

It will drastically increase the number of nurses holding doctorates. It will also increase the number of PhD and DNP graduates as a result of clarifying career paths.

The DNP degree will also strengthen undergraduate nursing education. We will have access to more clinical faculty who are teaching at the undergraduate and graduate levels. The quality of teaching will escalate, and the gap between education and practice will close.

Now... 2011

Dr. O'Connor, we discussed your nursing background and education last time we spoke. Could you describe your current position?

Currently I am Professor and Chair of the Nursing Graduate Program at Madonna University in Livonia, MI. In addition, I am the Program Director for the Doctor of Nursing Practice program. In the position, I oversee all of the nursing graduate programs, including the nurse practitioner program, the nursing administration program, and our post-MSN certificate programs. I lead the DNP specialty faculty team as well.

Dr. O'Connor, as a DNP program director, could you describe the progress of your program at Madonna University?

Our program at Madonna began in May 2009 with our first cohort of 21 post-MSN students. We deliver the 36 semester hour program using an executive model, with face-to-face sessions three times per semester on Friday/Saturday blocks, and the remainder of the program is delivered online. We admitted cohort 2 in May 2010 (17 students), and cohort 3 (12 students) in May 2011. We were pleased to graduate our first DNPs in May 2011. CCNE accreditation was attained in 2011, prior to our first graduating class.

Dr. O'Connor, could you please describe your perception of the progress of the DNP degree in general?

I think that general DNP program uptake has exceeded our predictions as a discipline; this is being fueled by external public and professional recognition of the unique knowledge base that nursing brings to solving pressing human health and healthcare organizational problems, and the fact that DNPs are visible in their leadership positions within health care in a variety of advanced roles including administration, advanced practice, health policy, and nursing education.

Dr. O'Connor, do you think the momentum of enrollment has increased over time? If so, why?

Yes, I think that continuing DNP program development and availability have sustained the early enrollment trends in both post-MSN and post-BSN programs.

Dr. O'Connor, how has Madonna University benefitted from having a DNP degree program?

The DNP is the first doctoral degree to be granted by Madonna University; as such, it has been rewarding to note the growth in scholarly activity across campus. Being seen as a full-spectrum nursing department has positively impacted our growth as a nursing department as well. Students like the fact that we have all levels of nursing students studying at Madonna University. The BSN students seek out the DNP students to speak in class, at commencement, etc. They look to them as mentors and role models and are proud to point them out to their families and friends.

Dr. O'Connor, what are some of the new challenges you face as a DNP program director?

Balancing the demand for increasing NP program admission with the desire to expand the DNP program is one challenge. Another is developing a transition model for post-BSN DNP models in a few years. Finally, maintaining sufficient faculty members to adequately supervise all the DNP final projects among their other competing demands. DNPs in the field are helping here as adjunct faculty members serving on committees.

Dr. O'Connor, how do you think the DNP degree has affected nursing education since you became a DNP program director?

The availability of more doctorally prepared nurses in our area makes obtaining doctorally prepared faculty easier!

Dr. O'Connor, do you agree with the AACN's recommended target date of 2015 for the DNP degree as entry into practice for advanced practice registered nurses? If so, how do you recommend we continue to strive toward this goal?

I do agree with this goal; schools that can move immediately to the post-BSN model should do so; others can continue the post-MSN models; new graduate students are seeking the DNP degree as entry-level preparation. Continue to help remove regulatory barriers to schools of nursing to offer professional doctoral degrees to preserve educational opportunity for advanced practice roles to meet consumer demand. Continue to lobby for scholarship money for DNP students to study full time and enter the job market quickly.

Dr. O'Connor, what is your advice to nurses and potential students regarding the DNP degree?

Run, do not walk to the best DNP program you can find and take the plunge. You will amaze yourself with the positive impact on your career, with your impact on our profession, and with your enhanced impact on our healthcare system. Loretta Ford, founder of the NP role, cautioned nurses to "be in a hurry—there is no time to waste!" Heed the call. Take action now. Knowledge is power. Become a DNP and help unleash the power of nursing practice.

SUMMARY

- Although the evolution of doctoral education in nursing to a practice-focused doctorate has been discussed since the 1970s, the adoption of the Doctor of Nursing Practice (DNP) degree has evolved over the last decade.
- Early discussions regarding a DNP degree seemed to focus on the advantages and disadvantages of a practice doctorate in nursing.
- Early arguments against the DNP degree included the following:
  - "A new nursing degree will add to the public's confusion about educational requirements in nursing" (Dracup & Bryan-Brown, 2005, p. 279).
  - Practice doctorates "will threaten the already tenuous supply of nurses who pursue a PhD" (Dracup & Bryan-Brown, 2005, p. 279).
  - The DNP degree will "enlarge the gap that already exists between academic and clinical nursing and increase discord within the profession" (Dracup & Bryan-Brown, 2005, p. 280).
- Accurate information about the DNP degree and entry into practice needs to be disseminated. Currently, the master's degree is still required for entry into practice for advanced practice registered nurses. However, the DNP degree has sparked concern among advanced practice registered nurses regarding eligibility to practice (Sperhac & Clinton, 2004).
- There is confusion regarding titles. The ND, DNS, DrNP, DNP, and DNSc degrees have all been referred to as practice doctorates in the past (Sperhac & Clinton, 2004).
- Increasing educational preparation of APRNs to doctorate level will convey a level of competence to legislators and facilitate increased scope of practice and privileges (Sperhac & Clinton, 2004).
- The nursing professoriate has finally achieved senior ranks in academia in leading universities. The AACN has stated that additional education is needed for DNP graduates to pursue roles in education (Chase & Pruitt, 2006).
- Chase and Pruitt (2006) also related concerns regarding titling and licensure. It was noted that although the DNP is an academic degree, it remains unclear how certifying bodies will credential DNP graduates.
- The lack of course work devoted to the development of the discipline of nursing was noted to be a concern. The variance that exists among current DNP degree curricula and outcomes was also noted (Chase & Pruitt, 2006).
- Concerns regarding the addition of nurse-residency programs to the DNP degree course work have been raised (Chase & Pruitt, 2006).
- Counterarguments for the DNP program were also noted in the literature:
  - The DNP degree will not enlarge the gap that exists between academic and clinical nursing but will instead do the opposite. In fact, this degree will "bridge the practice–research chasm that has haunted nurses professionally" (Burman, et al., 2005, p. 463). Further, this degree may "bring together

the spectral ends of the continuum of professional life: The academician researcher and the clinician" (Burman, et al., 2005, p. 463).

- The DNP degree will not force nurses to choose between a research doctorate and a practice doctorate. This choice already occurs frequently, and claims that this will worsen with a practice doctorate are unsubstantiated. "Nurse educators should be able to be clinicians, at the highest degreed level, with or without a mantle of research layered over their shoulders" (Burman, et al., 2005, p. 463).

- "The DNP gives nursing the opportunity to reconceptualize what advanced practice nursing is and should be to develop the core sciences of true advanced nursing practice" (Burman, et al., 2005, p. 464).

- Increased educational preparation will meet the needs of a complex healthcare environment. This complex healthcare environment requires a knowledge base that integrates a growing set of skills and level of expertise (Sperhac & Clinton, 2004).

- With the adoption of the DNP degree, there has been an increase in the number of nurses returning to school for doctoral work (Hathaway, et al., 2006).

- The DNP degree fosters the theory–research–practice feedback loop, which has been a goal of nursing for years (Hathaway, et al., 2006).

■ The AACN maintains an updated program list of all approved DNP programs across the country. This list continues to grow as new programs are developed. This list may be accessed at http://www.aacn.nche.edu/dnp/program-schools. At the time of this writing, 153 programs existed, with 160 programs in development.

■ Although variations may exist among programs with regard to length, clinical components, and course structure, the content and length of programs should be somewhat unified for DNP programs to establish credibility.

■ In an effort to decrease ambiguity regarding curriculum development, the National Organization of Nurse Practitioner Faculties (NONPF) has designed curriculum templates for DNP programs to help guide course development. These templates may be accessed at http://www.nonpf.com/associations/10789 /files/DNP-NPCurricTemplates0907.pdf.

■ New DNP graduates will help to meet the need for clinical faculty positions. However, this will require a paradigm shift among universities and nursing faculties.

■ The success, productivity, and enthusiasm of current DNP graduates will also help to determine whether others continue to pursue this degree. It is imperative that DNP graduates publish their doctoral work after graduation to share their contributions to nursing from a practice-oriented perspective.

■ It is acknowledged that additional clinical hours will be required to achieve the DNP Competencies outlined by NONPF. Therefore, many DNP programs have integrated "residencies" or "role immersion" experiences that focus specifically on the skills outlined by the NONPF Competencies and the AACN's *Essentials of Doctoral Education for Advanced Nursing Practice.*

- In 2010, the American Association of Colleges of Nursing published *The Doctor of Nursing Practice: A Report on Progress.* This report confirmed that 2015 remained the target date for adoption of the DNP degree as entry into advanced nursing practice.
- The DNP degree enables nursing to continue to serve societal needs, such as caring for chronically ill, complex populations and persons with health disparities.
- The practice of nursing is "based on a social contract that acknowledges professional rights and responsibilities as well as mechanisms for public accountability" (ANA, 1995, p. 3).
- The knowledge and expertise acquired in a DNP program assist graduates in meeting the changing needs of society. DNP graduates' preparation enables them to utilize information technologies, provide evidence-based practice, develop healthcare policies, and provide leadership in an effort to meet the societal needs of a multicultural, complex healthcare environment.
- Whether fulfilling roles as leaders, clinicians, researchers, educators, or an integration of these roles, DNP graduates are on the cutting edge of shaping the future of nursing education and healthcare delivery.

REFLECTION QUESTIONS

1. How do you think the early arguments for and against the DNP degree have shaped the growth of the degree?
2. Which set of arguments is most compelling for you?
3. What do you think will increase credibility of the DNP degree?
4. Do you think DNP graduates should fulfill the current need for additional nursing faculty? If so, how should this occur?
5. Do you believe the current momentum of enrollment in DNP programs will continue? If so, what will ensure this momentum?
6. Do you think "nurse residencies" are necessary in DNP programs? What would you hope to gain from a "nurse residency"?
7. Do you think DNP graduates are and will continue to fulfill current societal needs? If so, in what ways?

REFERENCES

American Association of Colleges of Nursing (AACN). (2006a). *Essentials of doctoral education for advanced nursing practice.* Retrieved from http://www.aacn.nche.edu/publications/position /DNPEssentials.pdf

American Association of Colleges of Nursing (AACN). (2006b). *Doctor of nursing practice roadmap task force report.* Retrieved from http://www.aacn.nche.edu/dnp/roadmapreport.pdf

American Association of Colleges of Nursing (AACN). (2010). *The doctor of nursing practice: A report on progress.* Retrieved from http://www.aacn.nche.edu/leading-initiatives/dnp/DNPForum3-10.pdf

American Association of Colleges of Nursing (AACN). (2011). Nursing shortage fact sheet. Retrieved from http://www.aacn.nche.edu/media-relations/fact-sheets/nursing-faculty-shortage

American Nurses Association (ANA). (1995). *Nursing's social policy statement.* Washington, DC: Author.

American Nurses Association (ANA). (2010). *Nursing's social policy statement* (2nd ed.). Washington, DC: Author.

Brown, M., Draye, M., Zimmer, P., Magyary, D., Woods, S., Whitney, J., et al. (2006). Developing a practice doctorate in nursing: University of Washington perspectives and experience. *Nursing Outlook, 54*(3), 130–138.

Burman, M., Hart, A., & McCabe, S. (2005). Doctor of nursing practice: Opportunity amidst chaos. *American Journal of Critical Care, 14*(6), 463–464.

Chase, S., & Pruitt, R. (2006). The practice doctorate: Innovation or disruption? *Journal of Nursing Education, 45*(5), 155–161.

Clinton, P., & Sperhac, A. M. (2009). The DNP and unintended consequences: An opportunity for dialogue. *Journal of Pediatric Health Care, 23*(5), 348–351.

Dracup, K., & Bryan-Brown, C. (2005). Doctor of nursing practice—MRI or total body scan? *American Journal of Critical Care, 14*(4), 278–281.

Hathaway, D., Jacob, S., Stegbauer, C., Thompson, C., & Graff, C. (2006). The practice doctorate: Perspectives of early adopters. *Journal of Nursing Education, 45*(12), 487–496.

Edwardson, S. R. (2010). Doctor of philosophy and doctor of nursing practice as complementary degrees. *Journal of Professional Nursing, 26*(3), 137–140.

Florczak, K. L. (2011). Research and the doctor of nursing practice: A cause for consternation. *Nursing Science Quarterly, 23*(1), 13–17.

Greiner, A. C., & Knebel, E. (Eds.). (2003). *Health professions education: A bridge to quality.* Washington, DC: National Academies Press.

Institute of Medicine (IOM). (2010). *The future of nursing: Leading change, advancing health report recommendations.* Washington, DC: National Academies Press. Retrieved from http://www.iom.edu/Reports/2010/The-Future-of-Nursing-Leading-Change-Advancing-Health.aspx

Mundinger, M., Kane, R., Lentz, E., Trotten, A., Tsai, W., Cleary, P., et al. (2000). Primary care outcomes in patients treated by nurse practitioners or physicians: A randomized trial. *Journal of the American Medical Association, 283*(1), 59–68.

National Association of Clinical Nurse Specialists (NACNS). (2009). *Core practice doctorate clinical nurse specialist competencies.* Retrieved from http://www.nacns.org/docs/CorePracticeDoctorate.pdf

National Organization of Nurse Practitioner Faculties (NONPF). (2010). *Clinical education issues in preparing nurse practitioner students for independent practice: An ongoing series of papers.* Washington DC: Author.

Newman, M. (1975). The professional doctorate in nursing: A position paper. *Nursing Outlook, 23*(11), 704–706.

Sperhac, A., & Clinton, P. (2004). Facts and fallacies: The practice doctorate. *Journal of Pediatric Health, 18*(6), 292–296.

Tracy, C., & Fang, D. (2010). *Special survey on vacant faculty positions for academic year 2010-2011.* Washington, DC: American Association of Colleges of Nursing. Retrieved from http://www.aacn.nche.edu/IDS/pdf/vacancy10.pdf

Vincent, D., Johnson, C., Velasquez, D., & Rigney, T. (2010). DNP-Prepared nurses as researchers: Closing the gap between research and practice. *The American Journal for Nurse Practitioners, 14*(11/12), 28–33.

The Certification Question: Where Are We?

■ Karen McBroom Butler ■

■ Introduction

The American Association of Colleges of Nursing (AACN) advocates for the Doctor of Nursing Practice (DNP) to be the entry-level degree for all advanced practice registered nurses (APRNs) by the year 2015. DNP graduates should be prepared using essential advanced academic content, compared to master's-prepared APRNs, and DNP competencies should reflect this higher level of preparation (AACN, 2006). To date, AACN supports national certification for all APRNs but at the time of this writing (mid-2011) it does not recognize a certification exam that distinguishes between the master's-level competencies and advanced DNP competencies.

Certification of graduates of nursing educational programs serves to ensure excellence in nursing practice. The American Nurses Credentialing Center (ANCC), which is a subsidiary of the American Nurses Association, is the "largest and most prestigious nurse credentialing organization in the world" (ANCC, 2011) and has certified more than a quarter million nurses since 1990. Offering nursing certification in almost 30 different specialties, ANCC reports that more than 80,000 advanced practice registered nurses are currently certified (ANCC, 2011).

Currently, there is no national certification standard or requirement for graduates of Doctor of Nursing Practice (DNP) programs. In 2007 the ANCC commissioned a task force of thought leaders to examine and make recommendations about certification of nurses holding the DNP degree. The task force developed a survey that was sent to selected leaders of nursing organizations, including certifying agencies, and then to nursing stakeholders. Based on the results of this survey, the task force made recommendations to the ANCC Commission on Certification. The following information comes from the ANCC DNP Survey Results release on the ANCC website (2008).

■ ANCC DNP Survey Results

There were 4,284 survey responses received (ANCC, 2008). Demographic characteristics of the respondents are available on the ANCC website and are summarized here. The majority of the respondents were white, non-Hispanic (92%), and female (94.3%). More than two-thirds (69.6%) were between the ages of 40 and 59 years. There were 3,060 respondents (71.4%) who stated they worked in an advanced practice role. Of these, 76.7% stated they were nurse practitioners, 11.9% nurse–midwives, 10.8% clinical nurse specialists, and less than 1.0% nurse anesthetists.

In terms of entry to practice, the majority held a BSN (54.8%), 16.5% obtained a diploma, and 19.2% obtained an associate's degree. The highest educational preparation attained for the vast majority (70.3%) was a master's degree, with 22.6% holding a doctorate. A total of 245 respondents (7%) indicated that their highest educational preparation was the DNP.

The major question asked by the survey was, "What do you envision as the desired future for certification of nurses holding the DNP degree in the year 2015?" The majority of respondents (59.7%) stated a preference for a single comprehensive certification exam at the end of the educational program, with DNP degrees required for entry into all areas of advanced practice nursing. Over 40% stated that staged certification was preferable, and students who enter accredited DNP programs as registered nurses should sit for national certification exams one or more times during their DNP program in addition to a final examination upon completing the program (ANCC, 2008).

When asked about what should be done now, slightly more than 50% thought that certifying bodies should start creating separate DNP- and master's-level certification exams. Another quarter of respondents thought certifying bodies should wait and see what happens, and the remainder thought that certifying bodies should begin creating a single certification exam at the DNP level by moving the current master's-level exams to the doctoral level (ANCC, 2008).

The opportunity for open-ended comments resulted in a vast and diverse profile of the views and concerns related to the DNP and to certification of DNP graduates. Many were grateful for the opportunity to provide input, and others were misinformed or confused about issues related to the DNP (ANCC, 2008).

ANCC intends to continue to communicate and work with stakeholders to assure them that their interests will be considered in the development of a DNP certification process, that there will be a reasonable period of time to transition to accommodate current students and faculty, and that current practitioners will be grandfathered in both licensing and certification requirements if there are changes in those areas (ANCC, 2008).

■ American Board of Comprehensive Care

There is at least one certification process underway that falls outside of the national testing arena. An e-mail sent in March 2008 to nursing deans and directors notified them of a newly created group called the American Board of Comprehensive Care (ABCC). This information can also be found in a press release on the ABCC website (2008). The e-mail states that to distinguish DNP graduates who have achieved a high level of competence in comprehensive care, the Council for the Advancement of Comprehensive Care (CACC) and the National Board of Medical Examiners (NBME) have created a certifying exam that will be offered to confirm advanced clinical competency. CACC, founded in 2000, is using the ABCC as its certifying body. Advanced practice registered nurses with national certification in an advanced practice nursing specialty and a Doctor of Nursing Practice degree are eligible to take the certification exam beginning in November 2008. The exam itself is derived from the test pool of the United States Medical Licensing Examination (USMLE) Step 3 exam for MD licensure candidates. Successful DNP candidates will be designated as Diplomats in Comprehensive Care by the ABCC.

The American Association of Colleges of Nursing (AACN, 2008) responded to its members stating there is an understanding that this exam will be voluntary and available only to DNP graduates who are APRNs and have already received certification and licensure from the appropriate groups. In addition, this exam is an independent development effort designed to document the attainment of a unique body of knowledge regarding nursing practice. It may be used by APRNs who wish to validate that they have acquired knowledge reflective of the demands of clinical interventions at the advanced level. The AACN agreed to work with the CACC to both monitor their work and determine if the exam will further efforts to clarify APRN scope of practice authority and assess its usefulness for ensuring competence to practice. This certifying examination is not intended for all DNP graduates, nor is it to be used for regulatory purposes that may conflict with the national initiatives for DNP certification.

■ Conclusion

Currently there are no new answers to how, when, and where DNP graduates will be certified. The ANCC currently provides certification in almost 30 specialties, and these certification exams are likely to be around at least through the transition to the 2015 DNP requirement, if not longer. Nursing leaders are currently working to determine the best way to validate DNP graduates' advanced skills, knowledge, and abilities. In the meantime, current certification avenues are available, and information about new DNP graduate certification possibilities will be communicated when it becomes available.

REFERENCES

American Association of Colleges of Nursing (AACN). (2006). *Doctor of nursing practice roadmap task force report.* Retrieved from http://www.aacn.nche.edu/dnp/roadmapreport.pdf

American Association of Colleges of Nursing (AACN). (2008). *AACN letter in response to DNP certification exam.* Retrieved from http://www.aacn.nche.edu/dnp/responseletter.pdf

American Board of Comprehensive Care (ABCC). (2008). *Council for the Advancement of Comprehensive Care and National Board of Medical Examiners announce new certification examination for doctors of nursing practice.* Retrieved from http://www.businesswire.com/news/home/20080402006367/en/Council-Advancement-Comprehensive-Care-National-Board-Medical

American Nurses Credentialing Center (ANCC). (2008). *ANCC DNP survey results released.* Retrieved from http://www.nursecredentialing.org/Headlines/DNPSurveyResults.aspx

American Nurses Credentialing Center (ANCC). (2011). *About ANCC.* Retrieved from http://www.nursecredentialing.org/FunctionalCategory/AboutANCC.aspx

■ Relevant Doctor of Nursing Practice Websites

The Doctor of Nursing Practice degree continues to be a dynamic, innovative degree. Although the most recent and accurate information regarding this degree has been presented in this text, this information continues to evolve. Therefore, a list of relevant websites is provided below to assist readers in accessing the most up-to-date information regarding the Doctor of Nursing Practice degree.

- List of frequently asked questions (FAQs) about the Doctor of Nursing Practice degree:
  http://www.aacn.nche.edu/dnp/faqs

- American Association of Colleges of Nursing (AACN) Position Statement on the Practice Doctorate in Nursing:
  http://www.aacn.nche.edu/dnp/position-statement

- AACN *Essentials of Doctoral Education for Advanced Nursing Practice*:
  http://www.aacn.nche.edu/publications/position/DNPEssentials.pdf

- AACN DNP Roadmap Task Force Report:
  http://www.aacn.nche.edu/dnp/roadmapreport.pdf

- AACN letter in response to DNP certification exam:
  http://www.aacn.nche.edu/dnp/responseletter.pdf

- DNP programs list:
  http://www.aacn.nche.edu/dnp/program-schools

Index

A

AACN. *See* American Association of Colleges of Nursing

ABCC. *See* American Board of Comprehensive Care

academic pathways. *See also* scholarship
  to DNP degree, 21–22
  tips for pursuing, 167

academic websites, 139

accountability, principle of, 197

accreditation requirements, 10

ACNP. *See* American College of Nurse Practitioners

activism. *See* political activism

Advance for NPs and PAs (blog), 315

advanced nursing practice
  as competency, 61
  definition of, 62, 158–159
  difference between advanced practice nursing and, 61–62, 95
  DNP, LLC/DNPPD outcome survey correlations, 270
  Essentials of doctoral education for, 18 (*See also Essentials of Doctoral Education for Advanced Nursing Practice* (AACN))

advanced practice nurses (APNs), 62

advanced practice nursing
  definition of, 62, 95, 265
  difference between advanced nursing practice and, 61–62, 95

advanced practice registered nurse–friendly culture, 274

advanced practice registered nurses (APRNs)
  APRN Consensus Model for, 60, 63, 95
  certification of, 329
  collaboration with, 123
  compensation for, 311
  definition of, 62
  educational preparation of, 311
  graduate educational requirements for, 219
  grandfathering of, 27, 218–219
  information technology use by, 69–71
  requirements for DNP degrees, 267

Advancing the Nation's Health Needs, NIH Research Training Programs (National Academy of Sciences), 12–13

adverse events, preventable, 10

advertising, 290

advocacy
  avenues for involvement in, 143–144
  case scenario, 151–153
  DNP involvement in, 131–156
  in health care, 16–17
  health policy and advocacy-related journals, 138
  health policy and advocacy-related textbooks, 140
  health policy and advocacy-related websites, 139
  information sources for, 154
  role of DNP in, 147–148, 151
  role of nursing profession in, 147, 150
  through education, 142–143
  through research, 143
  tips for becoming informed and involved, 137–144
  tips for getting started in, 154
  workplace involvement, 142–143

affiliative leadership, 42

African-American nurses, 135

Ahmed, Stephanie, 267

AJN. See American Journal of Nursing

alumnae associations, 134

AMA. *See* American Medical Association

American Academy of Nurse Practitioners, 239

American Association of Colleges of Nursing (AACN)
  on CACC certification for DNP graduates, 331
  characterization of DNS degrees, 8
  on Clinical Nurse Leader (CNL) role, xi

Commission on Collegiate Nursing
    Education (CCNE), 10
curriculum standards for DNP degree, 59–60
definition of advanced nursing practice,
    158–159
definition of nursing practice, 30
definition of scholarship, 109
DNP Programs list, 325, 333
DNP Roadmap Task Force, 218, 333
*The Doctor of Nursing Practice, A Report on
    Progress*, 316–317, 326
Doctoral Education Conference, 9
*Essentials of Doctoral Education for Advanced
    Nursing Practice*, 4, 12, 13, 14–18, 20, 21,
    25, 30, 36, 60, 158, 333
External Reaction Panel, 9
Journal of Professional Nursing, 138
key differences between DNP and PhD/
    DNS/DNSc programs, 6
*Position Statement on the Practice Doctorate
    in Nursing*, xi, 4, 9, 30, 157, 333
recommendations for DNP degree, xv, 9, 29,
    30, 256, 311, 323
response to AMA, 239–240
response to DNP certification exam, 333
on specialty-focused competencies, 19
*Standards for Establishing and Sustaining
    Healthy Work Environments*, 74–75
support for national certification for APRNs,
    329
Talking Points, 239–241
Task Force on the Practice Doctorate,
    5, 8–9, 26
website, 139
American Association of Critical-Care Nurses, 139
American Association of Nurse Practitioners, 139
American Board of Comprehensive Care (ABCC),
    331
American Cancer Society, 139
American College of Nurse Practitioners
    (ACNP)
    "Policy Institute," 140
    recommendations regarding nurse
        practitioner DNP education, 239
American Heart Association, 139
American Journal of Nursing (AJN), 134, 138
American Medical Association (AMA)
    Resolutions
    nursing responses to, 239–241
    Resolution 211 (A-06), 237–238, 259
    responses to, 238
    update, 241

American Nurses Association (ANA)
    approved nursing specialties, 68
    Code of Ethics for Nurses, 182, 184, 188–190,
        192, 197
    *Code of Ethics for Nurses with Interpretive
        Statements*, 211
    Commission on Nursing Research, 24
    definition of nursing, 61–62, 264–265
    discrimination in, 135
    Guide to the Code of Ethics for Nurses, 192
    history of, 134
    and NOPHN, 135
    Nurses Strategic Action Team (N-STAT), 141
    Nursing's Social Policy Statement, 132, 143, 153
    Online Journal of Issues in Nursing (OJIN),
        138
    Political Action Committee (ANA-PAC), 141,
        144, 146
    response to AMA, 239
    support for Equal Rights Amendment, 136
    support for suffrage, 135
    website, 139
American Nurses Credentialing Center (ANCC),
    329, 330
American Nursing Informatics Association
    (ANIA), 73
American Psychological Association (APA),
    110–111, 118
ANA. *See* American Nurses Association
analytical methods for evidence-based practice
    (EBP), 15–16, 60
ANCC. *See* American Nurses
    Credentialing Center
Anderson Cooper 360°, 140
ANIA. *See* American Nursing
    Informatics Association
APA. *See* American Psychological Association
APNs. *See* advanced practice nurses
appearances, 296
application, scholarship of, 168
applied ethics, 182–183, 209
APRN Consensus Model, 60, 63, 95
APRN Consensus Workgroup, 63
APRNs. *See* advanced practice registered nurses
Aquinas. St. Thomas, 183
Aristotle, 183
Arkansas, 236–237
Ashley, JoAnn, 136
Association of Faculties of Pediatric Nurse
    Practitioners, 239
AuD. *See* Doctor of Audiology
authorship, 117–118

autonomy
  definition of, 186–187
  personal, 186–187, 210
  principle of, 186–187
awareness
  public awareness about DNP degree, 283
  self-awareness, 40, 45, 93
  social awareness, 40

B

Beals's rules, 293–294, 303
Beckler, Becky, 146
Behler, Sheila, interview with, 86–89
"The Belmont Report," 116, 186, 210
beneficence, 187, 210
bioethics
  definition of, 185, 210
  history of, 185–186
  principles relevant for DNP graduates, 185–187
birth control, 136
Bishop, Catherine S., 267
Blanchard, Ken, 43
blogging
  Advance for NPs and PAs blog, 315
  ethical perils of, 197
  self-marketing through, 297
Boston University, 7
"The Bottleneck Proposal" (Klemczak), 146–147
branding
  for DNP graduates, 289–299, 303
  reasons for developing a brand, 290
  vs. marketing, 289–291
Brewster, Mary, 135–136
business cards, 298
Butts, Janie, interview with, 204–209

C

CACC. *See* Council for the Advancement of
    Comprehensive Care
candor, principle of, 196
capstone projects, 112–119
caring
  definition of, 185
  ethic of care, 185
caring competencies, 38–39, 56
Carnegie, Dale, 278
case scenarios
  of DNP graduates, 72–73
  of DNP graduates as nurse educators, 169–174
  ethical scenarios, 199–203
  of evidence-based practice, 66–67

of interprofessional collaboration, 76–78
of involvement in healthcare policy and
    advocacy, 151–153
of leadership and collaboration, 48–51
Case Western Reserve University, 8
casuistry, 184, 210
Catherine of Siena, 225
CCNE. *See* Commission on Collegiate
    Nursing Education
CDC. *See* Centers for Disease Control
    and Prevention
Center for Nursing Leadership, 38–39
Centers for Disease Control and Prevention (CDC)
    National Center for Health Statistics
        (NCHS), 131
    Tuskegee Syphilis Study (or Experiment),
        185–186
certification, 329–332
Chambers, Oswals, 227
change
    *The Future of Nursing, Leading Change,
        Advancing Health* (IOM), xi–xii
    leadership steps for, 46–47
chatting, 197
CIT. *See* computer information technology
Clarian Health, 205
clinical competence, 44
clinical doctorate, 266. *See also* practice doctorate
clinical hours, recommended minimum, 316
Clinical Nurse Leader (CNL) degree, xi, 4
clinical practice. *See also* nursing practice
    curriculum standards related to, 60–61
    evidence-based (*See* evidence-based practice)
    improvement with technology, 69–71
    leadership in, 49, 50–51
    nursing faculty in, 171–173
    in partnership with research, 168–169
    scholarship in, 15–16, 60, 120
    theories applicable to, 104
    tips for mentoring in, 81
    use of "doctor" in, 250, 256
clinical prevention
    definition of, 18
    DNP, LLC/DNPPD outcome survey
        correlations, 270
clinical scholarship
    DNP, LLC/DNPPD outcome survey
        correlations, 269
    for evidence-based practice (EBP), 15–16, 60
clinicians
    expert, 59–99
    interviews with, 82–94

Clinton, Bill, 186
CNL. *See* Clinical Nurse Leader
CNN, 140
coaching, 42
Code of Ethics for Nurses (ANA)
    principles of, 184
    provisions of, 188–190
    purposes of, 188
    as resource, 182
    and social networks, 197
    as standard, 188–190, 211
    website, 188, 192
Code of Ethics for Nurses (ICN)
    principal elements, 190–191
    principles of, 184
    as resource, 182
    and social networks, 197
    as standard, 190–191, 211
    website, 192
Code of Ethics for Nurses with Interpretive Statements (ANA), 211
codes of ethics, 182, 209. *See also specific codes*
collaboration
    across teams and disciplines, 43–44
    with APRNs, 123
    case scenarios for, 48–51
    challenges to, 74–76
    characteristics that may promote, 44
    choosing committees, 114–115
    curriculum standards for, 36
    definition of, 43, 74
    DNP, LLC/DNPPD outcome survey correlations, 270
    DNP graduates working with others, 43–46
    interprofessional, 17, 61, 73–78, 96, 270
    key components for, 74–75
    for leadership, 41
    networking for research and scholarship, 123–125
    preparation for, 35–58
    qualities for success, 44–45
    between researchers and clinical practitioners, 168–169, 313
    responsible partnering, 197
    tips for building bridges, 76
    true, 74–75, 76
    types of communication that fosters, 75
Columbia University, 7, 9
commanding leadership, 43
Commission on Collegiate Nursing Education (CCNE), 10
Committee on the RWJF Initiative on the Future of Nursing (IOM), 12, 30, 159

committees, 114–115
common morality, 182
communication
    Beals's rules for, 294
    business cards, 298
    for collaboration, 44
    elevator pitch, 295
    introductions, 294–295
    for leadership, 41
    OAR aids for, 296
    pamphlets, 298–299
    recommendations for conversing with others at networking events, 296–297
    sample pamphlet for DNP-prepared nurse practitioners, 305–307
    speaking publicly about DNP degree, 276–278
    thank-you notes, 299
    tips for speaking publicly about DNP degree, 278
    types that foster collaboration, 75
community involvement, 297
community leadership, 49–50
comparative ethics, 182–183
compassion, 41, 75–76, 183
compensation
    for DNP graduates, 269, 311
    salary benefits, 85, 88, 93
competencies
    caring competencies, 38–39, 56
    clinical competence, 44
    Core Practice Doctorate Clinical Nurse Specialist (CNS) Competencies (NACNS), 13–14, 20–21, 31, 60
    for DNP degree, 6
    essential for mentoring, 79–80
    Essentials of Doctoral Education for Advanced Nursing Practice (AACN), 4, 5, 12, 13, 14–18, 20, 21, 30, 36
    interpersonal, 44
    National CNS Competency Task Force Organizing Framework and Core Competencies, 20
    Practice Doctorate Nurse Practitioner Entry-Level Competencies (NONPF), 4, 12, 13–14, 19–21, 30, 36, 60, 61
    specialty-focused, 19
computer information technology (CIT), 107. *See also* information technology
computer software, 69, 70
Computers, Informatics, Nursing journal, 73
Connecticut, 236–237
conscientiousness, 183
consultants, ethical, 179–213

consulting others, 224
context, personal, 226
continuing education, 140–141
coordination, 76
coping strategies, 229–239
*Core Practice Doctorate Clinical Nurse Specialist
    (CNS) Competencies* (NACNS)
    as curriculum guide, 13–14, 20–21, 31, 315
    related to clinical practice, 60, 61
costs of health care, 10
Council for the Advancement of Comprehensive
    Care (CACC), 331
credibility, 75
critical theory, 184–185, 210
*Crossing the Quality Chasm, A New Health
    System for the 21st Century* (IOM), 11, 68–69
Crowley, Karen, 267
C-SPAN, 140
culture, advanced practice registered
    nurse–friendly, 274
Curie, Marie, 3
curriculum development, 4, 9–10, 312
curriculum standards, 13–22, 59–60, 158–159
    ethics curriculum for, 208
    for healthcare policy and advocacy,
        132–133, 153
    for leadership and collaboration, 36
    related to clinical practice, 60–61
curriculum templates, 315, 325
Cutler Institute for Health and Social Policy
    (Edmund S. Muskie School of Public
    Service), 139

D

da Vinci, Leonardo, 207
decision making
    about whether to pursue DNP degree, 217–232
    consulting others for, 224
    ethical decision-making model, 193–194,
        198–199
    guidelines for, 227
    for leadership, 39
    listening after, 227–228
    practical tools for, 220–224
    questions to guide, 227
    spiritual approaches to, 224–229
    spiritual tools for, 228–229
Decision Matrix Analysis, 223
decision-making research, 219–220
democratic leadership, 42
demonstration, 276
deontology, 183–184, 210

descriptive ethics, 182–183, 210
Detroit Medical Center, 120
diffusion, 292
Diffusion of Innovation Theory, 292–293, 303
discernment, 183
discrimination, 135
Disney, Walt, 59
distance education, 69
diverse opportunities, 166
diversity, 39, 45
DNP. *See* Doctor of Nursing Practice
DNP Programs list (AACN), 325, 333
DNP Roadmap Task Force (AACN), 218, 233
DNP Roadmap Task Force Report (AACN), 333
"DNP Talking Points," 239
DNPPD. *See* Doctors of Nursing Practice
    Professional Development, Inc.
DNS. *See* Doctor of Nursing Science
DNSc degree, 311
"doctor" (term), 234, 259, 265–266
"doctor" (title)
    on business cards, 298
    case scenario, 243–244
    debate over, 237–241
    history of, 234
    personal experiences with, 257–259
    restrictions regarding nurses with doctorates
        being addressed as "doctor," 236–238, 256
    tips for using, 257–259
    use of, 85, 89, 93, 233–234, 247–250, 252–253
Doctor of Audiology (AuD) degree, 236
Doctor of Education (EdD) degree, 5, 7, 157
Doctor of Nursing Practice (DNP) degree
    AACN recommendations for, xv, 9, 29, 30,
        256, 311, 323
    advice to candidates, 27
    capstone project, 112–119
    for clinicians, 95
    competencies for, 6
    *Core Practice Doctorate Clinical Nurse
        Specialist (CNS) Competencies*
        (NACNS), 13–14, 20–21, 31, 60
    current trends, 266–270
    curriculum, 4, 9–10
    curriculum development, 312
    curriculum standards, 13–22, 59–60, 315
    curriculum templates, 315, 325
    deciding to go back to school for, 217–232
    definition of, 4, 30, 266
    development of, xi, 208, 320
    differences between DNP degree and, 9–10
    differences between PhD degree and, 4–5, 6
    drivers for, 12–13, 234–236

educating healthcare professionals about,
275–277, 282–283
educating nurses about, 273–275, 282–283
educating others about, 263–288
educating patients about, 270–273
*Essentials of Doctoral Education for Advanced
Nursing Practice* (AACN), 4, 5, 12, 13,
14–18
ethics curriculum, 208
evolution of, 5, 9–10, 24–26, 28, 254–255, 322
expectations for theory, research, and
scholarship, 101–129
final DNP project, 112–119
focus of, 5
future challenges, 321
future directions, 27, 309–327
growth of, xii, 9, 26, 29, 252, 254–255, 312, 314
impact on nursing education, 255, 309,
321, 323
impact on nursing practice, 280
living with the decision to pursue, 229–230
motivation to return to school for, 90, 217–232,
245, 279
nursing debate regarding, 310–313
objectives, 6
overview, 3–33
pathways to, 21–22
*Practice Doctorate Nurse Practitioner
Entry-Level Competencies* (NONPF),
4, 12, 13–14, 19–21, 30, 36, 60, 61
as practice-focused, 30
professional issues, 215
program assessment and evaluation, 6
program comparisons, 267–269
program development, 315
program faculty, 6
program growth, xii, 9, 26, 29, 252, 254–255,
312, 314
program length, 163–164
program of study, 6
program outcome, 6
Programs list (AACN), 325, 333
public awareness about, 283
public speaking about, 276–278
purpose of, 9
Dagmar Raica on, 51–55
rationale for, 10–13, 95, 239–241, 320
reasons for pursuing, 230, 269, 295
recipe for, 4
recommendation for, xv
recommended minimum hours for, 316
relevant facts, 218–219
requirements for APRNs, 219

and research, 105–108
resources for, 6
responses to, 246
scholarly projects, 112–119
societal needs for, 317–318
student enrollments, 161, 315–316, 322
students, 6
as terminal degree, 30, 62
and theory, 102–104
tips for educating healthcare professionals
about, 277
tips for educating nurses about, 275
tips for educating patients about, 273
tips for speaking publicly about, 278
university/college program comparisons,
267–269
ways to cope with the stressors of pursuing,
229–230
websites, 333
Dr. Williams' vision for, 24–26, 28
Doctor of Nursing Practice (DNP) graduates
academic roles, 159
age of, 268
ANCC DNP Survey Results, 330
author's personal journey, 94–95
branding yourself, 289–307
case scenarios, 72–73, 169–174, 199–203
certification for, 329
as clinicians, 59–99, 74–76, 171–173
collaboration with others, 43–46, 73–78
collaboration with PhD graduates, 29
demographics of, 268
diverse opportunities for, 166
as educators, 157–178, 272–273, 285
as ethical consultants, 179–213
as ethicists, 179
as expert clinicians, 59–99
gender of, 268
as graduate education faculty, 165–166
in healthcare policy and advocacy,
131–156, 155
impact on health care, 283
income/salary, 269
on information highway, 71–72
information technology use by, 72–73
marketing for, 289–307, 302
as marketpreneurs, 291
as mentors, 78–81, 96
as novices, 78–80
as nurse educators, 169–174
as nursing faculty, 169–171, 171–173
nursing support for, 246–247
opportunities for role modeling, 274–275

as political activists, 137
practice areas, 268
practice settings, 269
as practitioner-researchers, 313
recommended activities for, 148, 150
research by, 119–123
resources for, 192
responsibilities of, 215
role in advocacy and health and social policy, 147–148, 151
role transition for, 1, 22–23, 31, 246, 249
sample pamphlet for, 305–307
scholarship by, 108–119, 119–123
self-marketing for, 289–307, 302
strategic leadership with, 163–164
tips for getting started in advocacy and healthcare policy, 154
tips for marketing yourself, 299
tips for pursuing careers in academia, 167
tips for using "doctor" title, 258
as undergraduate education faculty, 165
unique strategies for, 294–299
work environments, 268
Doctor of Nursing Practice (DrNP) degree, 30, 311
The Doctor of Nursing Practice, A Report on Progress (AACN), 316–317, 326
Doctor of Nursing Science (DNS, DNSc, DSN) degree
differences between DNP degree and, 5, 6
evolution of, 5
future of, 311
history of, 7–8
as research degree, 8, 30
research requirements, 8
Doctor of Pharmacy (PharmD) degree, 235
Doctor of Philosophy (PhD) degree
collaboration between PhD and DNP graduates, 29, 313
differences between DNP degree and, 4–5, 6, 266
first in nursing, 7
future of, 311
as research-focused, 30, 266
doctoral education in nursing
Essentials of Doctoral Education for Advanced Nursing Practice (AACN), 4, 5, 12, 13, 14–18
evolution of, 5–10, 30
future directions, 27
history of, 7–8, 26
practice-focused, 4–5, 7–8, 10–13
research-focused, 4–5, 8

Doctors of Nursing Practice, LLC (DNP, LLC)
history of, 280
impact on informing others about DNP degree, 284–285
interview with co-founder David G. O'Dell, 279–285
mission of, 280
progress and growth of, 284
purpose of, 280–281
role in educating others about DNP degree, 282
venues to educate others about DNP degree, 285
Doctors of Nursing Practice, LLC/Doctors of Nursing Practice Professional Development, Inc. (DNP, LLC/DNPPD)
outcome study, 266–270
outcome study development team, 267
outcome study genesis, 267
Doctors of Nursing Practice Professional Development, Inc. (DNPPD), 281
"Dr." (title). *See* "doctor"
dream reflection, 229
dress, 296
Dreyfus Model of Skill Acquisition, 78
DrNP. *See* Doctor of Nursing Practice
Duke Center for Health Policy, Law and Management, 139

E

EBM. *See* evidence-based medicine
EBNP. *See* evidence-based nursing practice
EBP. *See* evidence-based practice
eCode of Ethics, 196–197
EdD. *See* Doctor of Education
Edison, Thomas, 131
editors, query letters to, 116
Edmund S. Muskie School of Public Service, Cutler Institute for Health and Social Policy, 139
education. *See also* nursing education; patient education; public education
about DNP degree, 263–288
courses and continuing education, 140–141
deciding to go back to school, 217–232
DNP graduates as educators, 157–178
DNP-prepared educators, 163–164
ethics education, 206–208, 209
graduate, 165–166
involvement through, 142–143
motivation for returning to school, 90, 217–232, 245, 279

through demonstration, 276
undergraduate, 165
eHealth Code of Ethics, 192, 197
eHealth Ethics Initiative, 192
electronic medical records (EMRs), 195–196
elevator pitches, 295, 303
Emerson, Ralph Waldo, 157
Emory University, 23
emotional intelligence, 38, 39, 40, 257–258
empathic listening, 277, 286
empathy, 41–42, 45, 46
EMRs. *See* electronic medical records
Epocrates, 70
Equal Rights Amendment, 136
Essentials of Doctoral Education for Advanced Nursing Practice (AACN)
  as competencies important and relevant to nurse educators, 159
  as curriculum standards, 13–14, 36, 158
  as curriculum standards for clinical practice, 60, 61
  as curriculum standards for healthcare policy and advocacy, 132, 153
  DNP, LLC/DNPPD outcome survey correlations, 269–270
  establishment of, 30
  as guide for DNP program content, 4, 5, 12, 14, 314
  indicators of productive programs of nursing practice scholarship, 167–168
  and national initiatives, 159
  and other competencies, 20, 21
  recommendations for DNP program length, 163–164
  recommendations for graduate education, 165
  response to societal needs, 317
  summary, 14–18
  themes, 25
  website, 333
ethical concerns, 195–198
ethical conflicts, 194
ethical consultants
  DNP graduates as, 179–213
  resources for, 192
ethical dilemmas
  decision-making model for, 193–194, 198–199
  ethical decision-making model for, 198–199
  historically, 180–181
  scenarios, 199–203
ethical inquiry, 182–183

ethical leadership
  summary of, 195
  tools for, 192–195
  traits of, 193
ethical practice, professional, 206–208
ethical terms, 181–182
ethical theories, 183–185
ethicists, 179, 204–209
ethics
  applied, 182–183, 209
  basic review of, 181–185
  bioethics, 185–187
  of care, 185
  comparative, 182–183
  as competency area, 19–20
  definition of, 179, 181, 209
  descriptive, 182–183, 210
  and DNP degree development, 208
  feminist, 185
  meta-ethics, 182–183
  narrative, 184, 210
  normative, 182, 209
  nursing ethics, 187–192, 211
  perils of social networks, 197
  summary, 197–198
  telehealth, 195–198
  virtue, 210
  virtue ethics, 183
ethics education
  Dr. Butts/Dr. Rich on, 206–208
  significance of, 209
evidence-based medicine (EBM), 106
evidence-based nursing practice (EBNP), 106
evidence-based practice (EBP)
  analytical methods for, 15–16, 60
  barriers to, 64, 65, 96
  case scenario, 66–67
  in clinical practice, 63–67
  definition of, 63–64
  DNP, LLC/DNPPD outcome survey correlations, 269
  for DNP graduates, 66–67
  reducing barriers to, 65–66, 96
  research capabilities for, 105–108
  tips for practicing, 67
  tips for reducing barriers to, 66
Executive Nurse Fellowship Program (RWJF), 79–80
expert clinicians, 59–99

F

Facebook, 197
facilitators, 38
faculty availability, 314–315

faculty collaborators, 114–115
faculty shortage
      DNP graduates and, 159–162
      filling the gap, 162–166
      impacts on student enrollment, 161
      leadership and, 163
      strategies to reduce, 163–164
      vacancy rate, 161
Fairbanks Center for Medical Ethics, 205
fearlessness, 41
feminism movement, 136
feminist ethics, 185
FHEA. *See* Fitzgerald Health Education
      Associates, Inc.
Field, Sally, 233
final DNP projects
      choosing committees for, 114–115
      choosing topics for, 113–114
      expectations for, 112–119
      getting published, 115–116
Fitzgerald, Margaret, interview with, 300–302
Fitzgerald Health Education Associates, Inc.
      (FHEA), 300–301
5-Minute Clinical Consult (5MCC), 70
focal virtues, 183
Force Field Analysis, 220–221, 231
Four Ps, 293, 303
Franck, Carol, 146
future directions
      for DNP degree, 27, 309–327
      impact of DNP graduates on health care, 283
The Future of Nursing, Focus on Education
      (IOM), 12, 30
*The Future of Nursing, Leading Change, Advancing
      Health* (IOM), xi–xii

G

George, Nancy M., interview with, 132, 149–151
government-related websites, 139
GPO Access (website), 139
graduate education, 165–166. *See also* Doctor of
      Nursing Practice (DNP) degree
      requirements for, 316
grandfathering, 218–219
Grid Analysis, 223–224, 231
Grimes, Donald, 267
Guide to the Code of Ethics for Nurses (ANA), 192

H

Haggai, John, 101
health care
      advocacy in, 16–17
      costs of, 10
      online, 197

health care improvement
      aims for, 11
      technology for, 16, 60–61
health delivery systems, 19–20, 61
Health Insurance Portability and Accountability
      Act (HIPAA) (Privacy Rule), 195, 197
health policy. *See also* healthcare policy
      and advocacy-related journals, 138
      and advocacy-related textbooks, 140
      and advocacy-related websites, 139
      involvement in, 297–298
      recommended activities for DNPs, 148, 150
      role of DNP in, 147–148, 151
      role of nursing profession in, 147, 150
Health Policy Fellowship Program (RWJF),
      140–141
health professional association websites, 139
Health Professions Education, A Bridge to Quality
      (IOM), 11, 30, 35–36
Health Professions Education Committee (IOM)
      on DNP competencies, 11, 21
      *Health Professions Education, A Bridge to
            Quality,* 11, 30, 35–36
health promotion, 270
Healthcare Information and Management
      Systems Society (HIMSS), 73
healthcare policy
      for advocacy in health care, 16–17
      avenues for involvement in, 141–144
      case scenario, 151–153
      courses and continuing education for,
            140–141
      curriculum standards for, 132–133
      DNP, LLC/DNPPD outcome survey
            correlations, 269
      DNP involvement in, 131–156, 297–298
      Essentials of, 16–17
      health policy and advocacy-related journals,
            138
      health policy and advocacy-related textbooks,
            140
      health policy and advocacy-related websites,
            139
      information sources for, 154
      interview with Nancy M. George, 149–151
      interview with Jeanette Wrona Klemczak,
            145–148
      recommended activities for DNPs, 148, 150
      role of DNP in, 147–148, 151
      role of nursing profession in, 147, 150
      tips for becoming informed and involved,
            137–144
      tips for getting started in, 154

healthcare professionals
    awareness about DNP degree, 283
    education about DNP degree for, 275–277,
        282–283
    focal virtues of, 183
    parity among, 234–236
Heide, Wilma Scot, 136
HeLa cells, 180
Henry Street Nurses' Settlement, 135–136
HIMSS. *See* Healthcare Information and
    Management Systems Society
HIPAA. *See* Health Insurance Portability and
    Accountability Act
historical perspective
    on bioethics, 185–186
    on doctoral education in nursing, 7–8, 26
    on healthcare policy and advocacy, 133–137
    on nursing faculty shortage, 159–162
    on political activism, 153–154
Hoffman, Star Evangelista, 267
Hoisington, Tom, 146
homelessness, 131
honesty, 41, 196
hospital admissions, 10
human subjects concerns
    for DNP scholarly projects, 116–117
    Tuskegee Syphilis Experiment, 185–186
humility, 225
humor, 45

I

ICN. *See* International Council of Nurses
Ignatius of Loyola, 225, 226
independent practice, 19, 61
Indiana University School of Nursing, 205
informatics, nursing, 68, 73
information highway, 71–72
information literacy, 19–20, 60–61
information sources
    for becoming involved and informed, 138, 154
    on Internet, 196–197
    relevant DNP websites, 333
information systems, 16, 60–61, 269
information technology
    case scenario, 72–73
    in clinical practice, 67–73, 96
    computer information technology (CIT), 107
    curriculum standards related to, 60–61
    websites for, 73
informed consent
    description of, 210
    principle of, 186–187, 197

Initiative on the Future of Nursing (IOM),
    11–12, 30, 159
Institute of Medicine (IOM)
    aims for health care improvement, 11
    call for improved healthcare standards, 35
    Committee on the RWJF Initiative on the
        Future of Nursing, 159
    *Crossing the Quality Chasm, A New Health
        System for the 21st Century,* 11, 68–69
    To Err Is Human, xi, 10, 68–69
    The Future of Nursing, Focus on Education,
        12, 30
    *The Future of Nursing, Leading Change,
        Advancing Health,* xi–xii
    *Health Professions Education, A Bridge to
        Quality,* 11, 30, 35–36
    Initiative on the Future of Nursing, 12, 30, 159
    recommendations for DNP graduates, 59–60
    Scholars-in-Residence, 24
intelligence, emotional, 38, 39, 40, 257–258
internal review boards (IRBs), 114
International Council of Nurses (ICN), *Code of
    Ethics for Nurses,* 182, 184, 190–191, 192,
    197, 211
International Medical Informatics Association
    Special Interest Group on Nursing Informatics
    (IMIA-NI), 68
Internet. *See also* websites
    DNP graduates on, 71–72
    health policy and advocacy-related websites,
        139
    information seeking on, 196–197
    as information source, 138
    web-based resources, 107
Internet Healthcare Coalition, eCode of Ethics,
    196–197
interpersonal competencies, 44
interprofessional collaboration. *See also*
    collaboration
    case scenarios, 76–78
    in clinical settings, 73–78, 96
    DNP, LLC/DNPPD outcome survey
        correlations, 270
    for improving patient and population health
        outcomes, 17, 61
    tips for building bridges, 76
interviewing
    discussion points for, 295
    as DNP graduate, 295–296
    thank-you notes after, 299
interviews in this book
    with Sheila Behler, 86–89
    with Janie Butts, 204–209

with Margaret Fitzgerald, 300–302
with Nancy M. George, 149–151
with Frances Jackson, 251–256
with Jeanette Wrona Klemczak, 145–148
with Andrea Kwasky, 89–94
with Nancy O'Connor, 318–323
with David G. O'Dell, 279–285
with Linda Opsahl, 245–250
with Kathleen A. Payson, 82–86
with Dagmar Raica, 51–55
with Karen Rich, 204–209
with Carolyn A. Williams, 23–29
introductions, 294–295
IOM. *See* Institute of Medicine
IRBs. *See* internal review boards

J

Jackson, Frances
as Director, Oakland University DNP Program,
241, 243
interview with, 251–256
Johns Hopkins Hospital, 180
Joplin, Janis, 263
Journal of Nursing Scholarship, 138
Journal of Professional Nursing, 138
journal writing, 228–229
journalism, 297
journals
getting DNP scholarly projects published in,
116
health policy and advocacy-related, 138
professional, 138
query letters to editors of, 116
rejection rates, 119
justice, 187, 211

K

Kant, Immanuel, 179, 184
Kantianism, 183–184
Klemczak, Jeanette Wrona
"The Bottleneck Proposal," 146–147
interview with, 132, 145–148
response to AMA, 241, 242
and use of "doctor" (title), 244
knowledge explosion, 68
Kwasky, Andrea, interview with, 89–94

L

labels, 296
LACE network, 63
Lacks, Henrietta, 180, 181

leadership
affiliative, 42
attributes of, 37–41
caring competencies for, 38–39
case scenarios for, 48–51
in clinical practice settings, 49
coaching style, 42
commanding, 43
community, 49–50
as competency area, 19, 36
curriculum standards for, 36
definition of, 47
democratic, 42
description of, 37
dissonant styles, 42, 43
DNP, LLC/DNPPD outcome survey
correlations, 269
with DNP-prepared educators, 163–164
emotional intelligence competencies for, 39, 40
ethical, 193, 195
ethical tools for, 192–195
as facilitation, 38
and faculty shortage, 163
formal, 50–51
as mentoring, 39
organizational, 15, 269
pacesetting, 42–43
preparation for, 35–58
as professional, 38
for quality improvement, 15
Dagmar Raica on, 51–55
resonant styles, 43
steps for change, 46–47
strategic, 163–164
styles of, 41–43
systems, 15, 269
through role modeling, 38, 41, 48, 258–259
unexpected, 47–48
as visionary, 38, 41
visionary style, 41–42
vs. management, 47–48
legal issues regarding use of "doctor," 247–248
legislative websites, 139
Lentz, Elizabeth, 26
Leonardo da Vinci, 207
library literacy, 107
listening
after decision making, 227–228
empathic, 277, 286
literature reviews
reading research, 107–108
response to AMA Resolution 211
(A-06), 238

scholarship, 110
starting searches, 139
tips for reading nonresearch articles, 111

M

Madonna University, 319, 320–321, 322–323
Maine, 236–237
management
    definition of, 47
    vs. leadership, 47–48
manners, 296–297
marketing
    definition of, 289–290, 302
    for DNP graduates, 289–307
    Dr. Fitzgerald on, 301–302
    Four Ps of, 293, 303
    sample pamphlet for DNP-prepared nurse
        practitioners, 305–307
    strategies for, 292–299
    tips for self-marketing, 299
    tools for, 298–299
    vs. branding, 289–291
marketing plans, 301
marketpreneurship, 291, 303
Marquette General Hospital (Marquette, MI), 54
McGee, Anita Newcomb, 134–135
McMaster University
    evidence-based nursing initiative, 108
    Health Information Research Unit, 107–108
medical-related errors, 10
medicine, 265
meditation, 228
Mentor, 78
mentored research, 122–123
mentored scholarship, 121–122
mentoring
    competencies essential for, 79–80
    definition of, 78
    by DNP graduates, 78–81, 96
    as leadership attribute, 39, 41
    models of, 121
    steps that may foster successful relationships,
        80–81
    tips for, 81
mentors, 78, 121
meta-ethics, 182–183
Michigan (MI)
    Children's Special Health Care Needs
        program, 147
    restrictions regarding nurses with doctorates
        being addressed as "doctor," 236–237
    Strategic Plan for the Nursing Shortage, 147

Michigan Health Policy Forum, 146
Michigan Nursing Corps (MNC), 146–147, 148
Michigan State Loan Repayment Program, 147
Michigan State University, 146
middle-range theory, 103
MindTools (website), 220
mission statements, 291, 303
MNC. *See* Michigan Nursing Corps
moral reasoning, 182
morality, common, 182
morals, 181, 209
motivation
    as leadership attribute, 41
    for returning to school, 90
Mudinger, Mary O., 9–10
Mullin, Marlene, 155
multimedia resources, 140

N

NACGN. *See* National Association of Colored
    Graduate Nurses
NACNS. *See* National Association of Clinical
    Nurse Specialists
name badges, 296
narrative ethics, 184, 210
National Academy of Sciences
    *Advancing the Nation's Health Needs, NIH
        Research Training Programs,* 12–13
    recommendation for nonresearch nursing
        doctorate, 30
National American Woman Suffrage Association,
    135
National Association of Clinical Nurse Specialists
    (NACNS), *Core Practice Doctorate Clinical
    Nurse Specialist (CNS) Competencies,* 13–14,
    20–21, 31, 60, 315
National Association of Colored Graduate
    Nurses (NACGN), 135
National Association of Nurse Practitioners in
    Women's Health, 239
National Association of Pediatric Nurse
    Practitioners, 239
National Board of Medical Examiners (NBME),
    331
National Center for Bioethics in Research and
    Health Center (Tuskegee University), 186
National Center for Health Statistics (NCHS),
    131
*National CNS Competency Task Force Organizing
    Framework and Core Competencies,* 20
National Conference of Gerontological Nurse
    Practitioners, 239

National Council of State Boards of Nursing
APRN Advisory Committee, 63
National Doctors of Nursing Practice Conference,
281
National Health Interview Survey (NHIS), 131
National Health Policy Forum, 139, 146
National Institutes of Health (NIH), 12–13
National League for Nursing (NLN)
Governmental Affairs website section, 138
history of, 134, 135
website, 139
National Multiple Sclerosis Society, 139
National Organization for Public Health Nursing
(NOPHN)
curriculum templates for DNP programs,
315, 325
history of, 135
recommended minimum hours for nurse
practitioner students, 316
requirements for graduate degrees, 316
National Organization of Nurse Practitioner
Faculties (NONPF)
collaboration with AACN, 8, 9
curriculum standards for DNP degree, 59–60
*Practice Doctorate Nurse Practitioner
Entry-Level Competencies,* 4, 9, 12,
13–14, 19–21, 30, 36, 60, 61
Practice Doctorate Task Force, 13
recommendations regarding nurse
practitioner DNP education, 239
National Public Radio (NPR), 140
National Research Act, 186
National Research Council, 159
natural law theory, 183, 210
NBME. *See* National Board of Medical Examiners
NCHS. *See* National Center for Health Statistics
networking. *See also* collaboration
recommendations for conversing with others
at events, 296–297
for research and scholarship, 123–125
neutrality, 225–226
New Jersey, 134
New York, 134
New York Times, 140
New York University, 7
newspapers, 140
NHIS. *See* National Health Interview Survey
Nightingale, Florence
concept of nursing, 133
definition of nursing, 61–62
as political activist, 137, 153
NLN. *See* National League for Nursing
nonmaleficence, 187, 211

NONPF. *See* National Organization of Nurse
Practitioner Faculties
NOPHN. *See* National Organization for Public
Health Nursing
normative ethics, 182, 209
North Carolina, 134
NPR. *See* National Public Radio
N-STAT. *See* Nurses Strategic Action Team
"nurse" (title), 134
nurse educators
DNP *Essentials* and, 159
DNP graduates as, 157–178
nurse ethicists
definition of, 205–206
interviews with, 204–209
Nurse Practitioner Roundtable, 239
nurse practitioners
average salary, 162
DNP-prepared (*See* Doctor of Nursing
Practice (DNP) graduates)
nurse residencies, 309, 316
nurses. *See also* advanced practice nurses (APNs);
advanced practice registered nurses (APRNs)
awareness about DNP degree, 283
certification for, 329–332
education about DNP degree for, 273–275,
282–283
parity for, 234–236
registration of, 134
shortage of, 147, 160, 176
as social engineers, 8
support for DNP graduates, 246–247
training programs for, 133–134
Nurses Coalition for Action in Politics, 136
Nurses Strategic Action Team (N-STAT), 141
nursing. *See also* advanced nursing practice
Dr. Behler on, 87
codes of ethics for, 182
definition of, 61–62, 264
essential features of, 62
as functional specialty, 7
historical perspective on, 133–137
involvement in healthcare policy and advocacy,
131–156
Dr. Kwasky on, 91
Nightingale on, 61–62, 133
patient education about, 270–273
Dr. Payson on, 83
role in advocacy, 147, 150
role in health and social policy, 147, 150
scientific underpinnings for practice, 14
Nursing Doctorate (ND) degree, 5, 8, 311
Nursing Economic$, 138

nursing education
DNP degree and, 255
doctoral (*See* doctoral education in nursing)
evolution of, 319–320
history of, 7–8, 13, 133–134
nursing ethics, 187–192, 211. *See also* ethics
nursing faculty
availability of, 314–315
average age, 161
average salaries, 161–162
case scenarios, 169–174
in clinical practice, 171–173
filling the gap, 162–166
nursing leadership and, 163
promotion of, 166–169
at regional state universities, 173–174
at research-intensive state universities, 169–173
shortage of, 159–162
strategies to increase, 163–164
tenure for, 166–169
vacancy rate, 161
nursing informatics, 68, 73
nursing leadership, 163
nursing organizations. *See* professional nursing
organizations
nursing practice. *See also* advanced nursing
practice; advanced practice nursing;
clinical practice
Dr. Behler on, 87, 88
definition of, 30, 264–265
independent practice, 19, 61
influence of DNP degree on, 280
Dr. Kwasky on, 91
Dr. Payson on, 83
professional ethical practice, 206–208
scholarship skills relevant for, 109
scope of, 318
nursing research. *See* research
nursing shortage, 147, 160, 176
nursing theory. *See* theory
Nursing's Social Policy Statement (ANA), 132,
143, 153, 191–192

O

Oakland University (OU)
Coalition Meeting, 242–243, 253–254
DNP program, 82, 90, 254, 255
response to AMA, 241, 242–243, 259
and titling issue, 248
OAR communication, 296
O'Connor, Nancy, interview with, 318–323
O'Dell, David G., interview with, 267, 279–285

Odysseus, 78
Office for Human Research Protections (OHRP),
185
OJIN. *See Online Journal of Issues in Nursing*
online chatting, 197
online health care, 197
Online Journal of Issues in Nursing (OJIN), 138
Online Journal of Nursing Informatics, 73
Opsahl, Linda
case scenario, 243–244
interview with, 245–250
organizational leadership, 15, 269
organizations, professional. *See* professional
nursing organizations
O'Shaughnessy, Arthur William Edgar, 309

P

pacesetting, 42–43
PACs. *See* political action committees
Palmer, Sophia, 134
pamphlets, for DNP-prepared nurse practitioners,
298–299
sample, 305–307
partnerships, 41, 197
Parton, Dolly, 309
paternalism, 187, 210
patient care technology, 16, 60–61
patient education, 142–143
about DNP degree, 273, 282–283
about nursing, 270–273
Payson, Kathleen A., interview with, 82–86
PDAs. *See* personal digital assistants
Pearson, Linda, 236–237
"The Pearson Report," 236–237, 259
peer review, 118
personal autonomy, 186–187, 210
personal context, 226
personal digital assistants or PDAs, 69, 70, 71, 72
PharmD degree, 235
PhD degree. *See* Doctor of Philosophy degree
physician (term), 265
Planned Parenthood, 136
Plato, 183
policy
as competency area, 19–20
health policy and advocacy-related journals,
138
health policy and advocacy-related textbooks,
140
health policy and advocacy-related websites,
139
healthcare policy, 16–17, 131–156

Policy, Politics & Nursing Practice, 138
"Policy Institute" (ACNP), 140
political action committees (PACs)
    American Nurses Association Political Action
        Committee (ANA-PAC), 141, 144, 146
    Nurses Coalition for Action in Politics, 136
political activism
    history of, 153–154
    nursing involvement in, 135–137
    tips for becoming informed and involved,
        137–144
population health, 17, 18, 61
*Position Statement on the Practice Doctorate in
    Nursing* (AACN), xi, 9, 30, 157, 333
practice doctorate
    definition of, 266
    development of, 26
    drivers for, 12–13
    rationale for, 10–13
    tenure for, 166–168
    themes central to, 25
    title issues, 311
*Practice Doctorate Nurse Practitioner Entry-Level
    Competencies* (NONPF)
    as curriculum standards, 13–14, 36
    establishment of, 30
    as guide for DNP program content, 4, 12
    and other competencies, 19–21
    related to clinical practice, 60, 61
practice inquiry, 19–20
practice-focused doctorate
    evolution of, 4–5
    need for, 29
    Dr. Williams on, 27
prayer, 228
precepting, 80–81, 96
preventable adverse events, 10
prevention, clinical, 18, 270
principlism, 184, 210
privacy, as principle, 197
Privacy Rule. *See* Health Insurance Portability
    and Accountability Act
professional doctorate, 266. *See also* practice
    doctorate
professional issues, 215
professional journals, 138. *See also* journals
professional nursing association websites, 139
professional nursing organizations
    as avenues for involvement in healthcare
        policy and advocacy, 141
    formation of, 134–135
    ideas for involvement in, 142
    involvement in, 297

professionalism
    attributes of, 38
    Beals's rules for, 294
    definition of, 38
    ethical practice, 206–208
    in online health care, 197
    preparation for, 206–208
    self-marketing through, 297
    through collaboration, 76
promotion
    faculty promotion, 166–169
    health promotion, 270
    self promotion, 290
protégés. *See* mentoring
public awareness, 283
public education. *See also* education
    about DNP degree, 263–288
    for health policy, 297–298
    methods for, 285
    responsibility for, 270–276
public health nursing, 135
public policy. *See* healthcare policy
public speaking
    about DNP degree, 276–278
    self-marketing through, 297
    tips for, 278
publication
    authorship, 117–118
    getting DNP scholarly projects published,
        115–116
*Publication Manual of the American Psychological
    Association* (APA), 110–111
purpose of life, 226

Q

quality and quality improvement
    aims for health care improvement, 11
    as competency area, 19
    leadership for, 15
    as principle, 196
query letters to editors, 116

R

Raica, Dagmar, interview with, 51–55
reasoning
    definition of, 182
    description of, 209
    moral, 182
reflection
    dream reflection, 229
    journal writing, 228–229
regional state universities, 173–174

registered nurses (RNs). *See also* advanced practice registered nurses (APRNs); nurses
shortage of, 160, 176
registration of nurses, 134
rejection, 119
relationship management, 40, 42, 44
research
 beyond graduation, 119–123, 313
 concerns regarding DNP graduates and, 312
 decision-making research, 219–220
 definition of, 116
 DNP and, 105–108
 DNP graduates as practitioner-researchers, 313
 ethical inquiry, 182–183
 for evidence-based practice, 105–108
 expectations for, 101
 for final DNP projects, 112–119
 human subjects concerns, 116–117
 Internet information seeking, 196–197
 involvement through, 143, 144
 mentored, 122–123
 networking for, 123–125
 in partnership with clinical practice, 168–169
 scholarship skills relevant for nursing research and practice, 109
research reports, 110
research-focused doctorate
 evolution of, 4–5
 need for, 29
 Dr. Williams on, 27
research-intensive state universities, 169–173
residencies, 309, 316
respect for diversity, 45
responsible partnering, 197
Rich, Karen, interview with, 204–209
RNs. *See* registered nurses
Robert Wood Johnson Foundation (RWJF)
 Executive Nurse Fellowship Program, 79–80
 Health Policy Fellowship Program, 140–141
 Initiative on the Future of Nursing, 11–12, 30, 159
 policy forums, 146
Rogers, Everett, 292–293
role immersion experiences, 316
role modeling
 leadership through, 38, 41, 48, 258–259
 opportunities for, 274–275
 Dagmar Raica on, 53, 55
role transition, 1, 22–23
Rothert, Marilyn, 146
Rush University, 8
RWJF. *See* Robert Wood Johnson Foundation
Rymal, Christine, 290–291

S

salary benefits, 85, 88, 93, 269
sales, 290
Sanger, Margaret, 136
Schlotfeldt, Rozella M., 8
scholarship
 of application, 168
 categories of, 119
 choosing committees for final DNP projects, 114–115
 choosing topics for final DNP projects, 113–114
 clinical, 15–16, 60
 conceptual model of, 120
 criteria for authorship, 117
 definition of, 108–109, 119
 DNP, LLC/DNPPD outcome survey correlations, 269
 DNP and, 108–119
 DNP scholarly projects, 112–119
 expectations for, 101
 getting DNP scholarly projects published, 115–116
 mentored, 121–122
 networking for, 123–125
 research beyond graduation, 119–123, 313
 skills relevant for nursing research and practice, 109
 of teaching, 119, 120
 tips for reading nonresearch articles, 111
scientific foundation competency, 19, 60
scientific underpinnings for practice, 14
search, 107, 139. *See also* research
Sebastian, Julie G., 25
self-awareness, 40, 45
Self-Awareness for Nurses in the Interdisciplinary Environment, 93
self-exploration, 226
self-management, 40, 45, 46
self-marketing
 Beals's rules of, 293–294, 303
 for DNP graduates, 289–307
 Dr. Fitzgerald on, 301–302
 sample pamphlet for DNP-prepared nurse practitioners, 305–307
 strategies for DNP graduates, 294–299
 through community and professional involvement, 297
 tips for, 299
Sigma Theta Tau International Honor Society of Nursing, 138
social awareness, 40
social engineers, 8

social networks, 197
social policy
   Nursing's Social Policy Statement (ANA), 132
   recommended activities for DNPs, 148, 150
   role of DNP in, 147–148, 151
   role of nursing profession in, 147, 150
societal needs, 317–318
Socrates, 182
software programs, 69, 70
South Carolina University, 8
Spanish-American war, 134–135
specialty association websites, 139
specialty-focused competencies, 19
spiritual approaches to decision making, 224–229
spiritual direction, 229
spiritual tools for decision making, 228–229
stakeholders, 193–194
*Standards for Establishing and Sustaining Healthy
   Work Environments* (AACN), 74–75
standards of DNP programs. *See* Essentials
   of Doctoral Education for Advanced
   Nursing Practice
Stanhope, Marcia K., 25
strategic leadership, 163–164
stress management, 229–239
students
   as authors, 117–118
   enrollments, 161, 315–316, 322
   recommended minimum hours for, 316
suffrage, 135
systems leadership, 15, 269
systems thinking, 15

T

talk shows, 140
Teacher's College (Columbia University), 7
teaching. *See also* education
   scholarship of, 119, 120
team styles, 45–46
technology
   for clinical practice improvement, 69–71
   as competency area, 19–20
   computer information technology (CIT), 107
   DNP, LLC/DNPPD outcome survey
      correlations, 269
   for health care improvement and
      transformation, 16, 60–61
   information systems/technology, 16, 60–61
   information technology, 67–73, 96
   patient care technology, 16, 60–61
   telehealth technologies, 70
technophobia, 68–69

telehealth
   definition of, 70
   summary, 197–198
telehealth ethics, 195–198
telehealth technologies, 70
Telemachus, 78
telenursing, 195
television programs, 140
tenure, 166–169
terminology
   for educating others about DNP degrees,
      264–266
   ethics terms, 181–182
   for patient education about nursing, 273
textbooks, 139–140
thank-you notes, 299
*The Future of Nursing, Leading Change,
   Advancing Health* (IOM), xi–xii
theory
   critical theory, 184–185, 210
   definition of, 102–103
   DNP and, 102–104
   ethical theories, 183–185
   expectations for DNP graduates, 101,
      102–104, 125
   theories applicable to clinical settings, 104
Thinking Hats, 221–223, 231
time management, 120
titles, 233–261, 311. *See also* "doctor"; "nurse"
To Err Is Human (IOM), xi, 10, 68–69
transformation, 16
trust, 41, 44
trustworthiness, 183
truth holding, 38
Tuskegee Syphilis Study (or Experiment), 185–186
Tuskegee University National Center for Bioethics
   in Research and Health Center, 186
Twitter, 197

U

undergraduate education, 165
University of Colorado, 8
University of Detroit Mercy, 92
University of Kentucky, 9, 23, 24, 25–26
University of North Carolina at Chapel Hill
   (UNC, CH), 23, 24
University of Pittsburgh, 7
University of Tennessee Health Science Center
   College of Nursing, 280
university/college program comparisons, 267–269
U.S. Department of Health and Human Services,
   139

U.S. Health Policy Gateway (website), 139
U.S. House of Representatives, 139
U.S. Legislation & Votes (website), 139
U.S. Public Health Service, 185
U.S. Senate, 139
utilitarianism, 184, 210

V

values, 182, 209
Vermont, 236–237
Virginia, 134
virtue ethics, 183, 210
vision statements, 291–292, 303
visionary leadership, 41–42
visionists, 38, 41

W

Waddles, Charleszetta, 35
Wald, Lillian, 135–136
Wall Street Journal, 140

Walters, Barbara, 289
Warhol, Andy, xii
web-based resources, 107
websites
  health policy and advocacy-related
    websites, 139
  for information technology, 73
  personal, 299
  relevant DNP websites, 333
Williams, Carolyn A., interview with,
  23–29
women's suffrage, 135
workplace involvement, 142
World Health Organization, 139
writing
  journal writing, 228–229
  self-marketing through, 297

Y

Young, Marie G., 267